ATLAS OF Heart Failure

Cardiac Function and Dysfunction

THIRD EDITION

Editor

WILSON S. COLUCCI, MD

Professor of Medicine
Boston University School of Medicine;
Chief
Cardiovascular Medicine
Boston Medical Center
Boston, Massachusetts

Series Editor

EUGENE BRAUNWALD, MD, MD (Hon), ScD (Hon)

Distinguished Hersey Professor of Medicine
Faculty Dean for Academic Programs at
    Brigham and Women's Hospital and Massachusetts General Hospital
Harvard Medical School;
Vice President for Academic Programs
Partners HealthCare System
Boston, Massachusetts

Developed by Current Medicine, Inc., Philadelphia

CURRENT MEDICINE, INC.

400 MARKET STREET, SUITE 700 • PHILADELPHIA, PA 19106

Developmental Editor	*Elise M. Paxson*
Editorial Assistant	*Annmarie D'Ortona*
Cover Design	*William Whitman Jr.*
Design and Layout	*Jennifer Knight, John McCullough*
Illustrators	*John McCullough, Marie Dean, Wieslawa Langenfeld, Maureen Looney*
Assistant Production Manager	*Penny Weisman*
Indexing	*Holly Lukens*

Library of Congress Cataloging-in-Publication Data

Atlas of heart failure : cardiac function and dysfunction / editor, Wilson S. Colucci. - 3rd ed.
   p. ; cm.
  Includes bibliographical references and index.
  ISBN 1-57340-184-6 (alk. paper)
   1. Heart failure--Atlases. I. Colucci, Wilson S., 1949-
   [DNLM: 1. Heart Failure, Congestive--Atlases. 2. Heart--physiology--Atlases. 3.
  Heart--physiopathology--Atlases. WG 17 A88162 2002]
  RC685.C53 A85 2002
  616.1'29'00222--dc21

2001053786

ISBN 1-57340-184-6

Printed in Singapore by Imago Productions (FE) Ltd.

10 9 8 7 6 5 4 3
For more information please call 1 (800) 427-1796 or (215) 574-2266
or e-mail us at inquiry@phl.cursci.com

www.current-science-group.com

CONTRIBUTORS

CARL S. APSTEIN, MD
Professor of Medicine and Physiology
Boston University School of Medicine;
Attending Cardiologist
Boston Medical Center
Boston, Massachusetts

ROBERT J. CODY, MD
Professor
Department of Internal Medicine
University of Michigan Health System
Ann Arbor, Michigan

JAY N. COHN, MD
Cardiovascular Division
University of Minnesota Medical School
Minneapolis, Minnesota

WILSON S. COLUCCI, MD
Professor of Medicine
Boston University School of Medicine;
Chief, Cardiovascular Medicine
Boston Medical Center
Boston, Massachusetts

MARK A. CREAGER, MD
Associate Professor of Medicine
Harvard Medical School;
Director, Vascular Center
Brigham and Women's Hospital
Boston, Massachusetts

JORGE A. CUSCO, MD
Department of Cardiovascular Medicine
Brigham and Women's Hospital
Boston, Massachusetts

D. BRADLEY S. DYKE, MD
Lecturer
Department of Internal Medicine
University of Michigan Health System
Ann Arbor, Michigan

MICHAEL M. GIVERTZ, MD
Assistant Professor of Medicine
Department of Medicine
Harvard Medical School;
Co-Director, Cardiomyopathy and Heart
* Failure Service*
Brigham and Women's Hospital
Boston, Massachusetts

JOSHUA M. HARE, MD
Associate Professor of Medicine
Department of Medicine/Cardiology
Johns Hopkins University School of
* Medicine;*
Associate Director, Heart Failure and
* Cardiac Transplantation*
The Johns Hopkins Hospital
Baltimore, Maryland

ARNOLD M. KATZ, MD
Professor of Medicine (Emeritus)
University of Connecticut School of
* Medicine*
Farmington, Connecticut

TODD M. KOELLING, MD
Assistant Professor
Department of Internal Medicine
University of Michigan Health System
Ann Arbor, Michigan

CARL V. LEIER, MD
Overstreet Professor of Medicine and
* Pharmacology*
Division of Cardiology
The Ohio State University Medical Center
Columbus, Ohio

DONNA MANCINI, MD
Associate Professor
Department of Medicine;
Medical Director, Cardiac Transplantation
Columbia University
New York, New York

CONTRIBUTORS

ANJU NOHRIA, MD
Fellow
Cardiovascular Division
Brigham and Women's Hospital
Boston, Massachusetts

HENRY OOI, MB, MRCPI
Fellow
Department of Cardiology
Boston University School of Medicine;
Fellow
Boston University Medical Center
Boston, Massachusetts

DAVID A. ORSINELLI, MD
Associate Professor of Clinical Medicine
Department of Internal Medicine;
The Ohio State University
Director, Echocardiography Lab
Ohio State University Hospitals
Columbus, Ohio

MARC A. PFEFFER, MD, PHD
Professor of Medicine
Harvard Medical School;
Physician
Cardiovascular Division
Brigham and Women's Hospital
Boston, Massachusetts

DOUGLAS B. SAWYER, MD, PHD
Assistant Professor
Department of Medicine
Boston University School of Medicine
Boston, Massachusetts

MARK R. STARLING, MD
Professor of Internal Medicine
Associate Chief, Division of Cardiology
Director, Cardiology Training Program
University of Michigan Health System;
Chief, Cardiovascular Section
Veterans Affairs Medical Center
Ann Arbor, Michigan

MAT WILLIAMS, MD
Department of Surgery
Columbia University
New York, New York

JAMES B. YOUNG, MD, FACC
Medical Director
Kaufman Center for Heart Failure;
Head, Section of Heart Failure and Cardiac
* Transplant Medicine*
The Cleveland Clinic Foundation
Cleveland, Ohio

PREFACE

Heart failure is a common clinical syndrome that has enormous impact on the prognosis and lifestyle of patients.

In recent years, impressive strides have been made toward understanding the pathophysiology of heart failure at all levels, from molecular changes to the integrated circulatory system. It is now apparent that many forms of primary cardiomyopathy, such as hypertrophic cardiomyopathy and some forms of dilated cardiomyopathy, are genetic in origin, and rapid progress is being made in identifying specific molecular defects that cause a variety of inherited heart muscle diseases.

Likewise, it is now clear that profound secondary changes occur in previously normal myocardium in response to abnormal mechanical stresses and neurohumoral stimuli that result from common cardiovascular conditions such as myocardial infarction, valvular heart disease, and systemic hypertension. Collectively referred to as "remodeling," these secondary changes in myocytes, fibroblasts, and other constituents of the myocardium result in myocyte hypertrophy and apoptosis, alterations in the interstitial matrix, chamber enlargement, and abnormalities of systolic and diastolic pump function. These structural and functional changes determine the timing and extent of the myocardial dysfunction and thereby play a central role in defining the time course and severity of the clinical syndrome.

Advances in understanding the pathophysiology of heart failure have been paralleled by an impressive expansion in modalities available for treatment. Only a few years ago, a monograph dealing with this syndrome would have focused on therapies directed at the short-term improvement of hemodynamic function. Although short-term hemodynamic stabilization continues to be an important goal of the in-hospital management of patients with heart failure, it is increasingly apparent that hemodynamic improvement is only one aspect of successful long-term therapy.

There is now evidence that therapy of heart failure with at least two types of neurohormonal antagonists, converting enzyme inhibitors, and β-adrenergic blockers, improves clinical status and reduces mortality. Furthermore, it appears that the early treatment of patients with left ventricular dysfunction can slow or prevent the progression of disease and the development of heart failure. Several new factors, including inflammatory cytokines, endothelin, and oxidative stress, have been identified that have the potential to mediate the development of myocardial failure and have led to promising new therapeutic approaches.

This edition is divided into three sections. The first section provides a state-of-the-art review of the mechanisms that regulate normal myocardial function, beginning with molecular and cellular events in the cardiomyocyte and progressing to the level of tissue/organ mechanics and systemic circulatory regulation. In the second section, pathophysiology is presented in four chapters that address the etiology of the syndrome, the molecular and cellular basis of myocardial failure, myocardial remodeling, and the critical roles of the circulatory system and neurohumoral mechanisms in the pathophysiology of heart failure. The third section, which is devoted to the clinical management of patients with heart failure, has been expanded with the addition of three new chapters that address inhibitors of the renin-angiotensin system, β-blockers, and diastolic failure, respectively.

As understanding of heart failure advances, new approaches to the prevention and treatment of the syndrome will emerge. Conversely, it is likely that lessons learned from prevention and treatment trials will continue to foster insight into the mechanisms that determine this syndrome. The complexity of this intersection of basic and clinical information presents a challenge to both the clinician and the investigator but ultimately promises that additional exciting progress will occur in both arenas. We believe that this edition of the *Atlas of Heart Failure* will serve clinicians, investigators, and teachers who are interested in heart failure by synthesizing and presenting information that is relevant to all.

Wilson S. Colucci, MD

CONTENTS

MOLECULAR AND CELLULAR BASIS OF CONTRACTION

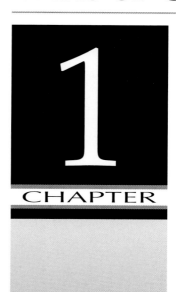

1

CHAPTER

Arnold M. Katz

The ability of the heart to meet the changing demands of the circulation involves three fundamentally different mechanisms [1]. The work of the heart can be regulated by changes in its ability to empty and fill (organ physiology), to utilize chemical energy for the performance of mechanical and osmotic work (cell biochemistry), and to replace its constituent parts (gene expression). Each of these control mechanisms operates over a different time course.

As an organ, the heart adjusts to changing preload (venous return) and afterload (arterial impedance) by length-dependent mechanisms: the Frank-Starling relationship, or Starling's Law of the Heart [2]. These physiologic mechanisms, which allow increased preload or afterload to augment the heart's ability to eject blood, provide beat-to-beat adjustments that enable the heart to meet short-term changes in hemodynamics and to equalize the outputs of the two ventricles.

The second mechanism relies on biochemical changes to modify the ability of individual cardiac myocytes to contract and to relax, and thus to alter the heart's ability to empty (inotropy) and fill (lusitropy). Most of these cellular mechanisms, which enable the heart to meet such sustained hemodynamic demands as those caused by exercise and emotion, influence the interactions between the cardiac contractile proteins by modifying the many membrane ion pumps, ion channels, and ion exchangers that regulate the inotropic and lusitropic properties of the heart [2]. The calcium fluxes involved in excitation-contraction coupling and relaxation, in turn, are influenced by a variety of signaling cascades. These cascades are initiated by the arrival of an extracellular signal, usually a chemical transmitter or hormone, at the cell surface, and generate a diverse group of intracellular messengers that modify cardiac function.

The third and most complex of the mechanisms by which the heart adjusts to the changing demands of the circulation involves growth abnormalities that modify gene expression in the cardiac cells. The resulting molecular changes provide long-lasting adjustments in response to such stimuli as endocrinopathies (*eg*, altered thyroid function), aging, and chronic hemodynamic overload. Although an understanding of this third mechanism is still in its infancy, rich and subtle molecular changes caused by growth abnormalities in the diseased heart are likely to play an important role in such common clinical conditions as heart failure [3].

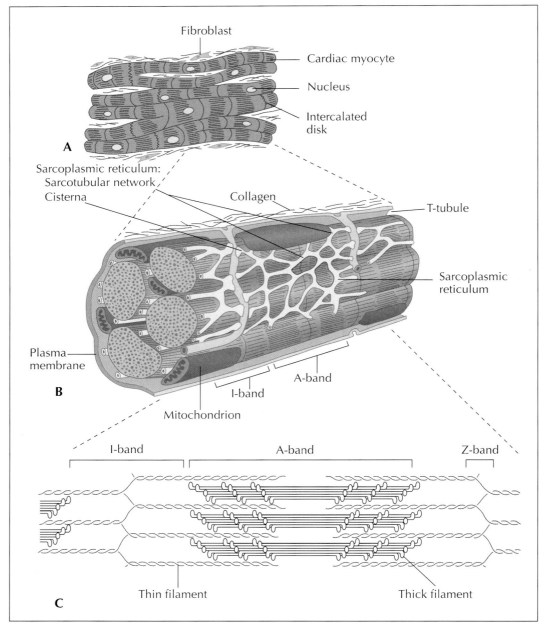

FIGURE 1-1. Structure of the heart. The heart is composed of both myocytes and nonmyoctes. **A,** Nonmyocytes include connective tissue cells (mainly fibroblasts), vascular smooth muscle cells, and endothelial cells. Whereas large cardiac myocytes make up most of the heart's mass, the majority of the cells of the heart (approximately 70%) are smaller nonmyocytes. The large, branched cardiac myocytes, which are enmeshed in a collagen network, are separated longitudinally by intercalated disks, which represent specialized cell-cell junctions. The intercalated disks provide strong mechanical connections between adjacent cells and contain gap junctions that provide low-resistance pathways for electrical conduction.

B, Cardiac myocytes that are specialized for contraction contain myofilaments whose organization in a regular array of thick and thin filaments gives rise to the characteristic striated appearance. Also prominent within these cells are two membrane structures: energy-producing mitochondria and the sarcoplasmic reticulum, which regulates cytosolic Ca^{2+} concentration. The latter is an intracellular membrane system that contains the calcium channels that initiate systole by delivering activator calcium to the myofilaments, and calcium pumps that, by removing calcium from the cytosol, dissociate this activator cation from its binding sites on the thin filament.

Myofilaments contain about 70% of the protein of the cardiac myocytes, and most of the membrane surface is found in the mitochondria. Other important membranes include the plasma membrane, which is continuous with the transverse tubular membranes (t-tubules) that extend toward the center of the cell and carry depolarizing currents into the myocardial cell.

C, Each sarcomere, which is delimited by two Z-bands, contains one A-band and two half I-bands. The A-bands are made up of thick, myosin-containing filaments into which thin filaments interdigitate from the adjacent two half I-bands. The latter are made up of actin and the regulatory proteins, tropomyosin and the troponin complex. Bisecting each Z-band is a lattice of axial and cross-connecting filaments that includes the overlapping ends of thin filaments from adjacent sarcomeres. (Part B *adapted from* Katz [3].)

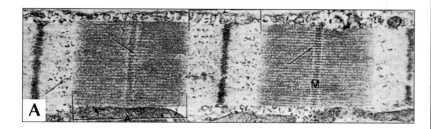

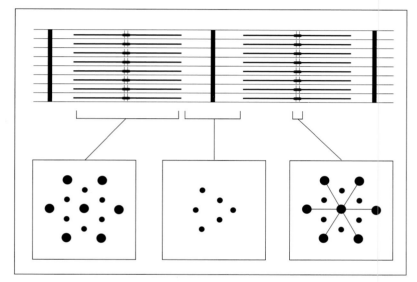

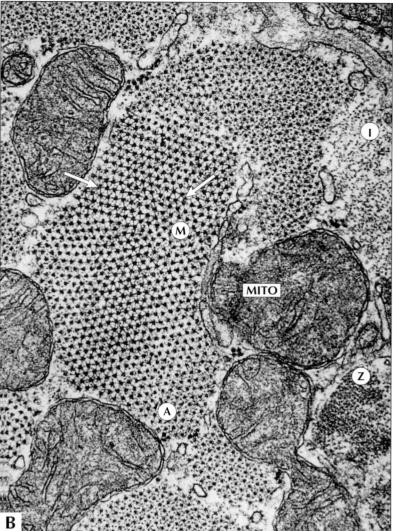

FIGURE 1-2. Sarcomere structure. **A,** A longitudinal section of two sarcomeres of cat atrial myocardium shows the characteristic cross-striations created by the regular array of myofilaments. The A-band (A) is made up of closely packed, myosin-containing thick filaments. In the center of the A-band is the M-band (M), an electron-dense region that contains thin radial filaments running transversely to the long axis of the sarcomere. The I-bands (I), which are made up of the thin actin-containing filaments, are bisected by the Z-bands. Glycogen granules are present in the cytoplasm and between myofilaments (*arrows*), and mitochondria are seen below. Cross-sections of the myofilament at different levels of one of the sarcomeres show relationships between the thick and thin filaments. The A-band is a hexagonal array of thick filaments containing thin filaments that lie at the trigonal points of the array. Thin filaments in the I-band, where thick filaments are absent, are less ordered. Thin radial filaments connect adjacent thick filaments within the M-band at the center of the A-band. **B,** A transverse section through a cat right ventricular papillary muscle shows myofilaments cut at the level of the M-band, A-band, and I-band. *Arrows* point to the radial filaments between the thick filaments in the center of the M-band. Several energy-producing mitochondria (MITO) are also seen. The Z-band (Z) at *lower right* appears as a dense network. (*Adapted from* McNutt and Fawcett [5].)

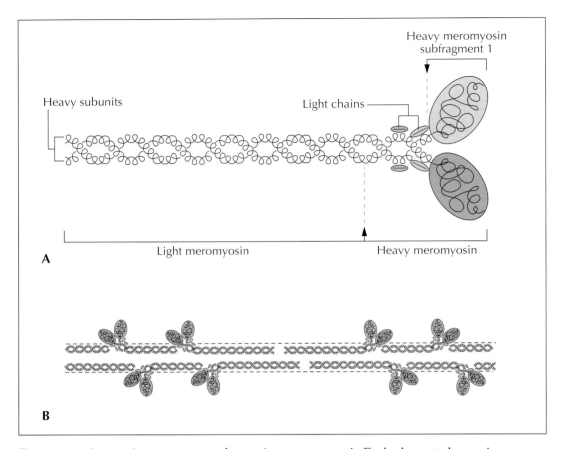

FIGURE 1-3. A myosin monomer and myosin aggregates. **A,** Each elongated myosin molecule consists of two heavy chains and two pairs of light chains. The "tail" of the molecule (*left*) is a coiled coil in which α-helical regions of the two myosin heavy chains are wound around each other. Each of the paired "heads" of the molecule (*right*) includes the globular region of one myosin heavy chain along with two myosin light chains. The latter, which are members of the same family of calcium-binding proteins that includes troponin C (*see* Fig. 1-4), play an as yet incompletely understood role in regulating contraction. Whereas enzymatic cleavage at the point indicated by the *lower arrow* yields heavy and light meromyosins, enzymatic cleavage of heavy meromyosin at the point indicated by the *upper arrow* yields the heavy meromyosin subfragment 1. Both the actin-binding and adenosine triphosphatase sites of myosin are within the myosin head, which corresponds to the cross-bridge that projects from the thick filament.

    B, The thick filament is an aggregate of individual myosin molecules. The "backbone" (*dashed lines*) is made up of the tails of the individual myosin molecules; the cross-bridges correspond to the myosin "heads," which have opposite polarities in the two halves of the thick filament (*right* and *left*). The bare area in the center of the thick filament is devoid of cross-bridges because of the "tail-to-tail" organization of myosin molecules. (*Adapted from* Katz [2].)

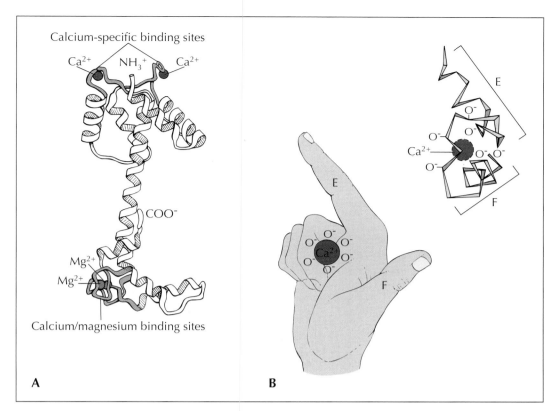

FIGURE 1-4. Troponin C. **A,** Ribbon representation based on x-ray crystallographic studies at 2.8-Å resolution shows the dumbbell-shaped molecule that contains four calcium-binding sites. The upper helical portions contain two calcium-specific binding sites, and the lower part of the molecule contains two nonspecific calcium/magnesium-binding sites. The latter probably have no role in excitation-contraction coupling, because the concentration of cytosolic Mg^{2+} is so much higher than that of Ca^{2+} that these sites remain occupied by Mg^{2+} during physiologic changes in cytosolic Ca^{2+} concentration. In skeletal troponin C, both calcium-specific sites bind calcium ions to initiate contraction. In cardiac troponin C, one of these sites has lost the ability to bind calcium, so that binding of only one calcium ion is required to initiate contraction.

B, Each calcium-binding site contains two α-helical regions (E and F) that are separated by a nonhelical loop. This structure, which localizes six oxygen atoms (O⁻) so that they tightly coordinate a calcium ion (Ca^{2+}), resembles a right hand and so is sometimes called an "E-F hand." (Part A *adapted from* Herzberg and James [6]; part B *adapted from* Katz [2].)

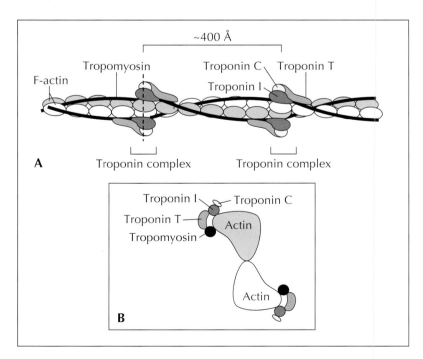

FIGURE 1-5. Structure of the thin filament. **A,** The "backbone" of the thin filament, seen in a longitudinal view, is F-actin which contains two strands of actin monomers (*light grey and white*). Troponin complexes, each made up of one molecule each of troponin C, troponin I, and troponin T, are distributed at approximately 400-Å intervals along the thin filament. Elongated tropomyosin molecules (*solid*) lie in the grooves between the two actin strands. **B,** A cross-section of the thin filament at the level where the troponin complexes are located shows probable relationships between actin, tropomyosin, and the three components of the troponin complex. The strength of the bond linking troponin I and actin varies, depending on whether Ca^{2+} is bound to troponin C. (*Adapted from* Katz [2].)

CONTRACTION AND RELAXATION

CONTRACTILE PROTEIN INTERACTIONS

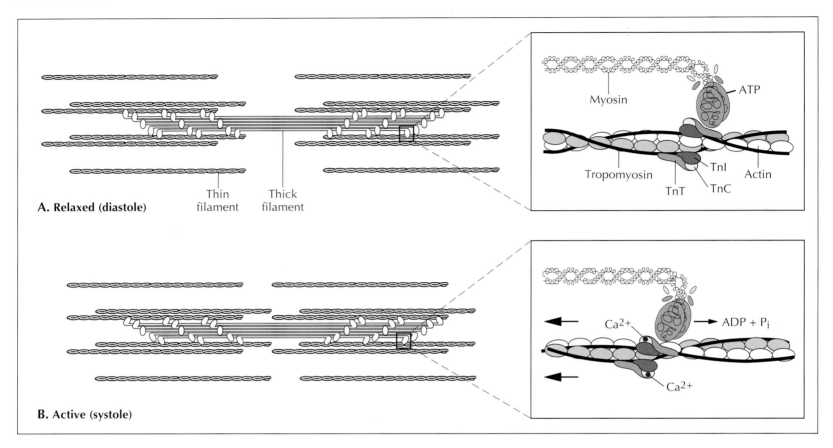

FIGURE 1-6. Cardiac contraction is brought about by interactions between actin in the thin filament and myosin cross-bridges that project from the thick filament. **A,** In relaxed muscle, where troponin C (TnC) is not bound to calcium, the "relaxed" conformation of the troponin complexes and tropomyosin prevents actin in the thin filament from interacting with the myosin cross-bridges. As a result, actin is unable to convert the chemical energy of the adenosine triphosphate (ATP) bound to the myosin cross-bridges into mechanical work.

B, In active muscle, Ca^{2+} bound to TnC has shifted the troponin complexes and tropomyosin to an "active" conformation that enables actin to interact with the myosin cross-bridges. Release of chemical energy when actin stimulates hydrolysis of myosin-bound ATP enables the cross-bridges to "row" the thin filaments toward the center of the sarcomere. TnI—troponin I; TnT—troponin T.

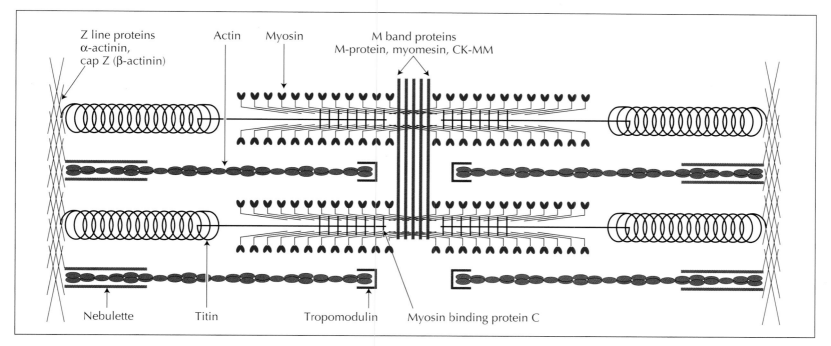

FIGURE 1-7. Cytoskeletal proteins found in the myofilaments are related to the thick and thin filaments, and the Z line. The giant protein, *titin*, which extends from the Z band into the thick filament, is connected to myosin near the center of the thick filament by myosin binding protein C. Those portions of the titin molecule that lie within the A band are quite rigid, while the regions found in the I band are more elastic. Several proteins make up the M bands, which are transverse structures that link the centers of the thick filament; these include M protein, myomesin, and the MM isoform of the enzyme creatine phosphokinase (CK-MM). Myosin binding protein C links adjacent thick filamants in the central region of the sarcomere. Proteins that support the thin filaments include *nebulette*, a protein related to skeletal muscle nebulin, which connects the ends of the thin filaments to the Z band, and *tropomodulin*, which caps the ends of the thin filaments. Proteins that connect the thick filaments to the Z line include α-actinin and cap Z (β-actinin). (*Adapted from* Katz [2].)

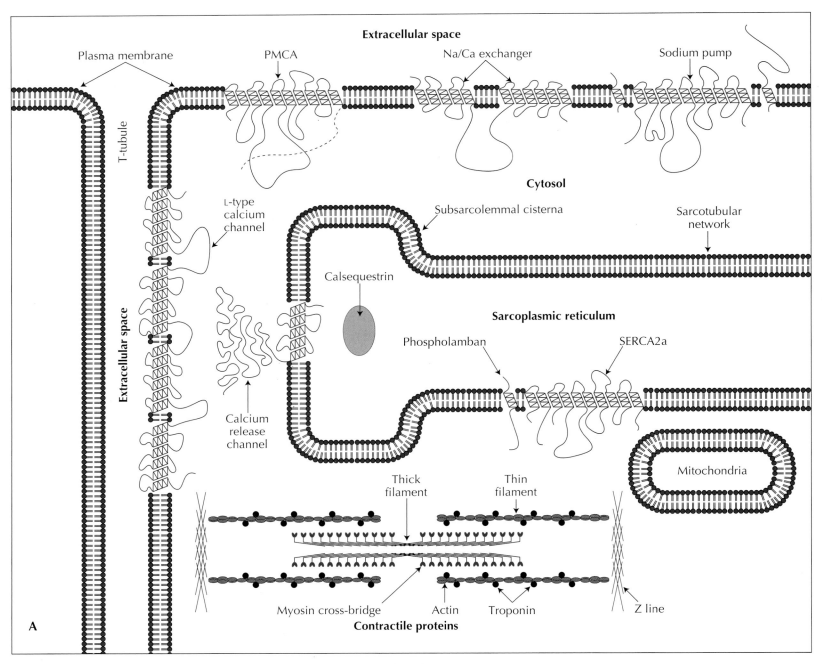

FIGURE 1-8. Key structures (**A**) and calcium fluxes (**B**) that control cardiac excitation-contraction coupling and relaxation. Calcium "pools" are in bold capital letters (**A**). (*continued*)

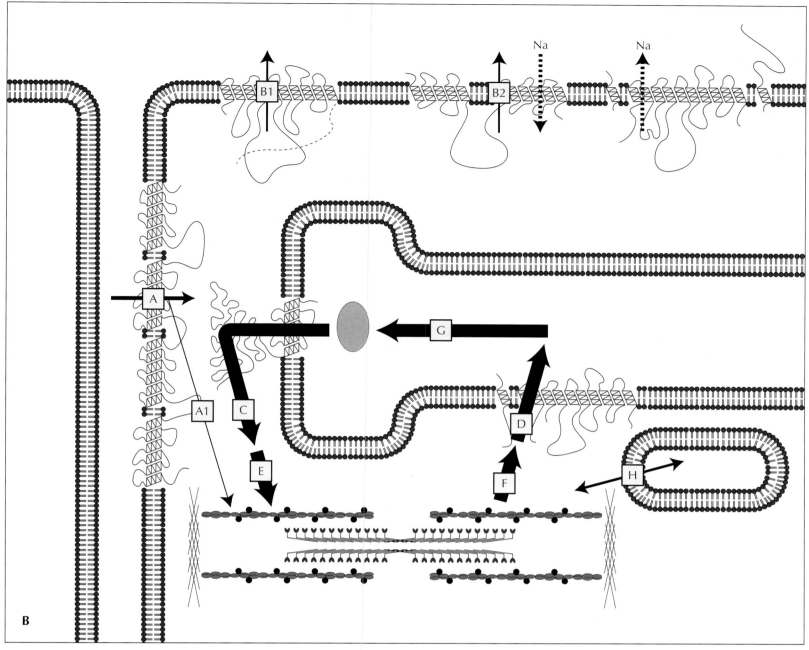

FIGURE 1-8. (*continued*) In **B,** the thickness of the arrows indicates the magnitude of the calcium fluxes, while their vertical orientations describe their "energetics": *down arrows* represent passive calcium fluxes; *up arrows* represent energy-dependent active calcium transport. Most of the calcium that enters the cell from the extracellular fluid via L-type calcium channels (*arrow A*) triggers calcium release from the sarcoplasmic reticulum; only a small portion directly activates the contractile proteins (*arrow A1*). Calcium is actively transported back into the extracellular fluid by the plasma membrane calcium pump ATPase (PMCA; *arrow B1*), and the Na/Ca exchanger (*arrow B2*). The sodium that enters the cell in exchange for calcium (*dashed line*) is pumped out of the cytosol by the sodium pump. Two calcium fluxes are regulated by the sarcoplasmic reticulum: calcium efflux from the subsarcolemmal cisternae via calcium release channels (*arrow C*) and calcium uptake into the sarcotubular network by the sarco(endo)plasmic reticulum calcium pump ATPase (*arrow D*). Calcium diffuses within the sarcoplasmic reticulum from the sarcotubular network to the subsarcolemmal cisternae (*arrow G*), where it is stored in a complex with calsequestrin and other calcium-binding proteins. Calcium binding to (*arrow E*) and dissociation from (*arrow F*) high-affinity calcium-binding sites of troponin C activate and inhibit the interactions of the contractile proteins. Calcium movements into and out of mitochondria (*arrow H*) buffer cytosolic calcium concentration. The extracellular calcium cycle is shown at arrows A, B1, and B2, while the intracellular cycle involves arrows C, E, F, D, and G. (*Adapted from Katz [2].*)

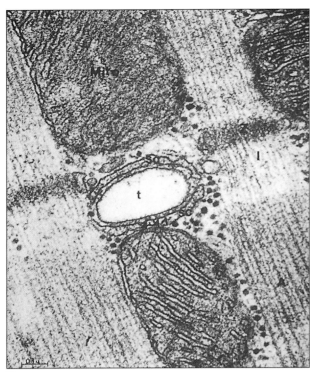

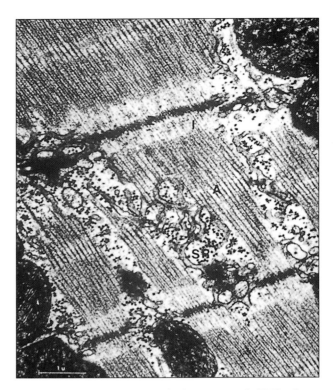

FIGURE 1-9. Cross-section of the triad in rat ventricular muscle. The large central structure is a cross-section of the transverse (t) tubular system, which is surrounded by two cisternae (sc), each of which partially envelops the t-tubule. The cisternal membrane does not contact the t-tubule; instead, excitation-contraction coupling depends on electron-dense "foot" proteins that lie between these two membranes (*arrows*). A—A-band; I—I-band; Mito—mitochondria; Z—Z-line. Scale bar = 0.1 μm. (*Courtesy of* Judy Upshaw-Earley and Ernest Page, Chicago, IL, and *adapted from* Katz [2].)

FIGURE 1-10. The sarcotubular network (SR) of rat ventricular muscle in a "grazing" section over the sarcomeres. The dark granules near this structure are glycogen. The faint linear structure composed of two parallel lines, crossing the SR (*lower right*), probably represents a microtubule. A—A-band; Mito—mitochon-dria; I—I-band; Z—Z-line. Scale bar = 0.1 μm. (*Courtesy of* Judy Upshaw-Earley and Ernest Page, Chicago, IL, and *adapted from* Katz [2].)

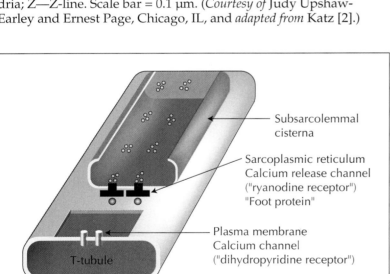

FIGURE 1-11. A dyad showing "foot proteins," now recognized to be the calcium release channels of the sarcoplasmic reticulum (also called "ryanodine receptors"), which lie in the subsarcolemmal cisternae immediately beneath sarcolemmal voltage-gated calcium channels in the t-tubule. These intracellular channels open when calcium crosses the plasma membrane through L-type channels (also called "dihydropyridine receptors"). (*Adapted from* Katz [2].)

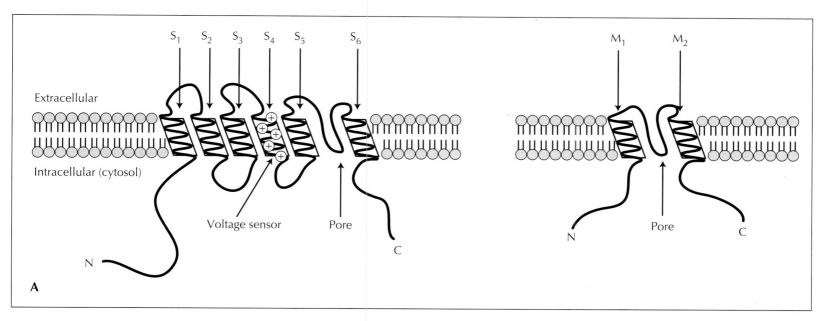

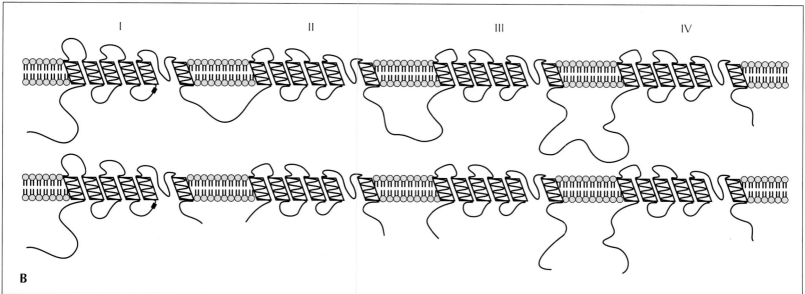

FIGURE 1-12. Domains involved in sodium, calcium, and potassium channels. **A,** The *left portion* shows the two types of domain found in voltage-gated ion channels. Each of the four domains that make up sodium channels, calcium channels, and outwardly rectifying potassium channels contains six transmembrane α-helices. The positively charged S_4 transmembrane α-helices in each of these domains provides the voltage sensor that responds to membrane depolarization by opening the channel. The "pore region" of the channel is made up of the S_5 and S_6 transmembrane α-helices and the intervening loop that "dips" into the membrane bilayer. The *right portion* shows inward rectifying potassium channels that are made of smaller domains that are homologous to the S_5 and S_6 transmembrane α-helices of the larger domain shown in **A**. This domain is largely a pore, made up of the M_1 and M_2 transmembrane α-helices along with the intervening loop. The absence of a charged transmembrane α-helix homologous to S_4 explains why the response of inward rectifying channels to membrane depolarization differs from that of channels made up of the larger domains depicted in the *left portion*.
B, The *top portion* illustrates sodium, calcium, and outwardly rectifying potassium channels as tetrameric structures made up of four homologous domains (numbered I to IV), each of which contains six transmembrane α-helices (see **A**). The *lower portion* shows that the outwardly rectifying potassium channels are also made up of four homologous domains, except that unlike the channels shown above, these domains are not linked covalently. Minor or β subunits (not shown), which include MinK and MiRP, contain a single transmembrane α-helix, and regulate channel function. (*Adapted from* Katz [2].)

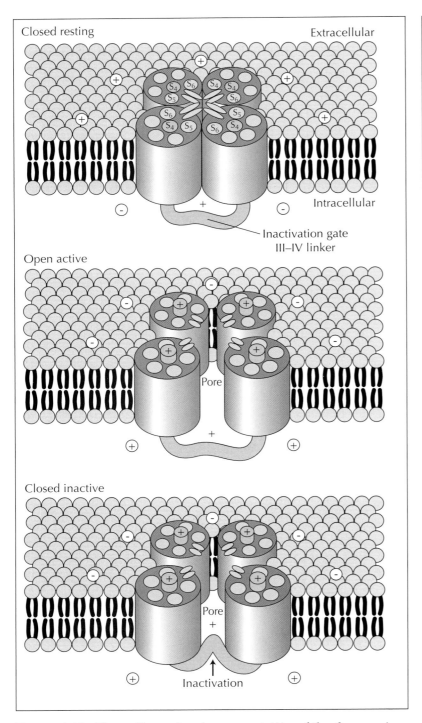

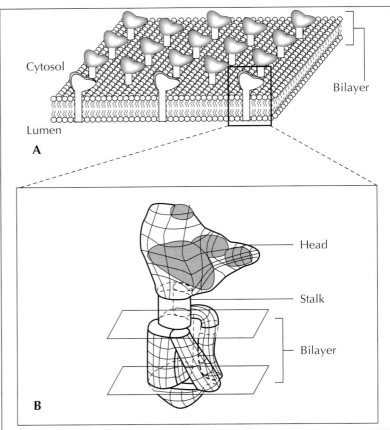

FIGURE 1-14. Orientation of the calcium pump in the sarcoplasmic reticulum. **A,** The sarcotubular network contains a densely packed array of calcium pump ATPase molecules. **B,** Each subunit of the calcium pump ATPase resembles a bird whose "head," which projects into the cytosolic space, contains both the ATP-binding and phosphorylation sites. (Part A *adapted from* Katz [2]; part B *adapted from* Toyoshima *et al.* [7].)

FIGURE 1-13. Three-dimensional representation of the three major states of a sodium or calcium channel. The S_5 and S_6 α-helical transmembrane segments along with the intervening peptide chains of the four domains surround the pore through which ions cross the lipid barrier in the core of the membrane. The S_1, S_2, and S_3 α-helical transmembrane segments (not labeled) allow the channel to interact with the bilayer. **A,** In the resting state, the pore is closed. **B,** The gating mechanism that opens the channel is provided by the four charge S_4 transmembrane segments (the m gates or voltage sensors) that shift their positions in response to membrane depolarization. **C,** The transition to the refractory state is brought about when the intracellular peptide chain that connects the III and IV domains (the h gate or inactivation particle) swings toward the membrane to occlude the pore. (*Adapted from* Katz [2].)

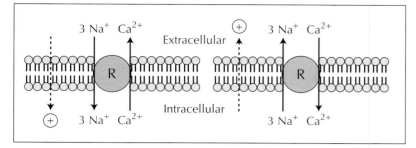

FIGURE 1-15. Reaction mechanism of the sodium-calcium exchanger. The exchanger, labeled "R," can move either three sodium ions or one calcium ion in either direction across the plasma membrane in exchange for either three sodium ions or one

calcium ion that cross the membrane in the opposite direction. Because a net movement of positive charge accompanies the flux of sodium, the sodium-calcium exchanger generates a small membrane current and so is electrogenic. The rates of sodium and calcium transported by the exchanger in either direction depend on the relative concentrations of these ions on the two sides of the membrane and on transmembrane potential. The positive inotropic effect of the cardiac glycosides, which directly inhibit the sodium pump, is mediated by the sodium-calcium exchanger. Because digitalis increases intracellular Na^+, the exchanger will carry more sodium and therefore less calcium out of the cytosol. By increasing cellular stores of calcium, this effect alone allows the cardiac glycosides to augment myocardial contractility. (*Adapted from* Katz [2].)

RESPONSES TO CHANGING ATP CONCENTRATION

DUAL ROLE OF ATP IN MYOCARDIAL FUNCTION

SUBSTRATE EFFECTS (ATP<1 µM)

Actomyosin ATPase (contractile proteins)

Ion pumps (sodium and calcium pumps)

ALLOSTERIC (REGULATORY) EFFECTS (ATP 0.1 TO >1 mM)

"Plasticize" actomyosin

Accelerate ion pumps (sodium and calcium pumps)

Accelerate ion exchanger (sodium/calcium exchange)

Accelerate ion fluxes

  Plasma membrane sodium and calcium channels

  Sarcoplasmic reticulum calcium release channels

Inhibit ATP regeneration

  Glycolysis

  Glycogenolysis

  Oxidative phosphorylation

FIGURE 1-16. Dual role of ATP in myocardial function. ATP has two fundamentally different effects on myocardial function. Substrate effects are seen at very low ATP concentrations, below 1 µM, which saturate the substrate-binding sites that provide energy for ion pumps and the contractile proteins. These substrate effects require that ATP be hydrolyzed to release its chemical energy. Because the free energy released during ATP hydrolysis (-δG) depends on the ratio [ATP]/[ATP] + [P_I], the energy made available by ATP hydrolysis is reduced by a fall in [ATP], and more importantly, by increases in [ADP] and [P_i]. ATP at much higher concentrations exerts quite different allosteric effects; these do not require that ATP be hydrolyzed and therefore can be mimicked by nonhydrolyzable ATP analogues. The allosteric effects seen at normal cytosolic ATP concentrations, which are in the millimolar range, generally stimulate ion pumps, ion exchangers, and ion channels; therefore, ATP can be regarded as a "lubricant" that increases both active and passive ion fluxes. Attenuation of these allosteric effects along with a decrease in the free energy released by ATP hydrolysis inhibits the calcium fluxes involved in both excitation and relaxation (see Fig. 1-8), and thereby reduces contractility and slows relaxation in the energy-starved heart. Because ATP binding to myosin cross-bridges also dissociates actin and myosin, a fall in ATP concentration directly inhibits relaxation of the contractile proteins. Other allosteric effects seen at normal levels of ATP slow energy production by inhibiting glycolysis, glycogenolysis, and oxidative phosphorylation. Attenuation of these inhibitory effects enables a decreased cellular ATP concentration to promote ATP regeneration in the energy-starved heart. ATPase—adenosine triphosphatase.

CELLULAR REGULATION

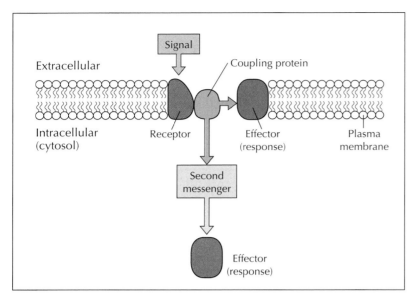

FIGURE 1-17. Most signals that impinge on the heart modify function by initiating complex multistep responses. For example, the signal generated by the arrival of a neurotransmitter at the extracellular side of the plasma membrane is commonly "recognized" when the transmitter molecule (ligand) binds with high affinity to a specific receptor. In most cases, the response to the signal requires that the ligand-bound receptor activate a coupling protein, which is a member of an extended family of GTP-binding proteins. By interacting *directly* with an effector molecule, *indirectly* by initiating the production of a second messenger, or both, the activated coupling proteins then evoke a response. Specificity in the responses to the many signals that influence cardiac function reflects the high affinity of the ligand for a specific receptor, the ability of a given ligand-receptor complex to activate a specific coupling protein, and the affinity of the activated coupling protein for specific effector systems in the cell.

PLASMA MEMBRANE RECEPTORS

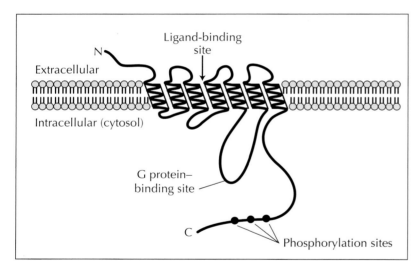

FIGURE 1-18. G protein–coupled receptors. These receptors contain seven transmembrane α-helices. Like many other proteins in the heart, these receptors are members of an extended family of membrane proteins that share a number of structural features. These include the seven transmembrane α-helices, a large N-terminal extracellular loop, a fatty acylation site within the bilayer, and a C-terminal intracellular loop containing phosphorylation sites. The most highly conserved peptide sequences are in the transmembrane segments, whereas diversity is greatest in the hydrophilic connecting loops. These receptors, which bind to catecholamines like norepinephrine, peptides like angiotensin II and endothelin, and lipid prostaglandins, participate in many signal transduction systems. When these receptors bind to their specific ligand, they interact with members of an extended family of GTP-binding coupling proteins, called G proteins, which allows the latter to stimulate or inhibit a variety of intracellular signaling systems.

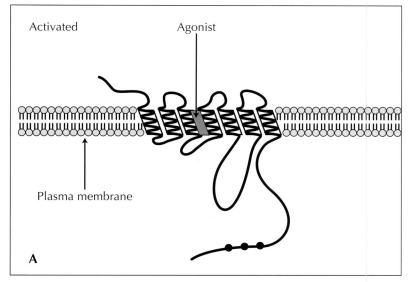

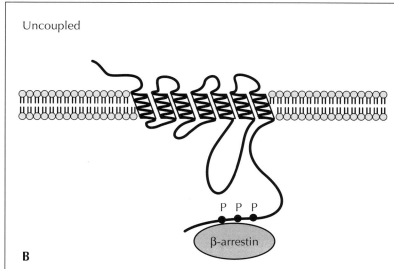

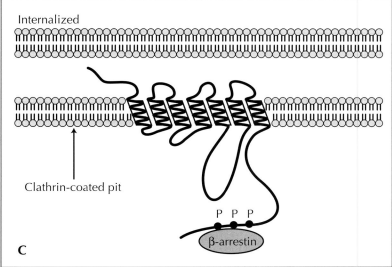

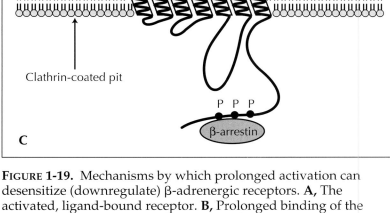

FIGURE 1-19. Mechanisms by which prolonged activation can desensitize (downregulate) β-adrenergic receptors. **A,** The activated, ligand-bound receptor. **B,** Prolonged binding of the receptor to its agonist stimulates a G protein–receptor kinase (GRK) called βARK (β-adrenergic receptor kinase) to catalyze the phosphorylation of the C-terminal intracellular peptide chain, which then binds a cofactor called β-arrestin that inactivates the receptor. **C,** Transfer of the phosphorylated receptors from the plasma membrane to clathrin-coated pits within the cell internalizes the receptors that, although structurally intact, can no longer interact with either their agonists or their G protein. Dephosphorylation (not shown), by allowing the internalized receptors to return to the plasma membrane, can resensitize the receptors. **D,** If the receptors remain internalized for a long period, they are digested by intracellular proteolytic enzymes. This mechanism, unlike uncoupling and internalization, is irreversible and so can be reversed only when new receptors are synthesized de novo. (*Adapted from* Katz [2].)

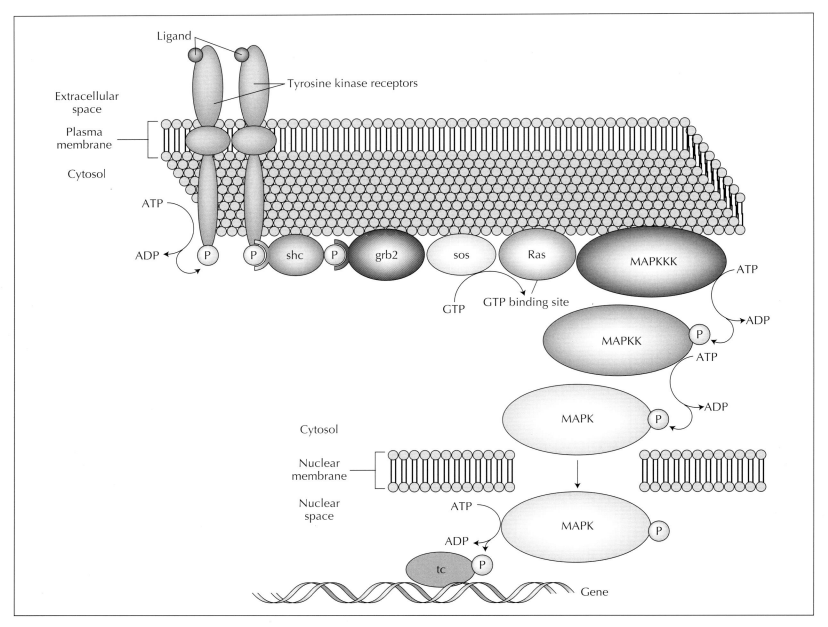

FIGURE 1-20. Proliferative responses. Proliferative responses are mediated by many different signal transduction pathways, including the MAP kinase pathway shown here. These signaling cascades utilize a GTP-binding coupling protein to activate a series of three serine–threonine kinase-catalyzed phosphorylations. The first two, catalyzed by MAP kinase kinase kinase (MAPKKK), and MAP kinase kinase (MAPKK), phosphorylate the next enzyme "down" the pathway. Phosphorylation of MAP kinase, the third in this series of kinases, allows this activated enzyme to enter the nucleus, where it activates nuclear transcription factors that evoke proliferative responses. There are at least three different MAP kinase pathways: the "classic" mitogenic pathway shown here, and two "stress-activated" MAP kinase pathways that phosphorylate transcription factors called JNK and p38. Mitogenic MAP kinases generally activate cell growth and proliferation and inhibit apoptosis, while stress-activated MAP kinases are usually pro-apoptotic and, in the case of p38, stimulate cytokine production. However, the cellular responses to these pathways are highly variable and depend both on cell type and the state of the cell.

The mitogenic MAP kinase pathway shown in this figure is coupled by the monomeric GTP-binding protein Ras, which is activated indirectly by a ligand-bound tyrosine kinase receptor. This pathway can also be activated by G protein–coupled receptors that are coupled to signaling molecules called $G_{\alpha q}$ or $G_{\beta \gamma}$, which are derived from the G proteins.

Proliferative signaling by the mitogenic MAP kinase pathway is initiated when a ligand, such as a peptide growth factor, binds to a tyrosine kinase receptor to activate a latent tyrosine kinase activity. This results in autophosphorylation, which creates a "docking site" on the receptor that binds, and then phosphorylates Shc, an "adaptor protein;" this creates another docking site on Shc, which adds Grb2 to a multiprotein aggregate that forms along the inner surface of the plasma membrane. This aggregate then activates Sos, a guanine nucleotide-exchange factor that exchanges Ras-bound GDP for GTP. The activated Ras-GTP complex stimulates Raf-1, a MAPKKK that phosphorylates and activates the MAPKK MEK-1, which then phosphorylates the MAP kinase (MAPK) ERK-2. Translocation of the latter to the nucleus allows the activated MAP kinase to phosphorylate nuclear transcription factors (tc) that interacts with specific DNA sequences. (*Adapted from* Katz [3].)

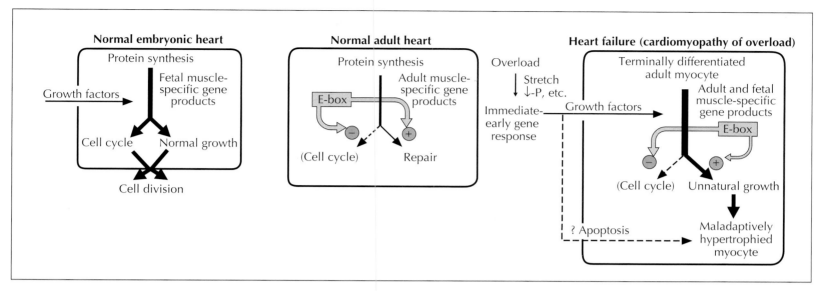

FIGURE 1-21. Differences in the overall growth patterns of proliferating myocytes of the embryonic heart, terminally differentiated myocytes of the adult heart, and maladaptively hypertrophied myocytes of the failing heart. In the embryonic heart, growth factors stimulate preferential synthesis of fetal protein isoforms, which, because it is matched to cell division, leads to the normal cell cycle. Withdrawal of the growth factors and binding of myogenic factors to the E-box in the terminally differentiated cells of the normal adult heart slows protein synthesis, inhibits the cell cycle, and favors the synthesis of adult muscle-specific gene products.

In the terminally differentiated cells of the normal adult heart, the slow rate of protein synthesis is appropriate for repair and renewal of cellular constituents. Overloading of the adult heart appears to initiate an unnatural growth response by activating an immediate-early gene response that renews growth factor stimulation, accelerates protein synthesis, and favors the expression of fetal muscle—specific gene products. In contrast to the embryonic heart, however, the cell cycle remains inhibited, so that the growth response of the overloaded adult cardiac myocytes is abnormal. Cell death in the overloaded heart, which probably plays an important role in the poor prognosis of patients with heart failure, may reflect, in part, the ability of some of the growth factors produced in the immediate-early gene response not only to stimulate protein synthesis, but also to cause programmed cell death (apoptosis). (*Adapted from* Katz [8].)

REFERENCES

1. Katz AM: Molecular biology in cardiology: a paradigmatic shift. *J Mol Cell Cardiol* 1988, 20:355–366.

2. Katz AM: *Physiology of the Heart*, edn 3. Philadelphia: Lippincott Williams & Wilkins; 2001.

3. Katz AM: *Heart Failure: Pathophysiology, Molecular Biology, Clinical Management*. Philadelphia: Lippincott Williams & Wilkins; 2000.

4. Katz AM: Congestive heart failure: role of altered myocardial cellular control. *N Engl J Med* 1975, 293:1184–1191.

5. McNutt NA, Fawcett DW: Myocardial ultrastructure. In *The Mammalian Myocardium*. Edited by Langer GA, Brady AJ. New York: Wiley; 1974:1–49.

6. Herzberg O, James MNG: Structure of calcium regulatory protein troponin C at 28Å resolution. *Nature* 1985, 313:653–659.

7. Toyoshima C, Sasabe H, Stokes DL: Three-dimensional cryo-electron microscopy of the calcium ion pump in the sarcoplasmic reticulum membrane. *Nature* 1993, 362:469–471.

8. Katz AM: The cardiomyopathy of overload: an unnatural growth response in the hypertrophied heart. *Ann Intern Med* 1994, 121:363–371.

PHYSIOLOGY OF MYOCARDIAL CONTRACTION

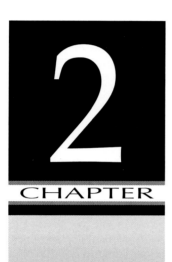

Mark R. Starling

The principal function of the heart is to propel oxygenated blood to the peripheral tissues to meet their metabolic demands. The systemic arterial and venous systems provide the conduits. The interaction of the left ventricle (LV) with the arterial and venous systems is therefore integral to the satisfactory performance of this vital function. It is important to understand how the normal heart functions and how it interacts with the systemic arterial and venous systems as a prelude to comprehending how it is affected by various pathologic conditions. This chapter provides a physiologic framework for understanding normal cardiac contraction and relaxation and the interaction of the LV with the systemic arterial and venous systems by developing seven basic concepts. Taken together, these concepts can be used to provide insight into abnormal cardiac mechanisms in pathophysiologic conditions.

First, the mechanics of cardiac contraction are examined by analysis of muscle models; isometric contraction, the force-velocity relation, and the force-velocity-length relation; the concept of length-dependent activation; the ultrastructural basis for Starling's law of the heart, differences between cardiac and skeletal muscle; and the sarcomere length-ventricular performance relation. Second, these concepts are carried into the intact heart by examining the determinants of contraction through analysis of the cardiac cycle and of LV dynamic geometry and the complex control of the intact circulation. Third, the concept of LV preload is examined through an analysis of LV diastolic properties, including the concepts of the importance of the pericardium and ventricular interaction, the regulation of venous return, and preload reserve and afterload mismatch.

Fourth, left ventricular contractility is analyzed using the time-varying elastance model to assess the effects of catecholamines and pharmacologic depressants on contractility and the interval-strength relationship. Fifth, LV afterload is defined and the contribution of arterial properties to afterload examined, as well as the effects of arterial impedance on LV contractility and ejection. Sixth, an assessment of myocardial energetics, using the myocardial oxygen consumption/pressure-volume area relationship as an approach to evaluating the efficiency of work performed by the contractile element, is presented. Finally, neural control of contractility is examined, the concept of "accentuated antagonism" defined, and the effects of neural reflexes on contractility presented.

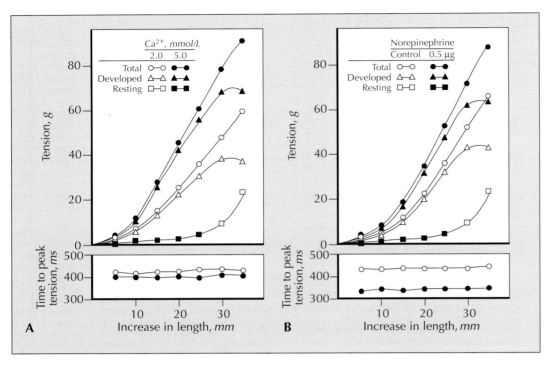

FIGURE 2-1. Muscle activity. Several muscle models have been proposed to describe this activity [1]. Each model is composed of three elements: a contractile element (CE), which is assumed to be freely distensible at rest but is capable of generating force and shortening with activation; one or two series elastic elements (SEs); and a parallel elastic element (PE). Whereas both the SE and PE are characterized by their length-tension curves, shortening of the CE is described by the relationship between force and velocity. During isometric contraction, the stimulated CE shortens, stretching the SE and thereby developing force in accordance with the stress-strain relationship of the SE. The rate of force development is therefore determined by the CE velocity and the stiffness of the SE. In the classic model, the passive length-tension curve defines the properties of the PE.

The relationship between developed and total tension generated at different muscle lengths at two calcium concentrations (**A**) and under control and enhanced contractile conditions produced by norepinephrine (**B**) in an isolated cat papillary muscle is illustrated. The resting length-tension curves are not altered by changes in contractile conditions, but with an increase in calcium concentration (**A**), there is an increase in both developed and total tension at each muscle length. In addition, at each muscle length the time to peak tension is shortened, demonstrating that an increase in tension development occurs in a shorter time, consistent with enhanced contractile element velocity. This is also true when norepinephrine is added (**B**), and the time to peak tension is achieved even more rapidly than with an increase in calcium concentration. (*Adapted from* Sonnenblick [2].)

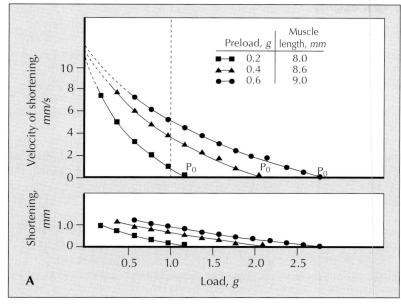

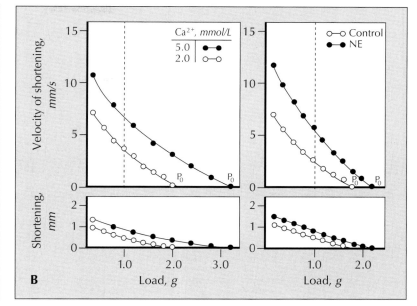

FIGURE 2-2. Preload force-velocity relationship. **A,** The effects of increasing preload, *ie*, initial muscle length, on the force-velocity and force-shortening relationships are shown to demonstrate several concepts [2]. First, with an increase in preload there is an increase in P_0 (isometric pressure), indicating an increase in isometric tension development consistent with the Frank-Starling mechanism. This is further illustrated for shortening by examining the effects of increasing preload on shortening and shortening velocity at the *dashed line*, representing a fixed afterload of 1.0 g. With increasing preload, there is an increase in both the extent and velocity of shortening. Second, extrapolation of the force-velocity relationship to V_{max} reveals that it is similar at all levels of preload, illustrating

that preload has little or no effect on contractile element velocity.

B, In contrast to the effects of initial muscle length, the effect of norepinephrine (NE) on the force-velocity and force-shortening relationships differs [2,3]. With administration of norepinephrine, there is an increase in the velocity of shortening for each afterload, as shown by the *dashed line*, for a load of 1.0 g. Isometric pressure increased as it did with an increase in preload. However, in contrast to the effects of changes in preload alone, extrapolation of the force-velocity relationship to zero load indicates there is an increase in V_{max} consistent with an increase in contractile element (CE) velocity. Consistent with enhanced CE velocity, there is an increase in shortening at each afterload. (*Adapted from* Sonnenblick [2].)

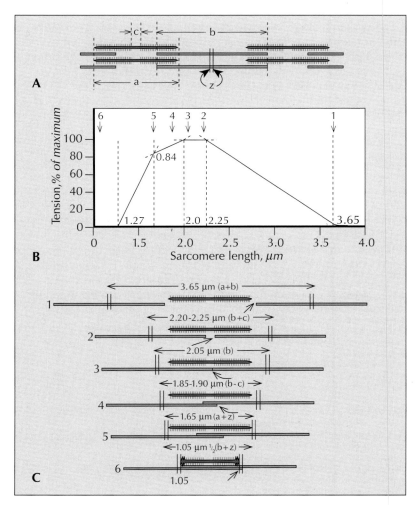

FIGURE 2-3. The Frank-Starling phenomenon. The capacity of the left ventricle to vary the force of contraction on a beat-to-beat basis is a function of sarcomere length and constitutes one of the major principles of cardiac function. It is generally referred to as the *Frank-Starling phenomenon*. This fundamental property of cardiac muscle is based on the length-tension relationship in which the force of contraction or extent of shortening is dependent on the initial muscle length. This, in turn, is dependent on the ultrastructural disposition of the thick and thin myofilaments of sarcomeres. The relationship between myofilament disposition and tension development in skeletal muscle is illustrated [4–6].

A, The myofilaments of the sarcomere are drawn to scale, where the thin filaments are 1.0 μm and the thick filaments are 1.6 μm in length. **B,** The relationship between the tension developed at specific sarcomere lengths in a single skeletal muscle fiber as a percent of the maximal tension is shown. The numbers shown across the *top* denote the specific break-points in the curve corresponding to the sarcomere lengths depicted in the diagram (**C**). Note that there is no overlap of the myofilaments at 3.65 μm to the far right of the tension curve. Optimal overlap of the myofilaments occurs at sarcomere lengths between 2.0 μm and 2.25 μm. As the sarcomere length falls below 2.0 μm, the thick and thin filaments begin to overlap to various extents. At approximately 1.25 μm, no tension is developed, because the thick and thin filaments are completely overlapped and compressed below the length of the thick filaments. The overlapping below 2.0 μm interferes with the formation of cross-bridges and therefore may alter the ability of the thick and thin filaments to bind calcium, reduce the sensitivity of the overlapping thick and thin filaments to calcium, or generate significant internal loads that impede shortening of the sarcomere. a—thick filament length; b—thin filament length; c—central region on thick filament without cross-bridges; z—Z-line attachments of thin filaments. (*Adapted from* Gordon *et al.* [6].)

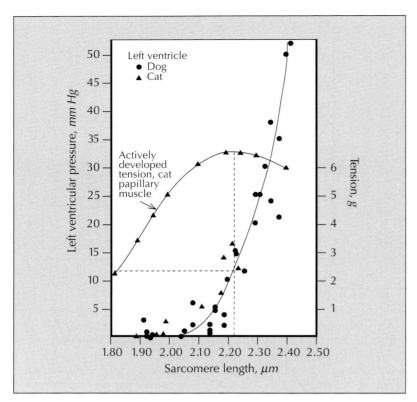

FIGURE 2-4. The relationship between midwall sarcomere length and filling pressure from the left ventricle (LV) is shown. When the LV is empty the sarcomere length averages 1.9 μm, but as the LV fills the sarcomere length increases. At a filling pressure of 12 mm Hg, the sarcomere length reaches approximately 2.2 μm. As illustrated in Figure 2-3, this is the optimal sarcomere length for force generation. Note that because of the stiffness of the passive elastic (PE) element, further distention of the LV causes a sharp increase in filling pressures as the PE element attempts to resist overextension of the sarcomere and prevent disengagement of the myofilaments. Remember also that as preload is increased into these ranges, the series elastic (SE) element becomes important and may contribute to the resistance to disengagement of the myofilaments.

The relationship between tension development in the cat papillary muscle over the same range of sarcomere lengths has been superimposed on the resting length-tension relationship. This confirms the information from Figure 2-3 demonstrating that the optimal sarcomere length for maximal tension development is approximately 2.2 μm. The *dashed lines* indicate that the apex of the active length-tension relationship occurs at the optimal filling pressure of 12 mm Hg when sarcomere length approximates 2.25 μm. (*Adapted from* Spotnitz *et al.* [7].)

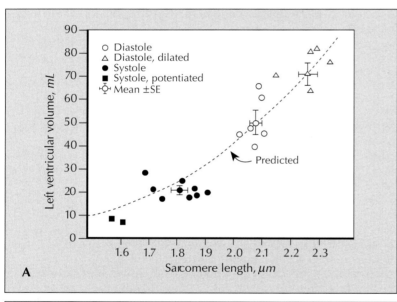

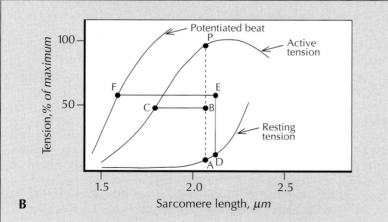

FIGURE 2-5. Ultrastructure-function relation. **A,** The relationship between left ventricular volume and midwall sarcomere length at end-diastole (*open circles*) and end-systole (*closed circles*) from an intact ejecting heart fixed *in situ* is shown [8]. The *open triangles* indicate the end-diastolic volume and sarcomere length after dilatation of the chamber, and the *closed squares* indicate potentiated end-systolic left ventricular volumes and sarcomere lengths.

B, The data from *panel A* have been used to construct the length-tension relationship [9]. The resting length-tension relationship and two active length-tension relationships are constructed. At 2.1 μm on the passive length-tension curve (Point A), indicating the end-diastolic sarcomere length, the maximal pressure (tension) generated under isometric conditions is represented by Point P. If shortening is allowed to occur in the ejecting heart at Point B, sarcomere length decreases to approximately 1.8 μm, which is indicated on the active length-tension curve at point C. On a potentiated beat, end-diastolic sarcomere length would increase along the passive length-tension curve to point D. Pressure (tension) would rise to point E, and ejection would occur to the potentiated end-systolic sarcomere length of 1.6 μm (Point F), defining a new active length-tension curve that is shifted to the left and has a steeper slope.

Thus, it can be extrapolated that in an actively ejecting normal heart, a sarcomere length change of approximately 13% would equate to an ejection fraction of approximately 50%. With a potentiated beat, the change in sarcomere length would increase to 21%, which would produce an ejection fraction of approximately 75%. (Part A *adapted from* Sonnenblick *et al.* [8]; part B *adapted from* Ross *et al.* [9].)

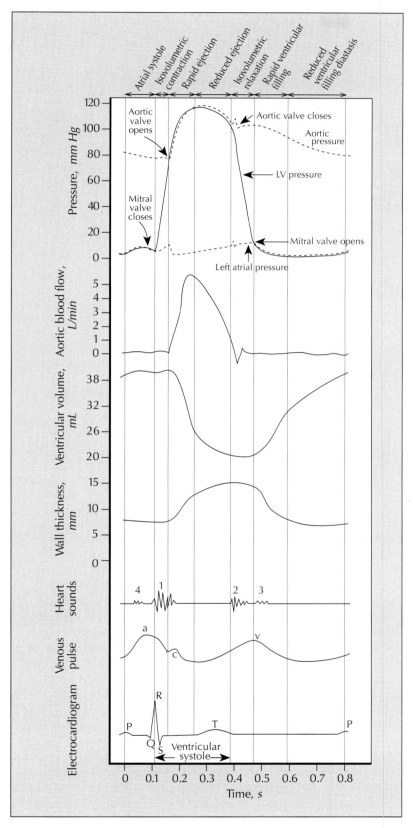

FIGURE 2-6. The events of the cardiac cycle. From *top* to *bottom*, aortic, left ventricular (LV), and left atrial pressure signals are shown, followed by the aortic flow signal, LV volume curve, LV wall thickness curve, heart sounds, the venous pulse, and the electrocardiogram. With electrical activation there is an abrupt increase in isovolumic LV pressure, followed by rapid ejection and sustained pressure elevation. Reduced ejection follows until closure of the aortic valve, achievement of zero flow, minimal volume, and maximal LV wall thickness, at which time diastolic events are initiated. The initial diastolic event, active LV pressure decline, is followed by rapid filling, which manifests as a rapid increase in LV volume and thinning of the LV wall, followed by diastasis. Diastole is completed with atrial contraction. (*Adapted from* Berne and Levy [10].)

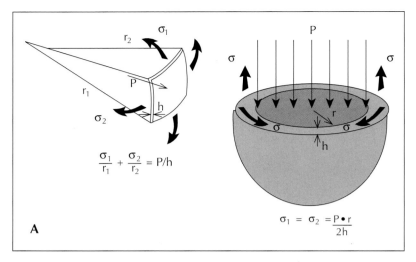

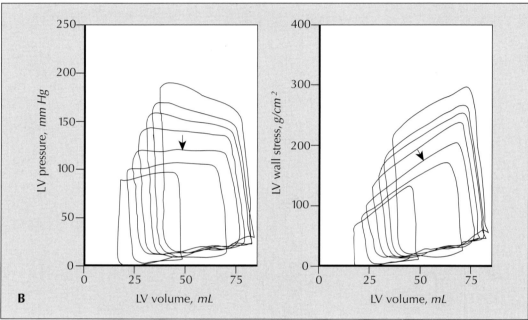

FIGURE 2-7. The heart compared with isolated muscle. In comparing the heart with isolated muscle, the heart's volume and pressure can be related to muscle length and tension [11]. In more complex formulations, the average circumferential wall stress (force per unit of cross-sectional area of wall) is related directly to the product of intraventricular pressure and radius, and inversely to wall thickness. In its simplest version, Laplace's law for a spherical ventricle is $\sigma = P \cdot r / 2h$, where r is the left ventricular (LV) radius at the endocardial surface, P is intraventricular pressure, and h is LV wall thickness.

As illustrated here in its general form for a thin-walled sphere, the law relates the various stresses to the internal pressure, P, by the equation: $\sigma/r_1 + \sigma/r_2 = P/h$, where σ_1 and σ_2 represent stresses acting on the surface perpendicular to each other, r_1 and r_2 represent the radii of curvature of the surface, and h represents the wall thickness.

However, the LV is not a thin sphere, but rather is more appropriately represented by an ellipsoid of revolution, which is thick-walled, where σ_1 and σ_2 are not equal. Therefore, two different stresses, meridional stress acting perpendicular to the short axis and circumferential stress acting perpendicular to the long axis and in the direction of the midwall circumferential fibers, can be expressed by equations $Pb/2h (1-h/2b)^2$ and $Pb/h [1-h/2b-b^2/2a^2]$, respectively [12].

In the calculation of meridional and circumferential stress (σ_m and σ_c, respectively), a and b represent the midwall semi-major and semi-minor axes, respectively. Thus, not only do the calculations of meridional and circumferential stress vary but they may vary in a nonlinear fashion with changes in LV geometry. In the ejecting LV, the extent and rate of shortening are analogous to the extent and velocity of shortening of isolated muscle. LV pressure during ejection is therefore closely related to afterload, although geometric factors must be considered in calculating wall forces in the heart. **B,** To illustrate this point, left ventricular (LV) pressure-volume and stress-volume loops generated over a wide range of loading conditions are shown. The *arrows* indicate the control pressure-volume and stress-volume loops [5,13]. The configuration of the stress-volume loops clearly differs from the pressure-volume loops because LV wall thickness and geometry are included in the calculation. Nevertheless, both relationships show linearity at end-systole. The diastolic pressure-volume and stress-volume relations both appear to be curvilinear over this range of loading conditions. Consequently, both pressure-volume and stress-volume relations provide the basis for assessing both LV systolic (contractile) and diastolic function in the intact heart. (*Adapted from* Ross [13].)

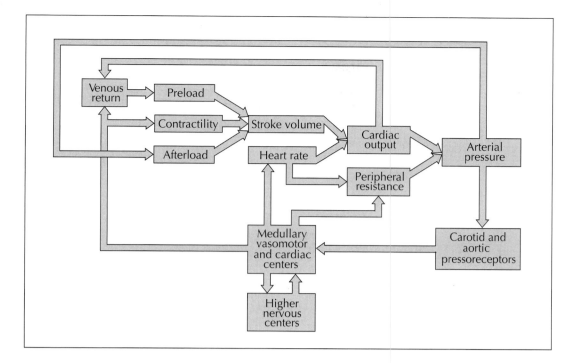

FIGURE 2-8. Interactions in the intact circulation. In the intact circulation, interaction of preload, contractility, and afterload in producing stroke volume is complex. Stroke volume combined with heart rate determines cardiac output, which, in turn, when combined with peripheral vascular resistance, determines arterial pressure for tissue perfusion. The characteristics of the arterial system also contribute to afterload. The interaction of these components with carotid and aortic arch baroreceptors provides a feedback mechanism to higher medullary and vasomotor cardiac centers and to higher levels in the central nervous system to affect a modulating influence on heart rate, peripheral vascular resistance, venous return, and contractility [14]. Heart rate changes may also influence contractility. Cardiac output and peripheral vascular resistance can modulate venous return. This complex interaction is intrinsically fine-tuned to regulate beat-to-beat changes and thereby adapt the system in response to demand. (*Adapted from* Badke and O'Rourke [11].)

PRELOAD

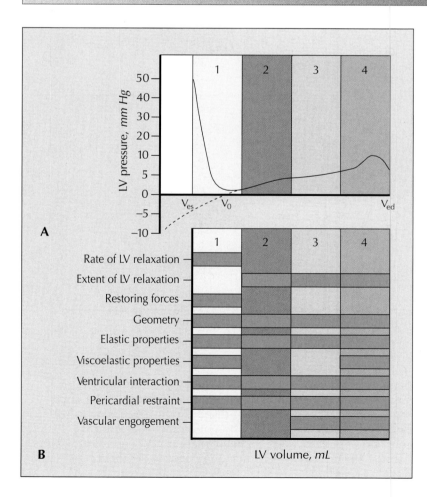

FIGURE 2-9. Left ventricular (LV) diastolic properties. **A**, LV diastole has four phases that include active relaxation during the period of isovolumic pressure decline (phase 1), rapid LV filling (phase 2), passive LV filling (phase 3), and the atrial contribution to LV filling (phase 4). LV relaxation begins at end-systolic volume (V_{es}) and is completed at end-diastolic volume (V_{ed}). V_0 represents the unstressed diastolic volume of the LV. **B**, The complex interaction of several factors can affect LV diastolic properties in different phases of diastole, and they include the rate of LV relaxation, the extent of LV relaxation, restoring forces of the LV, geometry of the LV, the elastic properties of the LV wall, the viscoelastic properties of the LV wall, right and left ventricular interaction, pericardial restraint, and vascular engorgement [15,16].

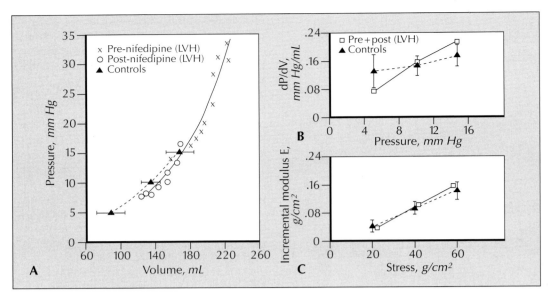

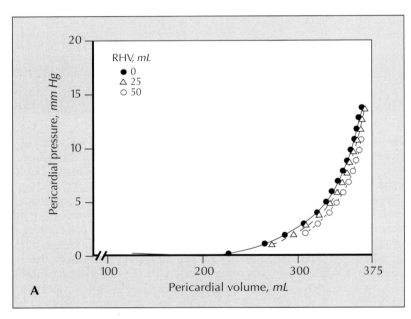

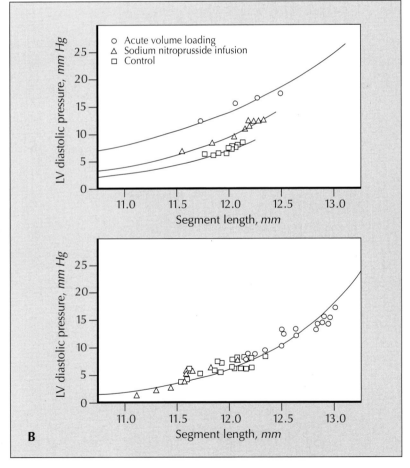

FIGURE 2-10. The use of left ventricular (LV) chamber stiffness and myocardial stiffness in differentiating the impact of pathologic processes (in this case, hypertrophy) on diastolic properties of the LV.

The plots of LV pressure versus volume in control subjects and patients with LV hypertrophy (LVH) before and after use of nifedipine are curvilinear, representing an exponential relationship between LV pressure and volume (**A**). When LV chamber stiffness is plotted against pressure, the relationship is linearized, and there is a distinct difference between the control subjects and patients with LVH, demonstrated by an increased slope in the LVH subjects consistent with increased stiffness of the LV chamber (**B**). In contrast, when myocardial stiffness is plotted against stress, there is no difference in the linear slope values between the control subjects and patients with LVH, indicating that the elastic stiffness of the muscle has not been affected by the hypertrophy process despite a significant change in the elastic stiffness of the LV chamber (**C**).

Therefore, LV chamber stiffness and myocardial stiffness can be used to differentiate the contribution of changes in myocardial properties to altered distensibility of the LV chamber. (*Adapted from* Mirsky [17].)

FIGURE 2-11. The pericardium has a substantial role in determining the left ventricular (LV) diastolic pressure-volume relationship. **A,** The pericardial pressure-volume relationship is uniquely bimodal [18]. This pericardial pressure-volume relationship was generated as right heart volume (RHV) was progressively increased from 0 to 50 mL. The pericardial pressure-volume relationships were little affected by right heart volumes. At low pericardial volumes, the pericardial pressure-volume relationship is quite flat, but it becomes extremely steep as pericardial volumes exceed approximately 225 mL. Therefore, the pericardial pressure-volume relationship has very little effect on LV diastolic properties at low volumes, but it can have a substantial restraining effect at high volumes.

B, To illustrate this point, LV pressure-segment length relations in conscious, chronically instrumented dogs were analyzed during acute volume loading with (*top*) and without (*bottom*) an intact pericardium [19]. With acute volume loading they were superiorly displaced, and with sodium nitroprusside they are inferiorly displaced toward the control level. With the pericardium removed, these relationships are not shifted superiorly, but they remain on a continuum despite the same sequence of volume loading and sodium nitroprusside infusion. Therefore, with acute cardiac dilatation the pericardium contributes substantially to the increase in LV diastolic pressure because of shifts in the LV diastolic pressure-segment length relationship. (*continued*)

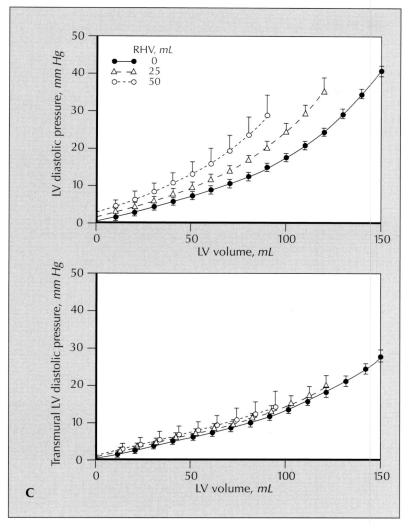

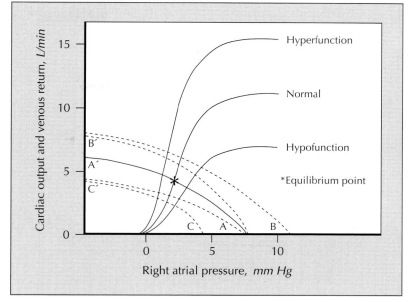

FIGURE 2-12. The regulation of venous return. The Y axis represents cardiac output and venous return, and the X axis represents right atrial pressure [20,21]. The *solid line* from A, on the X axis, to A′, on the Y axis, indicates the resting venous return curve. At A, the right atrial pressure is high enough to provide no pressure gradient from the peripheral tissue to the heart and, therefore, there is zero venous return. As right atrial pressure falls, the gradient from the peripheral tissues to the heart increases and venous return also increases. With superimposition of a normal cardiac output curve, the crossing of the cardiac output and venous return curves is the equilibrium point at which venous return to the heart from the peripheral tissues is matched with cardiac output from the heart to the peripheral tissues. With hypofunctioning of the heart, there is a shift in this equilibrium point to a higher right atrial pressure, thereby reducing venous return to the heart.

Parallel displacements of the venous return curve are consistent with changes in systemic venous pressure that may be attributable to changes in vasomotor tone, blood volume, interstitial fluid volume, intra-abdominal pressure, or muscle compression of the venous system. For example, with blood loss, the venous return curve shifts from the A-A′ curve to the C-C′ curve, and a lower equilibrium point is achieved at a lower right atrial pressure and cardiac output. The opposite effect is seen with an increase in blood volume or vasomotor tone. For example, with an increase in catecholamine activity seen with exercise, the venous return curve shifts from the A-A′ curve to the B-B′ curve. With hyperfunction of the heart associated with enhanced catecholamine activity, as with exercise, there is a greater venous return at a lower right atrial pressure to maintain cardiac filling during the demand for high output.

A different pattern of venous return curves results from alterations in peripheral vascular resistance at the arteriolar level. With a decrease in peripheral vascular resistance, the venous return curve shifts to the A-B′ curve, and with an increase in peripheral vascular resistance, the venous return curve shifts to the A-C′ curve. These changes in the venous return curve result from dilatation or constriction, respectively, of the systemic arterioles. Therefore, there is dynamic equilibrium between cardiac output and venous return, which is finely regulated on a beat-to-beat basis and with changes in demand, such as exercise, to maintain cardiac output and tissue perfusion.

FIGURE 2-11. *(continued)* This kind of upward displacement of the diastolic pressure-segment length or volume relationship is indicative of the restraining effect of the pericardium. This phenomenon can also be observed with dilatation of chambers of one side of the heart. **C**, The effects of increasing RHVs on the LV pressure-volume relationship have also been studied in canine hearts [18]. As RHVs are incrementally increased with the pericardium intact, LV pressures are also incrementally increased *(top)*. Over a comparable range of LV volumes, there is an upward displacement of the LV pressure-volume relationship due to ventricular interaction. As a consequence, for comparable LV volumes, LV pressures are disproportionately elevated and provide an inaccurate determination of LV filling pressure. In contrast, if transmural LV pressure, which takes into account both the LV pressure and pericardial pressure, is used, there are no differences in transmural pressure across the full range of right and LV volumes *(bottom)*, suggesting that transmural pressure represents a better measure of LV distending pressure. If right atrial pressure is substituted for pericardial pressure, then a simple approximation of transmural pressure can be calculated. (Parts A and C *adapted from* Hess *et al.* [18]; part B *adapted from* Shirato *et al.* [19].)

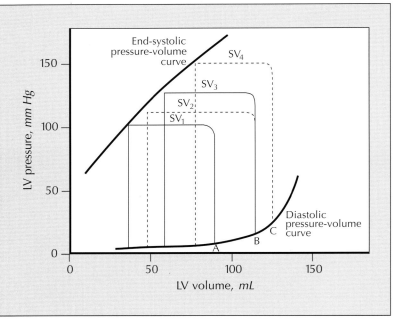

FIGURE 2-13. The concept of preload reserve and afterload mismatch. This concept was proposed by Ross [22] and demonstrated in studies by Lee *et al.* [23]. This concept provides a

possible explanation for the descending limb of the Starling curve.

An attempt to graphically depict this relationship in an intact circulation that is allowed to freely adapt to alterations in LV pressure and volume is shown here, assuming a single diastolic and end-systolic pressure-volume relationship. Starting at point A and following the *lower solid line* at a constant contractile state, SV_1 is generated. With volume loading alone, movement up the diastolic pressure-volume curve to point B occurs, and the *lower dashed line* is followed generating SV_2, which is greater than SV_1, indicating the presence of preload reserve. Similarly, with pressure loading there is an increase in end-diastolic volume and pressure to point B along the diastolic pressure-volume curve; the *upper solid line* is followed generating SV_3, which is equal to SV_1. Therefore, despite an increase in LV pressure, stroke volume is maintained owing to preload reserve. In contrast, with a further increase in LV pressure following the *upper dashed line*, stroke volume is decreased, as shown by SV_4, due to an afterload mismatch. Preload reserve is exhausted at point C on the diastolic pressure-volume curve and is therefore insufficient to compensate for the increase in afterload. This is consistent with the observations of Lee *et al.* [23] in conscious animals, indicating that preload reserve is substantial in the normal heart and it can compensate for increases in afterload on a beat-to-beat basis without changes in the passive diastolic pressure-volume relationship or contractility as long as venous return is adequate.

CONTRACTILITY

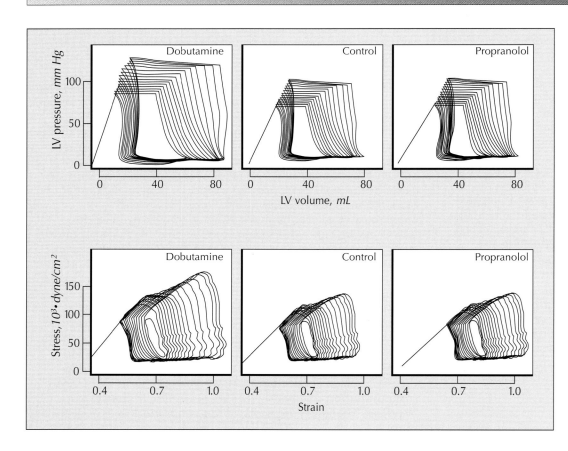

FIGURE 2-14. The effects of the β-agonist dobutamine and the β-antagonist propranolol on left ventricular (LV) contractility in the dog. By examining representative LV pressure-volume (*top*) and stress-strain (*bottom*) relationships, it is apparent that dobutamine increased the slope of the pressure-volume relation with very little change in the volume-axis intercept, and propranolol decreased the slope with no significant change in the volume-axis intercept. Similar observations were seen with the stress-strain relation. The slope of the LV end-systolic pressure-volume relationship is unique to the inotropic state. Both the LV pressure-segment length and stress-strain relationships provide similar information. (*Adapted from* Kaseda *et al.* [24].)

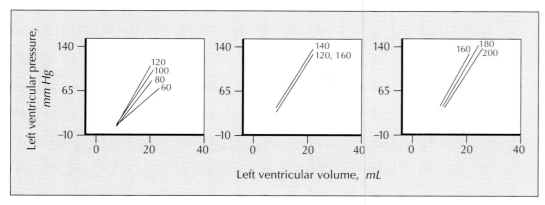

FIGURE 2-15. The effect of heart rate on the left ventricular (LV) end-systolic pressure-volume relationship (E_{es}) is shown from isolated, ejecting canine LV preparations to illustrate the interval-strength relationship [25]. Over a heart rate range from 60 to 120 bpm, the slope of E_{es} increased significantly from 3.5 to 5.3 mm Hg/mL (*left*). There was very little change in the average E_{es} above 120 bpm. Over the same heart rate range there is very little change in the volume-axis intercept, V_0. These changes are consistent with a positive inotropic effect such as that observed with catecholamines [26]. The interval-strength relationship in the isolated heart preparation is therefore similar to the interval-strength relationship documented in isolated muscle [2] or other preparations [27–30], which is indicative of the heart rate–dependence of contractility. (*Adapted from* Maughan *et al.* [25].)

AFTERLOAD

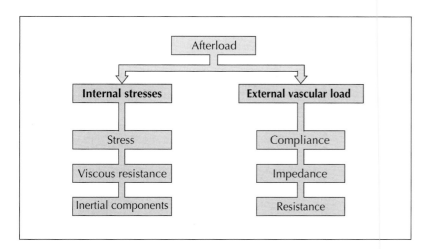

FIGURE 2-16. Afterload. The afterload against which the myocardium must work is composed of internal stresses, resistance, and inertial components. The external vascular load is composed of compliance, impedance, and resistance characteristics of the arterial vasculature. The components of stress, left ventricular (LV) pressure, mass, and geometry have been described. The viscous drag and inertial forces that must be overcome to generate blood movement are minor and are usually ignored. However, the characteristics of vascular load and their effects on LV ejection and contractility cannot be ignored because they contribute to the internal forces that the myocardium must carry during each contraction.

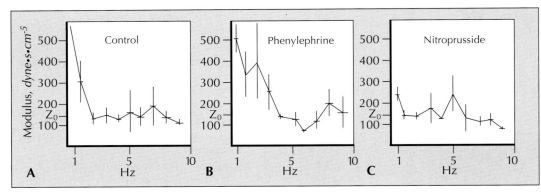

the second to tenth harmonic frequencies (Hz), which are indicative of wave reflections in the system.

A, Under control hemodynamic conditions, the input impedance falls from a high value at zero frequency (mean aortic pressure divided by a mean flow or vascular resistance) to a minimum and then oscillates around a mean characteristic impedance (Z_0) of approximately 140 dynes•s•cm^{-5}.

B, When phenylephrine is administered, the moduli for characteristic impedance rise to an average Z_0 of approximately 225 dynes•s•cm^{-5}, indicating increased wave reflections in the system.

C, Nitroprusside decreases these oscillations and characteristic impedance moduli. Similar observations have been reported in normal human systemic arterial vasculature [33,34]. It has also been demonstrated that heart rate and respiratory variation do not affect these quantitative measures of the systemic arterial vasculature [34]. (*Adapted from* Latham *et al.* [31].)

FIGURE 2-17. Arterial impedance. The average systemic arterial impedance moduli from normotensive baboons under control conditions and during phenylephrine and nitroprusside infusions are illustrated [31]. The *impedance* concept is an effort to present a quantitative description of the opposition to blood flow presented by the arterial vasculature [32]. Impedance should not be equated with *afterload*, which is a term that has been developed to describe the opposition to muscle shortening. Nevertheless, impedance can contribute to afterload through its influence on pressure, loading sequence, and geometry. Both resistance and compliance are properties of the arterial vasculature that contribute to, but are not equivalent to, total vascular impedance or opposition to blood flow.

Two specific terms, *input impedance* and *characteristic impedance*, have been used to differentiate the total opposition to blood flow: input impedance, if there were no wave reflections in the system; characteristic impedance, the average of impedance moduli over

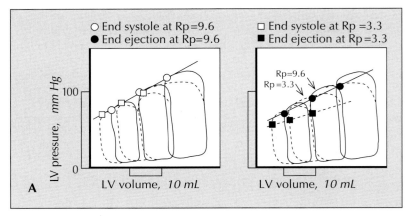

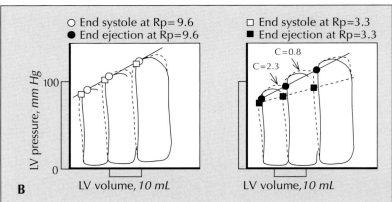

FIGURE 2-18. The effects of alterations in vascular characteristics on both left ventricular (LV) contractility (end-systole) and ejection (end-ejection). **A,** Systemic arterial resistance (Rp) was independently altered, and LV pressure-volume loops were generated over this range of resistance values. Whereas the LV end-systolic pressure-volume relationship (*left*) was not affected by these changes in arterial resistance, LV end-ejection (*right*) was greatly affected. At a higher resistance level, indicated by the *solid pressure-volume loops*, end-ejection appeared to be similar to end-systole (*left*). However, at reduced arterial resistance, indicated by the *dashed pressure-volume loops*, end-ejection (*right*) was substantially dissociated from end-systole (*left*). This indicates that changes in arterial resistance that exceed the expected variation in the normal vasculature *in situ* have little impact on the time of end-systole and this contractile index, but they have substantial effects on ejection characteristics of the LV.

B, In the same preparation, changes in arterial compliance (C) over a sixfold range were used to generate a wide range of LV loads. The end-systolic pressure-volume relations were not affected by these large changes in arterial compliance (*left*). In contrast, with reduced arterial compliance, represented by the *solid pressure-volume loops*, end-ejection (*right*) was similar to end-systole (*left*). When arterial compliance was substantially improved, as indicated by the *dashed pressure-volume loops* (*right*), there was a substantial dissociation of end-ejection from end-systole. This demonstrates, once again, a significant impact of changes in arterial characteristics on ejection characteristics of the LV but not the time of end-systole or this contractile index. (*Adapted from* Nishioka *et al.* [35].)

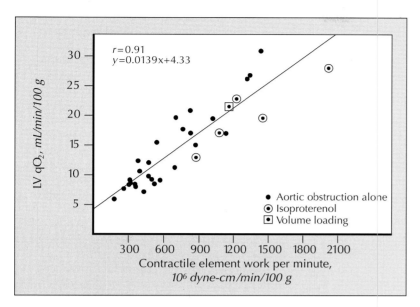

FIGURE 2-19. Formulation of muscle energetics. In 34 studies carried out in 23 dogs with various degrees of aortic obstruction, Britman and Levine [36] measured cardiac output, left ventricular (LV) and aortic pressures, heart rate, LV volume, coronary sinus blood flow, and coronary sinus oxygen extraction. They then compared LV oxygen consumption (LVqO$_2$) in mL/min/100 g of LV mass with contractile element work per minute in dynes•cm/min/100 g of LV weight. As shown here, over a wide range of loading conditions (volume loading) and contractile states (isoproterenol), contractile element work was the major determinant of myocardial oxygen requirements. They concluded that the ultimate formulation of muscle energetics must include consideration of the energy cost of resting cardiac muscle, excitation-contraction coupling, and isovolumic and ejecting work. (*Adapted from* Britman and Levine [36].)

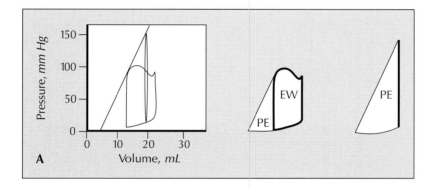

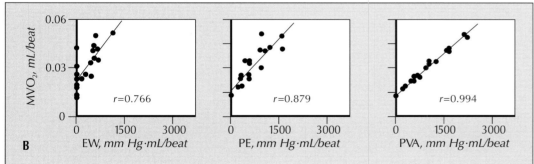

was defined in isovolumic and ejecting beats as the area enclosed by the LV end-systolic pressure-volume relationship, the diastolic curve, and the systolic portion of each pressure-volume trajectory, which differed from the definition used in the initial studies of Monroe and French [39]. It had two components in the ejecting beat, the external work (EW) performed and the potential energy (PE) stored within the contractile element to perform external work [40], whereas in the isovolumic beat only PE was stored in the contractile element.

B, When MVO$_2$ was regressed against EW, PE, or the PVA, there was a highly linear relationship between MVO$_2$ and the PVA. This indicated that neither external nor potential energy alone is sufficient for predicting MVO$_2$, but the PVA, which is the simple sum of EW and PE and reflective of the total potential work that can be performed by the contractile element, can reliably predict MVO$_2$ in a given heart under a stable set of contractile conditions. (*Adapted from* Suga *et al.* [37].)

FIGURE 2-20. Suga *et al.* [37,38] took the muscle-energetics concept into the pressure-volume plane. They regressed myocardial oxygen consumption (MVO$_2$) against the pressure-volume area (PVA) from isolated canine left ventricular (LV) preparations. **A,** The PVA

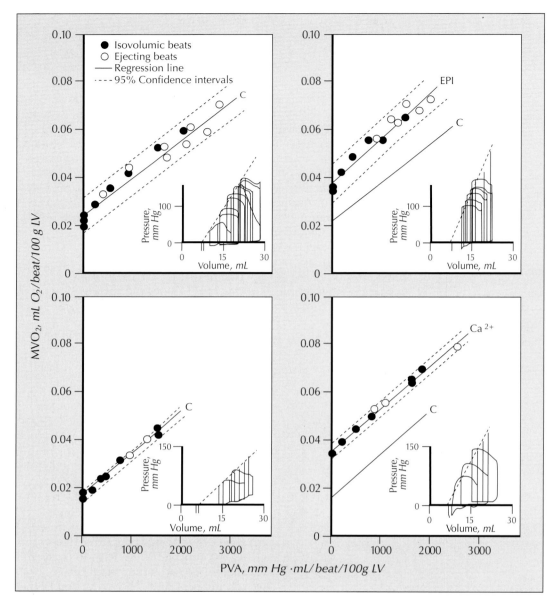

which reflects contractile efficiency, remained similar under the control and enhanced contractile conditions at approximately 30%. An increase in the Y-axis intercept reflects the increment in MVO_2 needed for excitation-contraction coupling, since basal metabolic rate should remain constant.

The incremental energy utilization for a given level of mechanical performance under the enhanced contractile state has been ascribed to the oxygen-wasting effect of inotropic agents. This oxygen-wasting effect has been related to the increased shortening velocity of the myocardium [43]. Others have ascribed the same effect to the augmented energetics for force-independent heat generation associated with calcium release and retrieval in the excitation-contraction coupling process [44].

The MVO_2/PVA relationship is unique in that it enables us to examine the mechanism for the augmented myocardial use of oxygen under enhanced contractile conditions. Because excitation-contraction coupling is known to require large amounts of energy at the sarcoplasmic reticulum and because both epinephrine and calcium augment calcium uptake by the sarcoplasmic reticulum, although by different mechanisms, the increase in MVO_2 needed during the enhanced contractile state probably results from the increase in energy utilization for excitation-contraction coupling produced by these positive inotropic agents. The constant efficiency observed in the MVO_2/PVA relationship indicates that the efficiency of energy conversion of the contractile machinery is constant over the wide range of loading conditions and contractile states employed in these studies. The independence of the slope and, therefore, contractile efficiency from the contractile state, has not, however, been observed in all *in situ* hearts [45,46]. Therefore, the MVO_2/PVA relationship is a concept that can provide new and useful insights into myocardial energy utilization in the intact LV. (*Adapted from* Suga *et al.* [42].)

FIGURE 2-21. In contrast to its independence of heart rate, because heart rate is included in this formulation [41] a positive inotropic agent has an important effect on the myocardial oxygen consumption (MVO_2)/pressure-volume area (PVA) relationship, as indicated here [42]. The same isolated canine left ventricular (LV) preparation was used to examine the relationship between MVO_2 and the PVA under control contractile conditions (C) and after either epinephrine (EPI) or calcium (Ca). These agents both increased the slope of the LV end-systolic pressure-volume relationship, a measure of LV contractility, by approximately 70%. The regression of MVO_2 on the PVA during the control and enhanced contractile states provided comparable slopes but an increase in the Y-axis intercepts with the enhanced contractile states. The reciprocal of the slope,

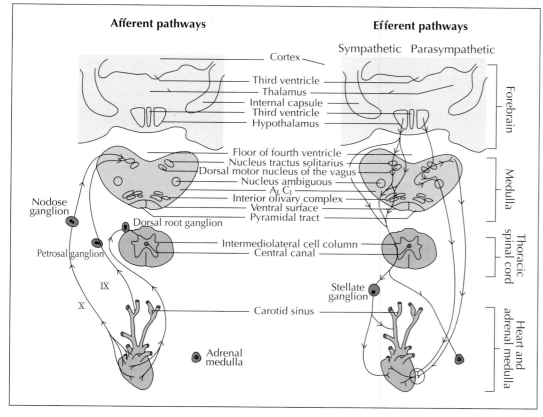

Afferent pathways

Efferent pathways

FIGURE 2-22. The cardiovascular sympathetic and parasympathetic afferent (*left*) and efferent (*right*) pathways. The sympathetic and parasympathetic preganglionic cells represent the final common pathway of neural impulses to the cardiovascular system. They receive excitatory and inhibitory impulses predominantly from the medullary centers. These centers may operate independently and are capable of regulating cardiac contractility and heart rate, arterial pressure, and regional blood flow distribution. Under normal conditions, their activity is influenced by higher centers, principally the

cerebral cortex. Tonic excitatory medullary center activity is constantly influenced by inhibitory impulses from cardiovascular mechano- and chemoreceptors. An increase in activity in the carotid sinus and aortic nerves, as well as the vagal afferent fibers from the heart, reflexly reduces neural activity in the efferent sympathetic fibers and augments efferent vagal activity.

The sympathetic preganglionic neurons lie in the intermedial lateral horns of the spinal cord, leave the spinal cord, synapse with the postganglionic neurons in the chain of ganglia on each side of the spinal cord, and send peripheral sympathetic nerves to the heart and blood vessels. Some preganglionic sympathetic nerve fibers pass directly through these chains to the adrenal medulla. The postganglionic sympathetic nerves originating from the right stellate ganglion are distributed primarily to the sinus node and right atrium and control heart rate, whereas those from the left stellate ganglion supply the left atrium and ventricle for control of contractility. Terminal sympathetic innervation of the heart is a plexiform structure extending around the muscle cells in close apposition to them. The ventricular myocardium is only sparsely innervated by parasympathetic nerves. (*Adapted from* Corr *et al.* [47].)

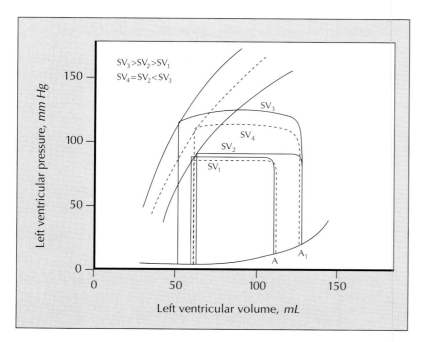

FIGURE 2-23. The effect of the postganglionic sympathetic and parasympathetic neural fibers on cardiac contractility has been described as "accentuated antagonism" [48–50], which is illustrated here. Starting at point A and following the *solid* and *dashed lines* under the basal contractile state where sympathetic activity is low and parasympathetic restraint is dominant, heightened activity of the parasympathetic system (*dashed line*) does not significantly affect contractility or depress stroke volume (SV_1). Heightened sympathetic neural activity, particularly from the left stellate ganglion, increases left atrial transfer function, thereby increasing left ventricular (LV) preload and moving on the passive diastolic filling curve from A to A_1, increasing stroke volume (SV_2). In addition, contractility is increased and pressure generation and shortening are improved, moving to a new LV pressure-volume relationship and enhancing stroke volume (SV_3).

During heightened sympathetic neural activity, an increase in parasympathetic neural activity becomes more apparent and decreases LV contractility, as indicated by a downward and rightward displacement of the LV pressure-volume relationship to the *dashed line*, with a reduction in stroke volumes (SV_4).

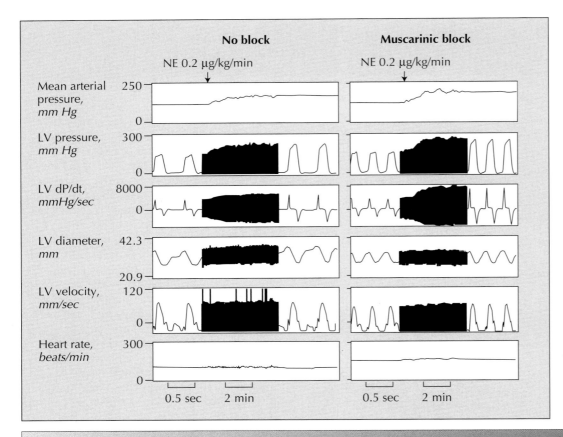

FIGURE 2-24. The steady-state effects of intravenous norepinephrine (NE) on mean arterial and left ventricular (LV) pressures, the rate of change of LV pressure (LV dP/dt), LV diameter and velocity of shortening, and heart rate before and after muscarinic blockade with atropine is shown from a conscious dog preparation. After muscarinic blockade there is a greater increase in LV pressure, LV dP/dt, and LV shortening velocity with norepinephrine. The parasympathetic nervous system can, therefore, exert a tonic inhibitory influence on inotropic responses to peripherally administered sympathomimetic amines. The striking augmentation of the inotropic potential of sympathomimetic amines by muscarinic blockade is probably mediated through the vagal release of acetylcholine, which may inhibit the action of sympathomimetic amines on the β-adrenergic receptor at a postsynaptic site. (*Adapted from* Vatner *et al.* [51].)

REFERENCES

1. Parmley WW, Sonnenblick EH: Series elasticity in heart muscle. *Circ Res* 1967, 20:112–123.

2. Sonnenblick EH: Force-velocity relations in mammalian heart muscle. *Am J Physiol* 1962, 202:931–939.

3. Burns JW, Covell JW, Ross J: Mechanics of isotonic left ventricular contractions. *Am J Physiol* 1973, 224:725–732.

4. Kentish JC, Wrzosek A: Changes in force and cytosolic Ca2+ concentration after length changes in isolated rat ventricular trabeculae. *J Physiol* 1998, 506:431–444.

5. Braunwald E, Sonnenblick EH, Ross J: Mechanisms of cardiac contraction and relaxation. In *Heart Disease: A Textbook of Cardiovascular Medicine*, edn 3. Edited by Braunwald E. Philadelphia: WB Saunders; 1988:383–425.

6. Gordon AM, Huxley AF, Julian FJ: The variation in isometric tension with sarcomere length in vertebrate muscle fibers. *J Physiol* 1966, 184:170–192.

7. Spotnitz HM, Sonnenblick EH, Spiro D: Relation of ultrastructure to function in the intact heart: sarcomere structure relative to pressure-volume curves of intact left ventricles of dog and cat. *Circ Res* 1966, 18:49–66.

8. Sonnenblick EH, Ross J, Covell JW, *et al.*: The ultrastructure of the heart in systole and diastole. *Circ Res* 1967, 21:423–431.

9. Ross J Jr, Sonnenblick EH, Covell JW, *et al.*: Architecture of the heart in systole and diastole: technique of rapid fixation and analysis of left ventricular geometry. *Circ Res* 1967, 21:409–421.

10. Berne RM, Levy MN: *Cardiovascular Physiology*, edn 3. St Louis: CV Mosby; 1977.

11. Badke FR, O'Rourke RA: Cardiovascular physiology. In *Internal Medicine*, edn 1. Edited by Stein JH. Boston: Little, Brown and Co.; 1983:407–423.

12. Mirsky I: Left ventricular stresses in the intact human heart. *Biophys J* 1969, 9:189–208.

13. Ross J: Applications and limitations of end-systolic measures of ventricular performance. *Fed Proc* 1984, 43:2418–2422.

14. Potts JT, McKeown KP, Shoukas AA: Reduction in arterial compliance alters carotid baroreflex control of cardiac output in a model of hypertension. *Am J Physiol* 1998, 274(suppl H):1121–1131.

15. Glantz SA, Parmley WW: Factors which affect the diastolic pressure-volume curve. *Circ Res* 1978, 42:171–180.

16. Gilbert JC, Glantz SA: Determinants of left ventricular filling and of the diastolic pressure-volume relation. *Circ Res* 1989, 64:827–852.

17. Mirsky I: Assessment of diastolic function: suggested methods and future considerations. *Circulation* 1984, 69:836–841.

18. Hess OM, Bhargava V, Ross J, *et al.*: The role of the pericardium in interactions between the cardiac chambers. *Am Heart J* 1983, 106:1377–1383.

19. Shirato K, Shabetai R, Bhargava V, *et al.*: Alteration of the left ventricular diastolic pressure-segment length relation produced by the pericardium. *Circulation* 1978, 57:1191–1197.

20. Rothe CF: Physiology of venous return: an unappreciated boost to the heart. *Arch Intern Med* 1986, 146:977–982.

21. Guyton AC, Jones CE, Coleman TG: Graphical analysis of cardiac output regulation. In *Circulatory Physiology: Cardiac Output and its Regulation*, edn 2. Edited by Guyton AC, Jones CE, Lobwan TG. Philadelphia: WB Saunders; 1973:237–252.

22. Ross J: Afterload mismatch and preload reserve: a conceptual framework for the analysis of ventricular function. *Prog Cardiovasc Dis* 1976, 18:255–264.

23. Lee JD, Tajimi T, Ptritti J, *et al.*: Preload reserve and mechanisms of afterload mismatch in normal conscious dog. *Am J Physiol* 1986, 250:H464–H473.

24. Kaseda S, Tomoike H, Ogata I, *et al.*: End-systolic pressure-volume, pressure-length and stress-strain relations in canine hearts. *Am J Physiol* 1985, 249:H648–H654.

25. Maughan WL, Sunagawa K, Burkhoff D, *et al.*: Effect of heart rate on the canine end-systolic pressure-volume relationship. *Circulation* 1985, 72:654–659.

26. Suga H, Sagawa K: Instantaneous pressure-volume relationships and their ratio in the excised supported canine left ventricle. *Circ Res* 1974, 35:117–126.

27. Mitchell JH, Wallace AG, Skinner NS: Intrinsic effects of heart rate on left ventricular performance. *Am J Physiol* 1963, 205:41–48.

28. Covell JW, Ross J, Taylor R, *et al.*: Effects of increasing frequency of contraction on the force-velocity relation of left ventricle. *Cardiovasc Res* 1967, 1:2–8.

29. Higgins CB, Vatner SF, Franklin D, *et al.*: Extent of regulation of the heart's contractile state in the conscious dog by alteration in the frequency of contraction. *J Clin Invest* 1973, 52:1187–1194.

30. Klautz RJ, Baan J, Teitel DF: The effect of sarcoplasmic reticulum blockade on the force/frequency relationship and systolic contraction patterns in the newborn pig heart. *Eur J Physiol* 1997, 435:130–136.

31. Latham RD, Rubal BJ, Sipkema P, *et al.*: Ventricular/vascular coupling and regional arterial dynamics in the chronically hypertensive baboon: correlation with cardiovascular structural adaptation. *Circ Res* 1988, 63:798–811.

32. Finkelstein SM, Collins VR: Vascular hemodynamic impedance measurement. *Prog Cardiovasc Dis* 1982, 24:401–418.

33. Nichols WW, Conti CR, Walker WE, Milnor WR: Input impedance of the systemic circulation in man. *Circ Res* 1977, 40:451–458.

34. Murgo JP, Westerhof N, Giolma JP, *et al.*: Aortic input impedance in normal man: relationship to pressure wave forms. *Circulation* 1980, 62:105–116.

35. Nishioka O, Maruyama Y, Ashikawa K, *et al.*: Effects of changes in afterload impedance on left ventricular ejection in isolated canine hearts: dissociation of end-ejection from end-systole. *Cardiovasc Res* 1987, 21:107–118.

36. Britman NA, Levine HJ: Contractile element work: a major determinant of myocardial oxygen consumption. *J Clin Invest* 1964, 43:1397–1408.

37. Suga H, Hayashi T, Shirahata M, *et al.*: Regression of cardiac oxygen consumption on ventricular pressure-volume area in dog. *Am J Physiol* 1981, 240:H320–H325.

38. Suga H, Yasumura Y, Nozawa T, *et al.*: Prospective prediction of O_2 consumption from pressure-volume area in dog hearts. *Am J Physiol* 1987, 252:H1258–H1264.

39. Monroe G, French GN: Left ventricular pressure-volume relationships and myocardial oxygen consumption in the isolated heart. *Circ Res* 1961, 9:362–374.

40. Suga H: External mechanical work from relaxing ventricle. *Am J Physiol* 1979, 236:H494–H497.

41. Suga H, Hisano R, Hirata S, *et al.*: Heart rate-independent energetics and systolic pressure-volume area in dog hearts. *Am J Physiol* 1983, 244:H206–H214.

42. Suga H, Hisano R, Goto Y, *et al.*: Effect of positive inotropic agents on the relation between oxygen consumption and systolic pressure-volume area in canine left ventricle. *Circ Res* 1983, 53:306–318.

43. Sonnenblick EH, Ross J, Covell JW, *et al.*: Velocity of contraction as a determinant of myocardial oxygen consumption. *Am J Physiol* 1965, 209:919–927.

44. Gibbs CL, Gibson WR: Isoprenaline, propranolol and the energy output of rabbit cardiac muscle. *Cardiovasc Res* 1972, 6:508–515.

45. Nozawa T, Yasumura Y, Futaki S, *et al.*: Relation between oxygen consumption and pressure-volume area of in situ dog heart. *Am J Physiol* 1987, 253:H31–H40.

46. Starling MR, Mancini GBJ, Montgomery DG, *et al.*: Relation between maximum time-varying elastance pressure-volume areas and myocardial oxygen consumption in dogs. *Circulation* 1991, 83:304–314.

47. Corr PB, Yamada KA, Witkowski FX: Mechanisms controlling cardiac autonomic function and their relation to arrythmogenesis. In *The Heart and Cardiovascular System.* Edited by Fozzard HA, Haber E, Jennings RB, *et al.* New York: Raven Press; 1986:1357–1371.

48. Levy MN, Martin PJ: Neural control of the heart. In *Physiology and Pathophysiology of the Heart*, edn 1. Edited by Sperilakis N. Boston: Martinus Nijhoff Publishing; 1984:337–354.

49. Levy MN: Sympathetic-parasympathetic interactions in the heart. *Circ Res* 1971, 29:437–445.

50. DeGeest H, Levy MN, Zieske H, *et al.*: Depression of ventricular contractility by stimulation of the vagus nerves. *Circ Res* 1963, 17:222–235.

51. Vatner SF, Rutherford JD, Ochs HR: Baroreflex and vagal mechanisms modulating left ventricular contractile responses to sympathomimetic amines in conscious dogs. *Circ Res* 1979, 44:195–207.

THE ETIOLOGIC BASIS OF CONGESTIVE HEART FAILURE

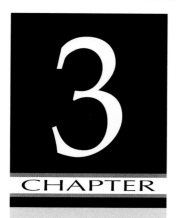

3

CHAPTER

Joshua M. Hare

Appropriate management of congestive heart failure requires recognition of the underlying etiologic basis. Currently, sequelae of ischemic heart disease are the most common causes of congestive heart failure in the United States. Mechanical causes of heart failure, which include coronary artery, valvular, and pericardial disease, must be diagnosed correctly in order to offer appropriate surgical therapy. Primary diseases of the myocardium, *ie*, cardiomyopathies, account for approximately 20% of cases of congestive heart failure [1]. Many systemic diseases, such as rheumatologic disorders, metabolic derangements, toxin exposures, and endocrinopathies, may affect cardiac function and present as a cardiomyopathy [2]. Although these secondary cardiomyopathies are rare, taken together they represent a significant proportion of new cases of dilated cardiomyopathy. As with mechanical causes, recognition of secondary cardiomyopathies is essential because treatment may result in the reversal of cardiac dysfunction.

Immunologic, molecular biologic, and genetic studies have helped to elucidate the etiologic basis of dilated cardiomyopathy. Among patients who present with new-onset dilated cardiomyopathy, approximately 10% have myocarditis [3,4]. Molecular biologic techniques have demonstrated that viral infection of the heart causing myocarditis can also lead to chronic dilated cardiomyopathy. In addition to coxsackie B virus, which is the most common cause of myocarditis, HIV represents a growing cause of myocarditis and dilated cardiomyopathy. Recent clinical and molecular biologic studies also have provided evidence that specific genetic defects may either directly cause or predispose to the development of dilated cardiomyopathy in another 20% to 35% of patients.

Despite the multiple different causes, left ventricular failure progresses by the common pathways of myocyte hypertrophy, fibrosis deposition, and left ventricular chamber enlargement. Abnormalities of function during systole, diastole, or both may contribute to diminished cardiovascular performance. This chapter presents a categorization of cardiomyopathic entities. The causes of cardiomyopathy that are potentially reversible if appropriately diagnosed and treated are emphasized.

A. CLASSIFICATION OF CARDIOMYOPATHIES

CLASSIFICATION BASED ON STRUCTURE OR FUNCTION OF VENTRICLE
Idiopathic dilated cardiomyopathy
Extramyocardial cardiomyopathy
Inflammatory heart disease
Secondary cardiomyopathy
Restrictive cardiomyopathy
Hypertrophic cardiomyopathy
Right ventricular cardiomyopathy
Nondilated cardiomyopathy

FIGURE 3-1. Classification of cardiomyopathies. Strictly defined, the term *cardiomyopathy* denotes a primary disorder of cardiac muscle not caused by coronary or valvular heart disease. Nevertheless, extramyocardial processes that cause heart failure frequently cause secondary changes in myocardial structure and function.

A, A general classification of cardiomyopathic processes based on observations in a large clinical series of patients followed over a 10-year period [2].

B. CLASSIFICATION OF CARDIOMYOPATHIES

INFLAMMATORY HEART DISEASE
Viral myocarditis
Idiopathic myocarditis
Giant cell myocarditis
Sarcoidosis
Eosinophilic myocarditis (hypersensitivity)
Infectious
  Lyme disease
  HIV
  Chagas' disease
Peripartum

EXTRAMYOCARDIAL CARDIOMYOPATHY
Coronary artery disease
Valvular heart disease
Congenital cardiac anomalies
Hypertension

SECONDARY CARDIOMYOPATHY
Endocrine
Rheumatologic
Nutritional
Toxic
Metabolic
Inherited
  Neuromuscular disorders
  X-linked
  Mitochondrial
  Familial dilated cardiomyopathy
  Storage diseases
  Disorders of cardiac energy metabolism
Tachycardia-induced cardiomyopathy
Hemochromatosis
Amyloidosis
Neoplastic

B, Subclassification of specific extramyocardial etiologies that can produce cardiomyopathy-like syndromes, inflammatory diseases of the heart, and specific secondary conditions that can manifest as dilated cardiomyopathy. Although most secondary cardiomyopathies are described in the literature as case reports or small series, in aggregate they may account for up to 50% of new cases of dilated cardiomyopathy [2].

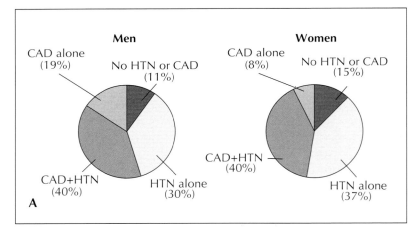

B. ETIOLOGIES OF CONGESTIVE HEART FAILURE

ETIOLOGY	PATIENTS, *n(%)*	NONISCHEMIC DISEASE WITH ETIOLOGY (%)
Ischemic	936(50.3)	
Nonischemic	925(49.7)	
No etiology provided	247(13.3)	
Etiology provided	678(36.4)	
Idiopathic	340(18.2)	(50.1)
Valvular	75(4.0)	(11.1)
Hypertensive	70(3.8)	(10.3)
Ethanol	34(1.8)	(5.0)
Viral	9(0.4)	(1.3)
Postpartum	8(0.4)	(1.2)
Amyloidosis	1(0.1)	(0.1)
Other/ unspecified	141(7.6)	(20.8)

FIGURE 3-2. The epidemiology of congestive heart failure in the United States. The Framingham Heart Study, which followed a cohort of 9405 Americans over a 40-year period, has provided valuable information regarding the etiologic basis of congestive heart failure in the United States [5]. **A,** Of 331 men and 321 women who developed heart failure, the majority had coronary artery disease (CAD) with or without hypertension (HTN), and approximately one third had HTN alone. At present, idiopathic dilated cardiomyopathy has replaced HTN as the second most important etiologic factor in the development of heart failure. CAD continues to be the most common risk factor for the development of heart failure in the United States.

B, Large treatment trials provide another valuable source of information about the causes of heart failure. Data are from a compilation of heart failure trials published between July 1989 and June 1990; categories are based on the presence or absence of significant ischemic heart disease [6]. In this analysis, 50% of cases were attributable to coronary disease; 18.2% of all patients and approximately 50% of those with nonischemic disease had idiopathic dilated cardiomyopathy. Less commonly, valvular heart disease, HTN, and excess alcohol consumption were identified as significant etiologic factors. (Part A *adapted from* Ho *et al.* [5]; part B *adapted from* Teerlink *et al* [6].)

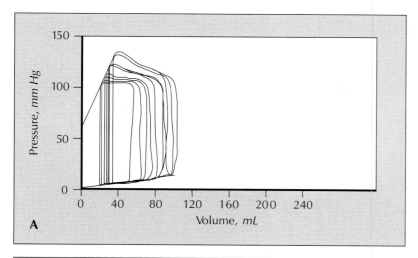

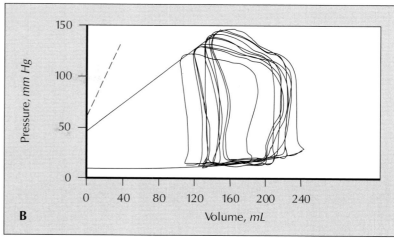

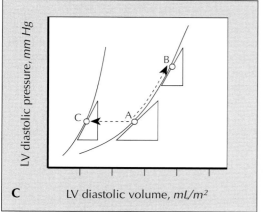

FIGURE 3-3. Systolic and diastolic heart failure. Abnormalities of ventricular function during systole, diastole, or both may produce congestive heart failure. Furthermore, the interaction of the heart with the circulation (*ie*, the loading conditions placed on the heart) is an important determinant of overall cardiovascular performance. Pressure-

volume diagrams can be used to characterize systolic dysfunction, altered diastolic compliance, and the influence of loading conditions on cardiac function.

A, A series of pressure-volume loops obtained from a patient with normal cardiac function. Each loop represents a cardiac cycle sampled during inflation of a balloon in the inferior vena cava to alter loading conditions. The slope of the end-systolic pressure-volume loop relationship (ESPVR, *solid line*) reflects end-systolic ventricular elastance, a relatively load-independent index of contractility. **B,** In dilated cardiomyopathy ventricular volumes are higher, and the ESPVR slope is reduced compared with normal (*dashed line*). Ventricular enlargement is a final common pathway in the heart with systolic impairment.

C, Diastolic dysfunction also may produce heart failure, either primarily or in conjunction with systolic failure. Myocardial ischemia, fibrosis, myocyte hypertrophy, elevated afterload, and pericardial constriction all may contribute to diastolic dysfunction [7]. The end-diastolic pressure-volume relationship (EDPVR) can be used to assess the passive properties of the ventricular chamber. The *operative volume stiffness* of the ventricle is defined as dP/dV (the slope of a tangent to the EDPVR), and the *compliance* of the ventricle is defined as the reciprocal of stiffness (*ie*, dV/dP). Alterations in diastolic function may occur because of increases in stiffness due to rises in chamber preload (A toward B) or actual shifts in the EDPVR (A toward C). Leftward shifts in the EDPVR can occur acutely with ischemia or chronically with fibrosis and hypertrophy. With such shifts, the EDPVR is steeper, and increments in volume produce an exaggerated rise in pressure. LV—left ventricular. (Parts A and B *courtesy of* David Kass, Baltimore, MD. Part C *adapted from* Gaasch *et al* [8].)

HEART FAILURE ASSOCIATED WITH CORONARY DISEASE

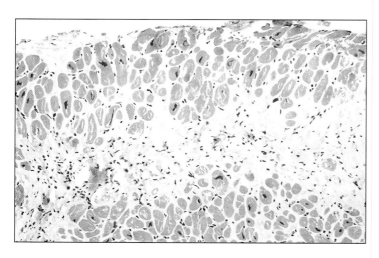

FIGURE 3-4. Histology of ischemic cardiomyopathy demonstrating replacement fibrosis. Myocyte hypertrophy occurs secondarily in response to increases in pressure or volume loads [9]. Fibrosis, the increased deposition of collagen, results from either repair of parenchymal myocyte injury (replacement fibrosis) or pathologic deposition in the interstitium. Histologic studies reveal that patients with ischemic cardiomyopathy display more replacement fibrosis but less myocyte hypertrophy than those with idiopathic cardiomyopathy. Depicted is a focus of replacement fibrosis in an endomyocardial biopsy sample obtained from a patient with ischemic cardiomyopathy. In one study, such foci were found to be 92% specific and 48% sensitive for a diagnosis of ischemic cardiomyopathy versus idiopathic dilated cardiomyopathy [10].

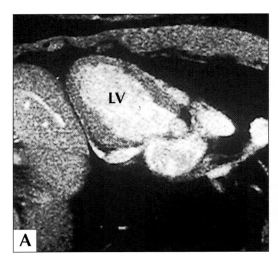

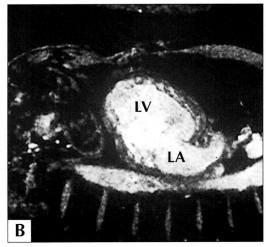

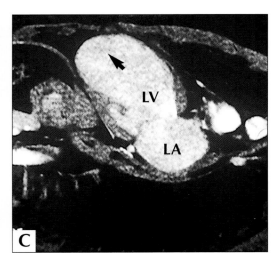

FIGURE 3-5. Magnetic resonance images depicting the normal left ventricle (LV; *panel A*), ischemic cardiomyopathy (*panel B*), and LV aneurysm (*panel C*). These images were obtained in the sagittal view through the LV. Ischemic cardiomyopathy may develop months or years after a myocardial infarction due to remodeling of the ventricle, a process affecting both infarcted and viable (*ie*, noninfarcted) segments. Although the contractile abnormality is focal, particularly early in the process, progressive ventricular enlargement and eventual failure of noninfarcted myocardium can lead to a state that clinically resembles idiopathic dilated cardiomyopathy. The ventricle shown here (*panel B*) is diffusely enlarged and more spherical than the normal ventricle. LV aneurysms (*arrow*) are large segments of ventricular wall composed of fibrous tissue. These areas exhibit paradoxical systolic expansion, which impairs ventricular function despite preserved function of the viable myocardium, and may lead to heart failure following large myocardial infarcts. About one half of patients with moderate to large aneurysms experience symptoms of heart failure with or without angina pectoris, and in such patients aneurysm resection may lead to a significant improvement in global LV function [11]. LA—left atrium. (*Courtesy of* Joachim Gaa and Robert Edelman, Boston, MA.)

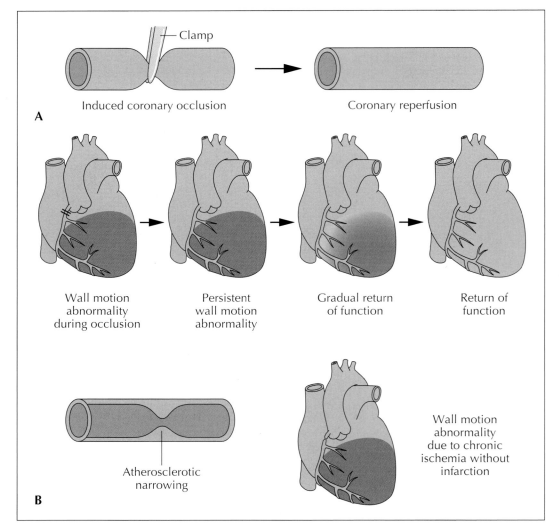

FIGURE 3-6. Stunned and hibernating myocardium. Both chronic myocardial ischemia and reperfusion of ischemic muscle may produce a reversible form of ventricular dysfunction. **A,** Stunned myocardium refers to left ventricular dysfunction after coronary reperfusion. Coronary occlusion, such as that occurring during acute myocardial infarction, may lead to regional dysfunction beyond the area of infarction. Despite restoration of flow, regional wall-motion abnormalities persist in these areas with viable myocytes. This process usually reverses over a period of several days after myocardial infarction. **B,** Hibernating myocardium results from chronic ischemia. Blood flow may be adequate to maintain myocyte viability, but may not be sufficient to support the full metabolic needs of normal contraction. After revascularization, myocardial function may significantly improve. (*Adapted from* Kloner *et al.* [12].)

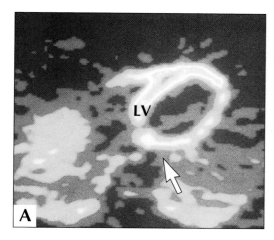 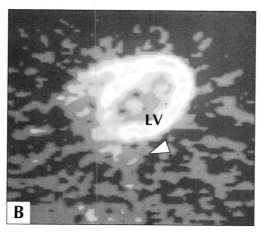

(*arrow*). **B,** The corresponding [18F]-fluorodeoxyglucose image demonstrates that metabolic activity is preserved in this region (*arrowhead*). After coronary bypass surgery, the patient experienced a dramatic improvement in left ventricular function. Other imaging techniques valuable in the assessment of hibernating myocardium include thallium imaging and dobutamine stress echocardiography. These techniques can predict, with 80% or greater accuracy, if there will be significant improvement in left ventricular function with revascularization. Recently, detection of viable myocardium with 201Tl scintigraphy has been shown to predict patient survival following coronary artery bypass surgery [13]. Therefore, patients may be considered as candidates for bypass surgery as an alternative to heart transplantation. (*Courtesy of* Henry Gewirtz, Boston, MA.)

FIGURE 3-7. (*See* Color Plate.) Positron emission tomogram demonstrating hibernating (viable but dysfunctional) myocardium in a patient with severe three-vessel coronary artery disease who presented with heart failure. In this technique, images are obtained after injection of isotopes that assess both myocardial perfusion and metabolic activity. In these images, active perfusion or metabolic activity appears yellow to red. **A,** A [13N]-ammonia scan demonstrating a large anterolateral perfusion defect

HEART FAILURE ASSOCIATED WITH VALVULAR LESIONS

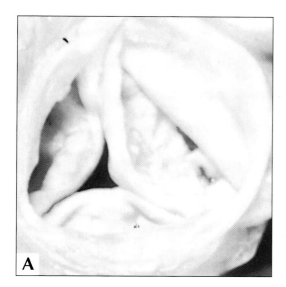 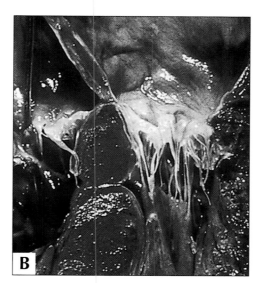 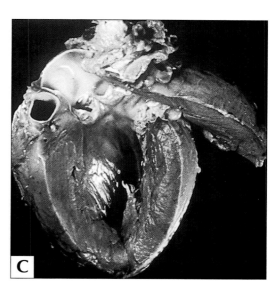

FIGURE 3-8. Heart failure associated with aortic valvular lesions. Heart failure represents a cardinal manifestation of both stenotic and regurgitant valvular heart disease. Aortic stenosis affects cardiac function by imposing progressively increasing systolic wall stress on the ventricle. Chronic aortic stenosis results in concentric left ventricular hypertrophy and fibrosis, and thereby increases wall thickness. The increase in wall thickness can initially restore wall stress to normal, but frequently heart failure ensues because of inadequate hypertrophy (afterload mismatch) or depression of myocardial contractility [14]. Heart failure may also reflect diastolic dysfunction due to increased diastolic stiffness. Heart failure in patients with aortic stenosis bodes a poor prognosis, with patients surviving only 1 to 1.5 years; however, it is generally responsive to valve replacement [15]. Aortic regurgitation imposes an excessive volume load on the ventricle. The rising end-diastolic volume increases diastolic wall stress and leads to eccentric hypertrophy of the left ventricle. The ventricle initially is capable of handling large volumes of regurgitant flow and generates an adequate forward flow without elevation of filling pressures. Heart failure usually ensues when end-diastolic volume continues to rise in the presence of a falling ejection fraction. The ratio of wall thickness to cavity diameter declines, wall tension increases, and further afterload mismatch occurs [14]. The end-systolic volume serves as a good index of prognosis: patients with volumes greater than 90 mL/m^2 generally have a poor operative mortality and fail to recover ventricular function. Ventricular dysfunction with exercise can be detected before the onset of symptoms and is an indication for surgery. Shown is a pathologic specimen from a patient in whom aortic stenosis (**A**) produced marked concentric ventricular hypertrophy (**B**). Also shown is a specimen from a patient with massive eccentric hypertrophy due to chronic aortic regurgitation secondary to healed bacterial endocarditis (**C**). Chronic aortic insufficiency produces the largest end-diastolic volumes of any heart condition, a condition termed *cor bovinum*. The weight of this specimen exceeded 1000 g. (*Courtesy of* Frederick J. Schoen, Boston, MA.)

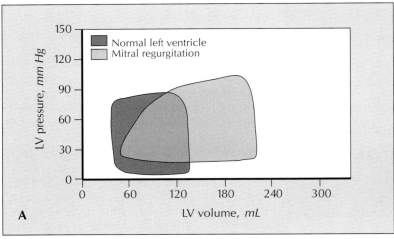

A

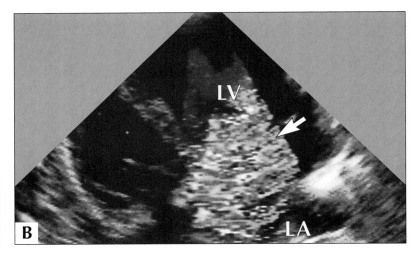

B

FIGURE 3-9. (*See* Color Plate.) Heart failure associated with mitral regurgitation. When mitral regurgitation is acute, it may produce symptomatic pulmonary edema as well as pulmonary hypertension and right heart failure. Mitral regurgitation can also cause chronic left ventricular (LV) dysfunction, which, if left untreated, can lead to the development of dilated cardiomyopathy. Incompetence of the mitral valve reduces ventricular afterload and increases the velocity of contractile element shortening; thus, the LV ejection fraction may be normal despite significant LV dysfunction. **A,** Pressure-volume diagram typical of mitral regurgitation. Ventricular volume decreases in early systole before opening of the aortic valve. After aortic valve closure, the ventricle continues to eject into the left atrium (LA), resulting in non-isovolumic relaxation. Contractility may be depressed in patients with mitral regurgitation as reflected by a diminished ratio of pressure to volume at the end-systolic point, an estimate of ventricular elastance (*see* Fig. 3-3). In chronic mitral regurgitation, the ventricle operates at a greater volume and, as with aortic regurgitation, ventricular size has proven to be predictive of impaired postoperative function. **B,** Echocardiogram with color Doppler depicting severe mitral regurgitation in a 70-year-old woman with a myxomatous mitral valve and a ruptured chordae. The Doppler jet demonstrates the systolic regurgitant flow-velocity from LV to LA (*arrow*). Ventricular enlargement has ensued with an LV end-diastolic dimension of 6.6 cm (normal range, 3.6 to 5.2 cm) and an LV end-systolic dimension of 4.2 cm (normal range, 2.3 to 3.9 cm). (Part A *adapted from* Kontos *et al.* [16].)

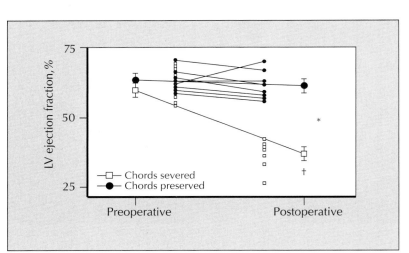

FIGURE 3-10. Paradoxically, dilated cardiomyopathy may appear to worsen after mitral valve replacement due to surgical transection of the subvalvular apparatus. Development of operative techniques for mitral repair and chordal preservation has largely eliminated this type of postoperative impairment of ventricular performance [17]. This graph shows the effect of chordal preservation on postoperative left ventricular (LV) ejection fraction. Patients received mitral valve replacement with or without preservation of the chordae tendineae. Only patients who had severance of their chordal structures experienced a decrease in ejection fraction with surgery (*asterisk* indicates *P*<0.05 between groups; *dagger* indicates *P*<0.05 before vs after mitral valve replacement). In this study, chordal preservation resulted in decreases in both diastolic and systolic volumes, as well as a decrease in end-systolic wall stress. In contrast, chordal transection led to an increase in both end-systolic volume and wall stress. (*Adapted from* Rozich *et al.* [17].)

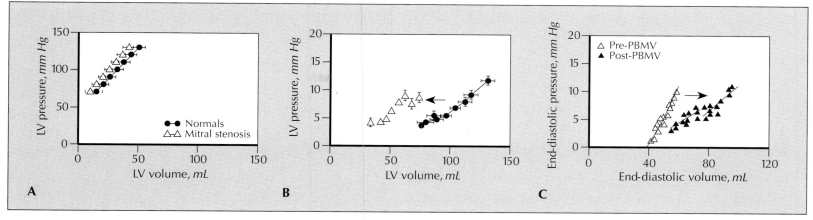

FIGURE 3-11. Diastolic dysfunction in mitral stenosis resulting primarily from the transvalvular gradient and subsequent pulmonary hypertension. Diminished cardiovascular performance has been associated with mitral stenosis. Liu *et al.* [18], using *in vivo* pressure-volume analysis, have demonstrated that cardiovascular impairment in mitral stenosis may be attributable, in part, to reduced diastolic compliance.

A, Comparison of the end-systolic pressure-volume relationship in normal subjects and patients with mitral stenosis. These relationships were very similar except for a small shift to lower volumes in the mitral stenosis group.

B, In contrast, the end-diastolic pressure-volume relationship (EDPVR) in patients with mitral stenosis demonstrates both a leftward shift to lower volumes and a slope increase indicative of reduced compliance.

C, The effect of percutaneous balloon mitral valvuloplasty (PBMV) on the EDPVR in mitral stenosis was used to assess the mechanism of this increase in diastolic stiffness. Immediately after valvuloplasty, the slope of the EDPVR indicated increased compliance, suggesting that the thickened, immobile valve apparatus exerted a mechanical constraining effect. The chamber compliance increased even further at 3 months of follow-up, approaching normal values. LV—left ventricular. (*Adapted from* Liu *et al.* [18].)

IDIOPATHIC DILATED CARDIOMYOPATHY

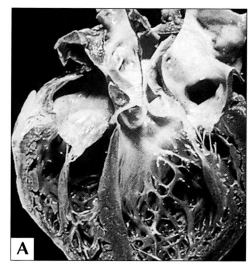

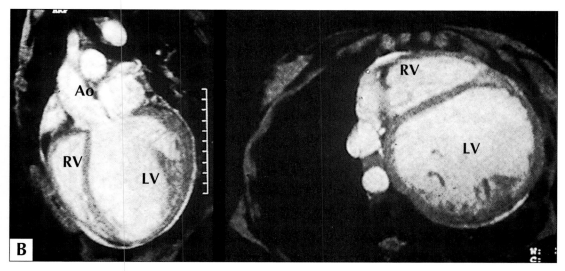

Figure 3-12. Idiopathic dilated cardiomyopathy. Idiopathic dilated cardiomyopathy, a diagnosis of exclusion, is the second most common cause of heart failure in the United States, following ischemic heart disease (*see* Fig. 3-2B). Among patients who present with dilated cardiomyopathy, up to half have specific underlying etiologies, which in many cases are treatable. In addition, it is becoming apparent that many cases previously labeled "idiopathic" may actually reflect prior myocarditis or genetic disease.

A, Gross appearance of the heart in idiopathic dilated cardiomyopathy. This condition leads to four-chamber dilatation and

hypertrophy. In this example, focal anteroseptal apical wall thinning was a result of an infarct of embolic origin. The coronary arteries were free of obstructive narrowing.

B, Magnetic resonance images of dilated cardiomyopathy in four-chamber (*left*) and short-axis (*right*) views. This imaging technique provides an excellent *in vivo* assessment of cardiac structure and function. Ao—aorta; LV—left ventricle; RV—right ventricle. (Part A *courtesy of* Frederick J. Schoen, Boston, MA; part B *courtesy of* Joachim Gaa and Robert Edelman, Boston, MA.)

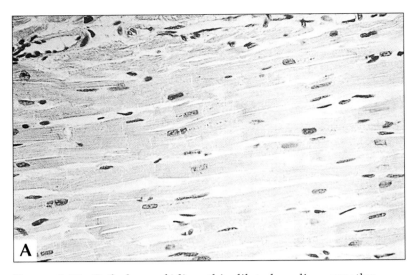

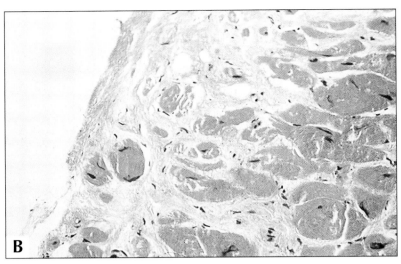

FIGURE 3-13. Pathology of idiopathic dilated cardiomyopathy. **A,** Histologic architecture of normal myocardium, demonstrating parallel alignment of uniformly sized myocytes without significant fibrosis. **B,** In contrast, the myocardium from a patient with idiopathic dilated cardiomyopathy demonstrates myocyte hypertrophy with variability in myocyte size and enlargement of nuclei. There is significant deposition of fibrotic tissue in the interstitium. (Part A *courtesy of* Evan Loh, Philadelphia, PA.)

INFLAMMATORY DISEASES OF THE MYOCARDIUM

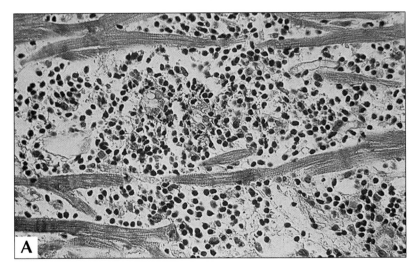

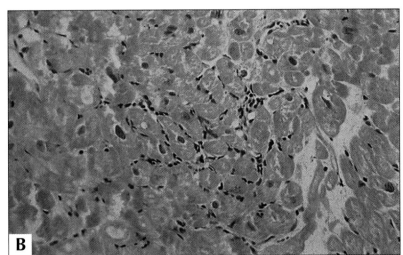

FIGURE 3-14. Histologic diagnosis of myocarditis. The Dallas Criteria [19] were formulated by a panel of cardiac pathologists, and have led to standardization of the histologic diagnosis of myocarditis by endomyocardial biopsy. **A,** As defined by the Dallas Criteria, a diagnosis of myocarditis requires the presence of both inflammatory infiltrates and evidence of myocardial necrosis.

B, Borderline myocarditis is defined as an inflammatory infiltrate without clear evidence of myocyte necrosis. These criteria were used as enrollment criteria in the Myocarditis Treatment Trial for the assessment of immunosuppressive therapy in patients with myocarditis. Interestingly, the degree of inflammation or the presence of myocyte necrosis does not necessarily indicate the presence of viral infection or provide prognosis [20].

As shown in Fig. 3-16C, enteroviral infection may cause severe ventricular dysfunction without inflammation. Furthermore, myocardial inflammation with or without myocyte necrosis may occur in nonviral disease processes (*see* Fig. 3-22). Despite the limitation of sampling error, endomyocardial biopsy remains the gold standard for the diagnosis of myocarditis [21]. It is hoped that the application of molecular and immunologic assays of myocardial tissue will enhance the clinical value of endomyocardial biopsy in the future. When endomyocardial biopsy is performed in centers that have experience with the technique, the incidence of major complications that require intervention or lead to patient death is less than 1% [22,23]. (*Courtesy of* H. Thomas Aretz for the Myocarditis Treatment Trial, Boston, MA.)

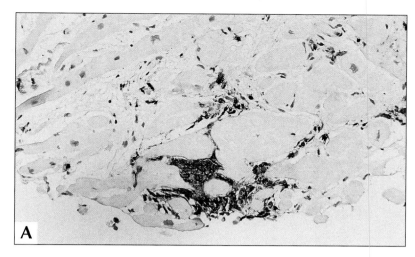

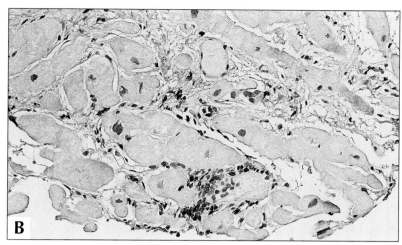

FIGURE 3-15. In addition to the Dallas criteria, immunohistochemical staining is valuable to characterize myocardial lymphocytic infiltration. Most human and animal myocarditis is characterized by infiltration with T cells that utilize the α-β T-cell receptor [24]. **A,** Immunohistochemical staining for CD3+ T cells (general T-cell surface marker). **B,** CD8+ T cells (cytotoxic/suppressor T cells) obtained from a patient with chronic active myocarditis. CD8+ T cells are commonly detected in human myocarditis. Immunohistochemical staining has the potential to play a role in distinguishing autoimmune from viral myocarditis because the former may be characterized by T cells that contain the γ-δ T-cell receptor as opposed to α-β T cells [24]. Immunopositive cells stain *black.* (*Courtesy of* R. Hruban, Baltimore, MD.)

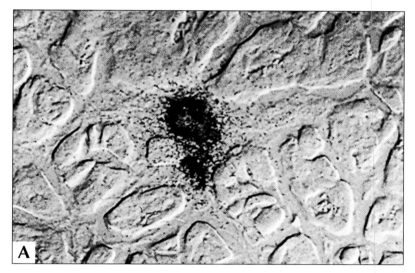

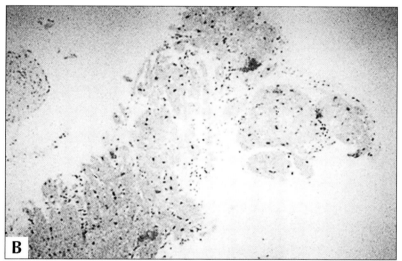

FIGURE 3-16. Viral myocarditis. Myocarditis accounts for approximately 10% of patients with new-onset congestive heart failure [3,25,26]. Enteroviruses of the Picornaviridae family have been implicated as the most common offending agents. Recent studies have implicated adenovirus as an additional myocarditis-causing virus that may affect pediatric patients more commonly than adults [27]. Molecular techniques such as polymerase chain reaction amplification [28] and *in situ* hybridization [29,30] have clearly demonstrated the presence of a viral genome in heart tissue from patients with acute myocarditis and in those with dilated cardiomyopathy, suggesting that viral myocarditis is a precursor to some cases of dilated cardiomyopathy.

A, Interference contrast microscopy (× 1000) demonstrating *in situ* hybridization of 35S-labeled coxsackievirus B3 cDNA to the myocardium of a patient with an 8-year history of chronic dilated cardiomyopathy. The autoradiographic silver grains localize to distinct infected myocytes. Kandolf [30] has found enteroviral infection in 17% of 47 patients with idiopathic cardiomyopathy.

B, The typical pattern of enteroviral infection in an adult patient with recurrent myocarditis presenting with severe heart failure. The autoradiographic silver grains localize to individual myocytes. Mononuclear cellular infiltration lies adjacent to infected myocytes. (*continued*)

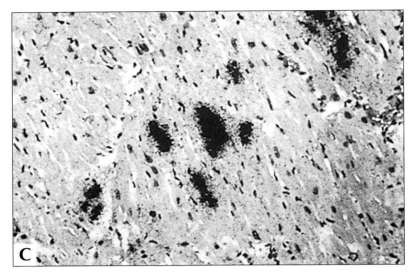

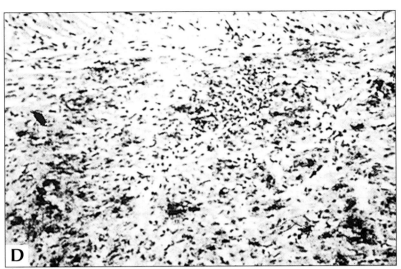

FIGURE 3-16. (*continued*) **C,** Early viral infection in a patient dying from fulminant heart failure. The high intensity of autoradiographic staining indicates a high copy number of replicating viral genomes. In this patient there is relatively little cellular inflammatory response, indicating that cardiac dysfunction may ensue from viral infection in the absence of inflammation.

D, Fulminant enteroviral infection with an inflammatory response in neonatal myocarditis. This section demonstrates extensive auto-radiographic staining, inflammatory infiltration, and progression of infection from inflamed to noninflamed areas, suggestive of cell-to-cell spread of the virus. (Part A *from* Kandolf [29]; parts B to D *from* Kandolf [30]; with permission.)

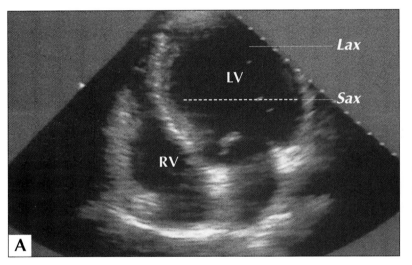

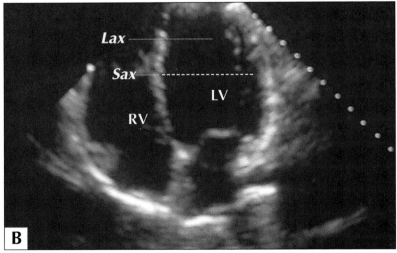

FIGURE 3-17. Ventricular chamber distortion in myocarditis. Myocarditis causes left ventricular enlargement and results in an increase in ventricular sphericity similar to that produced by postin-farction ventricular remodeling. Depicted are apical four-chamber echocardiograms from a patient with active myocarditis (**A**) and a

patient with a normal ventricle (**B**). In comparison with the normal ventricle, the ventricle affected by myocarditis is dilated and more spherical. The ventricular width at the short axis (Sax) has increased ralative to the length in the long axis (Lax). (*Courtesy of* Lisa Mendes for the Myocarditis Treatment Trial, Boston, MA.)

CLINICOPATHOLOGIC CLASSIFICATION OF MYOCARDITIS

	FULMINANT	ACUTE	CHRONIC ACTIVE	CHRONIC PERSISTENT
Left ventricular dysfunction	+++	++	++	-
Histology	Myo	Myo/BMyo	Myo/BMyo	Myo/BMyo
Response to immunosuppression	?	+/-	-	-
Natural history	Complete recovery or death	Incomplete recovery or DCM	DCM	Normal ventricular function

Minus signs indicates absent; *double plus signs* indicate moderate; *triple plus signs* indicate severe.

Figure 3-18. A clinicopathologic classification of myocarditis. Lieberman *et al.* [3] have proposed a clinicopathologic description of myocarditis with four presentations that are analogous to those of viral hepatitis. This characterization was based on 35 of 348 patients who underwent endomyocardial biopsy for evaluation of cardiac dysfunction. Fulminant myocarditis manifested as acute, severe congestive heart failure with a clear-cut flu-like prodrome and severe histologic evidence of inflammation and myocyte necrosis, leading to either death or complete recovery. This presentation may be associated with progressive myocardial damage caused by ongoing viral infection. Fulminant myocarditis patients have excellent long-term survival if they survive the index presentation [31].

Acute myocarditis was the most common presentation. Patients presented with minimally dilated hypokinetic ventricles with an indistinct onset of symptoms. Endomyocardial biopsy revealed either borderline (BMyo) or active (Myo) myocarditis. In this group, patients with BMyo responded to immunosuppressive therapy (prednisone and azathioprine) with improvement in ventricular function and regression of chamber dilatation [20]. As a group, however, patients with acute myocarditis tend to develop dilated cardiomyopathy [32] associated with increased mortality [31]. Patients who did not respond to therapy developed end-stage dilated cardiomyopathy (DCM). *Chronic active myocarditis* presented in a manner similar to active myocarditis. Patients experienced brief, dramatic but unsustained responses to immunosuppressive therapy and followed a slowly progressive course of deterioration to end-stage DCM. Initial histology revealed either borderline or active myocarditis and subsequent biopsies demonstrated the appearance of giant cells and extensive fibrosis. *Chronic persistent myocarditis* was characterized by ongoing myocardial inflammation in the absence of significant ventricular dysfunction. Patients had symptoms of palpitations or atypical chest pain. (*Adapted from* Lieberman *et al.* [3].)

FIGURE 3-19. Nuclear imaging in the diagnosis of myocarditis. Antimyosin ^{111}In scintigraphy is a useful modality for the initial evaluation of patients with suspected myocarditis. This image depicts diffuse global uptake of radiolabeled antimyosin antibody by the left ventricle (*large arrows*) in an anterior planar image. The apical region has been relatively spared (*small arrows*). This patient presented with a syndrome masquerading as myocardial infarction with chest pain and elevations in creatine kinase MB isoenzymes. The left ventricle was dilated and hypocontractile. *L* denotes the normal hepatic activity of the labeled antibody. Compared with endomyocardial biopsy, antimyosin antibody imaging was 83% sensitive and 53% specific for the diagnosis of myocarditis [33]. (*From* Narula *et al.* [34]; with permission.)

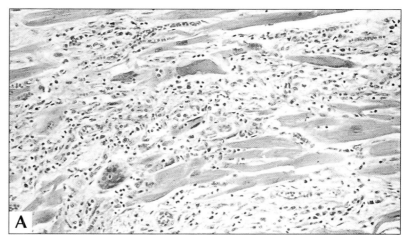

FIGURE 3-20. Giant-cell myocarditis and sarcoidosis. These two rare inflammatory diseases of the myocardium are distinguished by the presence of giant cells. **A,** Giant-cell myocarditis is characterized by lymphocytic infiltration, myocyte necrosis, and giant cells. Its course is slowly progressive yet insidious, and is often associated with ventricular arrhythmias or conduction system disease [3,35]. Giant-cell myocarditis has a very poor prognosis that may be improved by a cyclosporin-based immunosuppressive regimen or heart transplantation [36]. Rarely, giant-cell myocarditis may present as fulminant heart failure. (*continued*)

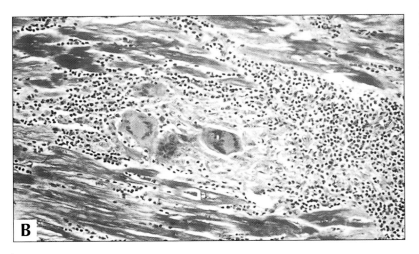

FIGURE 3-20. (*continued*) **B,** Section of left ventricular myocardium obtained at autopsy, demonstrating myocardial sarcoidosis. Myocardial sarcoidosis can be distinguished by the presence of true noncaseating granuloma within the myocardium. Approximately 5% of patients with sarcoidosis have clinically significant myocardial disease. However, involvement of the myocardium can be observed in 25% of autopsy cases [37]. The manifestations include cardiomyopathy, syncope, tachyarrhythmias, and sudden death. Patients may respond to corticosteroids and should be maintained on long-term, low-dose maintenance therapy [37]. (Part A *courtesy of* Frederick J. Schoen, Boston, MA; part B *courtesy of* Richard Mitchell, Boston, MA.)

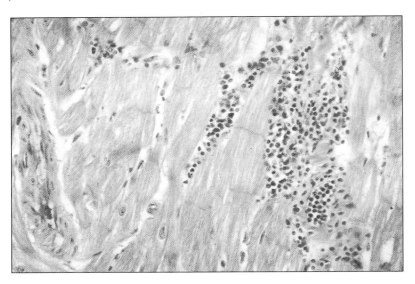

FIGURE 3-21. Hypersensitivity (eosinophilic) myocarditis. Some drugs, most commonly the sulfonamides, penicillins, and methyldopa, may cause an eosinophilic infiltration of the heart [38]. Typically, patients with hypersensitivity myocarditis present with the symptoms of an allergic drug reaction (*ie*, rash, fever, and eosinophilia) accompanied by cardiac symptoms, tachycardia, and electrocardiographic changes. Fulminant heart failure occurs rarely and is usually due to acute necrosis of the myocardium [39]. The presentation may also mimic myocardial infarction, with rises in creatine kinase MB fraction. Diagnosis can be achieved by endomyocardial biopsy, and management should include withdrawal of the offending medication and consideration of corticosteroid therapy. (*Courtesy of* Evan Loh, Philadelphia, PA.)

SPECIFIC CLINICAL CONDITIONS ASSOCIATED WITH A HISTOLOGIC DIAGNOSIS OF MYOCARDITIS IN 60 PATIENTS

CLINICAL CONDITION	PATIENTS, *n(%)*
Peripartum or postpartum	21(35)
HIV infection	17(28)
Chronic alcoholism	3(5)
Cocaine abuse	4(7)
Arrhythmias not associated with EF< 40%	4(7)
Familial cardiomyopathy	2(3)
Hyperthyroidism	2(3)
Systemic lupus erythematosus	2(3)
Sarcoidosis	2(3)
Restrictive cardiomyopathy	2(3)
Lyme disease	1(2)

FIGURE 3-22. The histologic prevalence of inflammatory heart disease in specific cardiomyopathies. Myocardial inflammation may play an important pathophysiologic role in several cardiomyopathic processes [40]. Felker *et al.* [41] have noted myocarditis in 78% of patients with peripartum cardiomyopathy. Furthermore, enteroviral RNA has been identified by the polymerase chain reaction in some patients with peripartum cardiomyopathy, indicating a viral etiology [28]. Myocarditis is also observed in patients who present primarily with arrhythmia or restrictive cardiomyopathy and in those with a history of drug exposure, endocrinopathy, or a familial predisposition to cardiomyopathy [40]. Myocarditis also plays a role in heart failure associated with rheumatologic illnesses, the prototype being systemic lupus erythematosus [42,43]. The most common cardiovascular manifestations of systemic lupus erythematosus include pericarditis (affecting 19% to 49% of patients) and Liebman-Sacks endocarditis. Approximately 10% of patients with systemic lupus erythematosus develop congestive heart failure, and 50% of these have myocarditis. Patients with systemic lupus erythematosus are also at increased risk for myocardial infarction on the basis of accelerated atherosclerosis or coronary arteritis, which may lead to the development of congestive heart failure. EF—ejection fraction. (*Adapted from* Herskowitz *et al.* [40].)

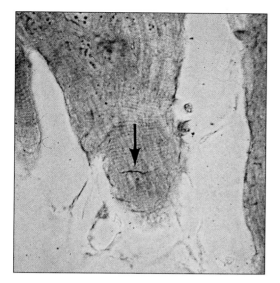

FIGURE 3-23. Detection of the spirochete *Borrelia burgdorferi* (*arrow*) in human myocardium (modified Steiner's silver stain). Lyme disease, a multisystem disorder caused by infection with *B. burgdorferi*, produces cardiac disease, notably arrhythmias and myocarditis, as a tertiary manifestation [44]. This infection is transmitted to humans from bites of ticks of the genus *Ixodes*. Here the spirochete is demonstrated in myocardium from a patient with a 4-year history of dilated cardiomyopathy and a serologic profile consistent with chronic Lyme disease. Despite therapy with ceftriaxone, the patient did not experience improvement in cardiac function. *Bar*=25 μm. (*From* Stanek *et al.* [44]; with permission.)

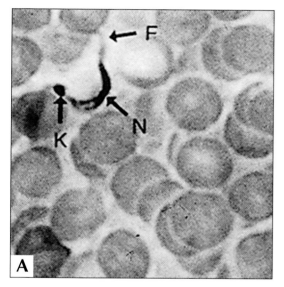

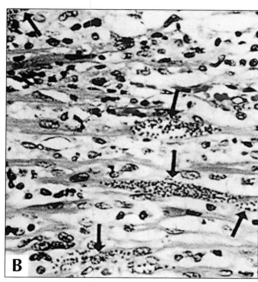

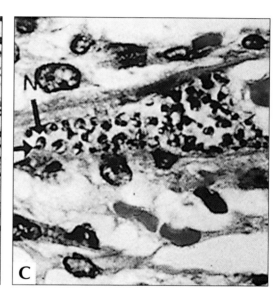

FIGURE 3-24. American trypanosomiasis (Chagas' disease). The most common infection of the heart worldwide is Chagas' disease, caused by the protozoan parasite *Trypanosoma cruzi*, which is spread by reduviid insects [45]. Infection with *T. cruzi* is endemic in Latin America and is now increasingly observed in the United States. Acute Chagas' disease is characterized by the systemic spread of the parasites to muscle, including myocardium. Two drugs, benznidazole and nifurtimox, shorten the acute phase of *T. cruzi* infection but achieve a cure in only 50% of patients. **A,** *T. cruzi* isolated from the blood of a patient with Chagas' disease. The trypomastigote is shown in mouse blood (Giemsa stain, × 2000). **B,** Histopathology of acute Chagas' myocarditis with a mononuclear infiltration. The *arrows* denote myocytes containing amastigote forms of the parasites (hematoxylin and eosin, × 360). **C,** High magnification of an infected myocyte (hematoxylin and eosin, × 900). F—flagellum; K—kinetoplast of amastigotes; N—nucleus. (*From* Kirchhoff [45]; with permission.)

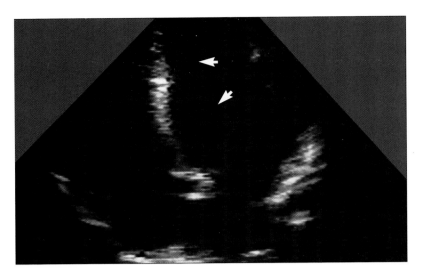

FIGURE 3-25. Chronic Chagas' disease. Patients chronically infected with *Trypanosoma cruzi* develop manifestations over a period of one to three decades [46]. Cardiac involvement is most common and manifests as biventricular enlargement, thinning of the ventricular walls, apical aneurysms (*arrows*), and mural thrombi. Clinically, patients experience heart failure, arrythmias, thromboembolic events, and sudden death. The prognosis of patients with Chagas' cardiomyopathy is worse than that of patients with idiopathic dilated cardiomyopathy [47]. Cardiac transplantation has often been followed by recurrence of *T. cruzi* infection [45]. Depicted is a four-chamber echocardiogram showing two left ventricular apical aneurysms, which are characteristic of chronic Chagas' disease [46,47].

SECONDARY CAUSES OF CARDIOMYOPATHY

ENDOCRINE CAUSES

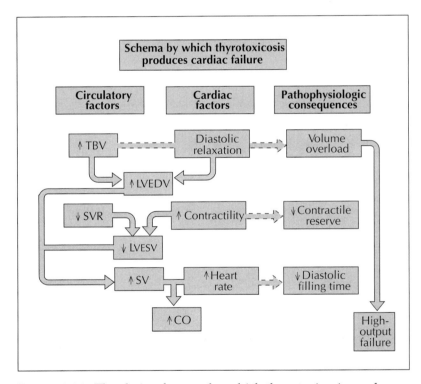

FIGURE 3-26. The chain of events by which thyrotoxicosis produces high-output cardiac failure. Excess circulating thyroxine influences both the vasculature and the heart, thereby affecting both cardiac

loading conditions and intrinsic cardiac function. Peripherally, thyrotoxicosis increases total blood volume (TBV), which increases preload, and decreases systemic vascular resistance (SVR), which decreases afterload. Thyroxine influences cardiac function by enhancing heart rate, increasing ventricular contractility, and lengthening diastolic relaxation. Therefore, baseline increases in cardiac performance associated with an increased volume load limit contractile reserve and may lead to heart failure and cardiac dilatation in about 6% of patients.

Risk factors for the development of congestive heart failure include age greater than 60 years and preexisting cardiac disease. A higher percentage of thyrotoxic patients also suffer from atrial fibrillation. Both congestive heart failure and atrial arrhythmias may respond favorably to treatment of hyperthyroidism.

Hypothyroidism also may produce dilated cardiomyopathy, which is reversible with therapy. Ladenson *et al.* [48] have recently reported a patient who experienced significant improvement in cardiac function during treatment for hypothyroidism. The clinical improvement was due to reversal of several molecular abnormalities associated with dilated cardiomyopathy (increased atrial natriuretic factor [ANF] and decreased α-myosin heavy chain and phospholamban). This case emphasizes that detection and treatment of thyroid, adrenal, and hypothalamic diseases in the patient with new-onset heart failure may lead to complete recovery of cardiac function. *Solid arrows* indicate direct effects; *dashed arrows* indicate potential consequences. CO—cardiac output; LVEDV—left ventricular end-diastolic volume; LVESV—left ventricular end-systolic volume; SV—stroke volume. (*Adapted from* Woeber [49].)

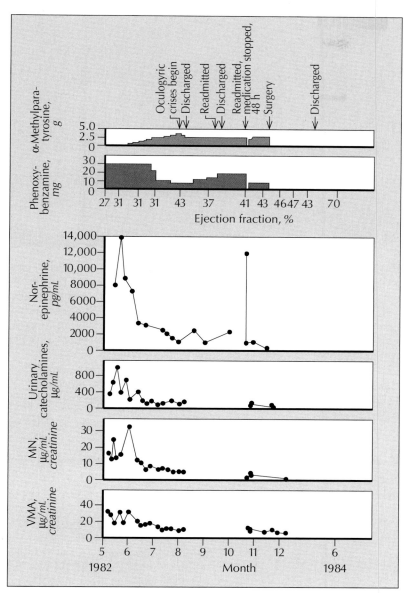

FIGURE 3-27. Reversal of dilated cardiomyopathy in pheochromocytoma. Several case reports document the development of dilated cardiomyopathy in patients with high levels of circulating catecholamines caused by pheochromocytoma [50–52]. A potential explanation for the pathophysiology of this lesion is that chronic adrenergic stimulation produces excessive activation of sarcolemmal calcium channels, increased cytosolic calcium, or accumulation of free radicals. Both increased calcium and free radicals may have toxic effects on the myocardium. Histologically, this lesion is characterized by myocyte vacuolization. Illustrated is the clinical course of a 12-year-old girl with pheochromocytoma and biventricular heart failure (initial ejection fraction, 27%). The patient was treated with α-methylparatyrosine and phenoxybenzamine before surgical resection of the tumor. Six months after surgery she had recovered normal ventricular size and function. MN—metanephrine; VMA—vanillylmandelic acid. (*Adapted from* Imperato-McGinley *et al.* [51].)

RHEUMATOLOGIC CAUSES

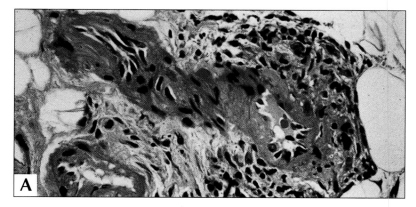

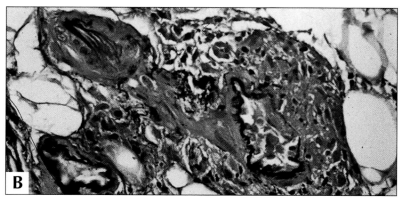

FIGURE 3-28. Necrotizing angiitis of a small intramural coronary artery in a patient with polyarteritis nodosa. Polyarteritis is a rare condition (incidence 6.3 in 100,00) that primarily affects the arteries of the kidney, peripheral nerves, skin, and abdominal viscera. Inflammation of the small branches of the coronary arteries represents a rare cause of cardiac microvascular disease and may produce myocardial infarction (often silent) and congestive heart failure. Depicted are sections of a right ventricular endomyocar-

dial biopsy specimen from a patient with polyarteritis nodosa, chest pain, an inferoposterior thallium perfusion abnormality, and normal epicardial coronary arteries.

A, A small intramural artery is surrounded with fibrinoid degeneration and cellular infiltration (hematoxylin and eosin, × 132). **B,** There is patchy destruction of the internal elastic membrane (elastica-van Gieson stain, × 132). (*From* Sugihara *et al.* [53]; with permission.)

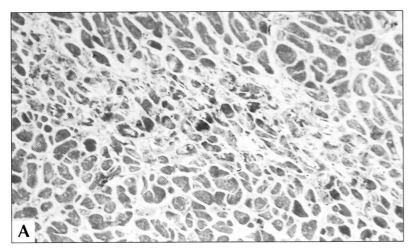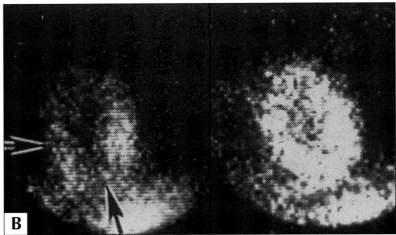

FIGURE 3-29. Myocardial involvement in systemic sclerosis. Microvascular vasoconstrictor abnormalities leading to myocardial fibrosis and left ventricular dysfunction are the hallmarks of scleroderma heart disease. The extent of myocardial fibrosis and contraction band necrosis predict the degree of left ventricular dysfunction [54].

A, Microinfarction with coagulation necrosis in the myocardium of a patient with systemic sclerosis (modified Masson's trichrome). The pathophysiology of the ischemic lesions appears to be microvascular disease similar to that observed in Raynaud's phenomenon [55]. Cardiac ischemia can be elicited by exposing patients with scleroderma to peripheral cold and detected as reversible thallium defects or transient segmental wall-motion abnormalities by echocardiography [55]. Kahan *et al.* [56] also have described impaired coronary flow reserve in response to dipyridamole in patients with systemic sclerosis.

B, Thallium scintigrams obtained from a patient with scleroderma obtained immediately after immersion of the patient's hand in ice water for 2 minutes (*left*) and after 3 hours of redistribution (*right*). Images were obtained in the 40° left anterior oblique view and demonstrate a septal and inferoapical perfusion defect (*arrows*) that completely resolved with redistribution. (Part A *courtesy of* Richard Mitchell, Boston, MA. Part B *from* Alexander *et al.* [55]; with permission.)

TOXIC AND METABOLIC CAUSES

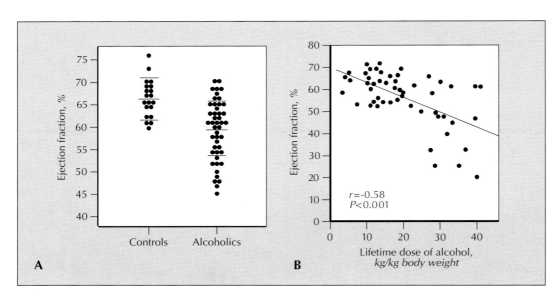

FIGURE 3-30. The toxic effects of alcohol consumption on cardiac function. Alcohol consumption has been implicated as an etiologic factor in approximately 5% of patients with nonischemic cardiomyopathy (*see* Fig. 3-2*B*). Urbano-Marquez *et al.* [57] have shown that fully one third of chronic alcoholics have cardiac dysfunction and that ethanol produces dose-related cardiac toxicity. **A,** Comparison of ejection fractions obtained by radionuclide ventriculography in 20 control subjects and 46 asymptomatic alcoholics in an outpatient rehabilitation program. The mean ejection fraction was 67% in the control subjects versus 59% in the alcoholic patients (*P*<0.001).

B, Correlation between total lifetime consumption of ethanol and left ventricular (LV) ejection fraction in 52 patients with alcoholism. In these patients, total lifetime consumption of alcohol was also positively correlated with LV mass (data not shown). Both relationships suggest a dose-related response to injury. Histologically, patients with alcoholic cardiomyopathy have changes indistinguishable from those of idiopathic cardiomyopathy, with interstitial and replacement fibrosis and myocyte hypertrophy. Alcoholics with early mild cardiac dysfunction may experience significant normalization in cardiac function if they abstain from alcohol consumption. (*Adapted from* Urbano-Marquez *et al.* [57].)

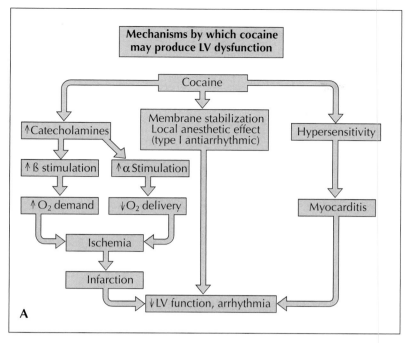

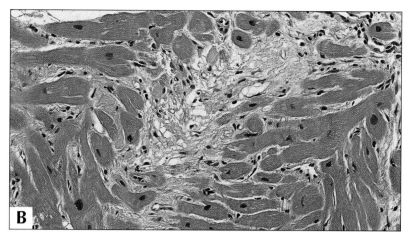

FIGURE 3-31. Schematic description of the potential mechanisms by which cocaine may produce cardiotoxicity and left ventricular (LV) dysfunction [58]. Cocaine, by inhibiting presynaptic reuptake of catecholamines, leads to increased β- and α-adrenergic stimulation. The former leads to increased heart rate and contractility and therefore to increased myocardial oxygen consumption. Increased α-adrenergic stimulation, on the other hand, causes rises in blood pressure and coronary vasoconstriction, thereby decreasing

oxygen delivery to the myocardium. The imbalance contributes to ischemia and possibly myocardial infarction. A second mechanism, that of decreased sodium transport leading to membrane stabilization or local anesthesia (a type I antiarrhythmic effect), may produce a negative inotropic effect that exceeds the positive inotropic effect of β-adrenergic stimulation. A third potential mechanism of LV dysfunction is that of hypersensitivity and myocarditis (*see* Fig. 3-22). Arrhythmias, QT and QRS prolongation, and sudden death occur due to LV dysfunction as well as to the direct type Ia effects of cocaine on the membrane. **B,** Histologic section obtained from a patient with dilated cardiomyopathy and chronic cocaine abuse. The section reveals replacement fibrosis, which may be a consequence of ischemia and microinfarction. (Part A *adapted from* Kloner *et al.* [58]; part B *courtesy of* R. Hruban, Baltimore, MD.)

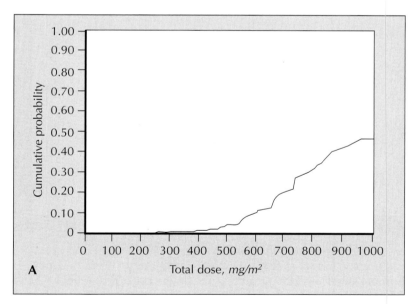

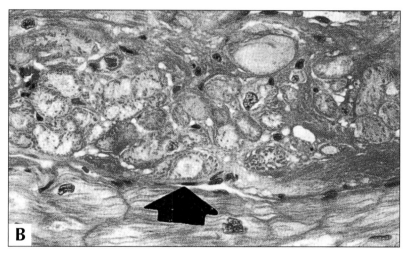

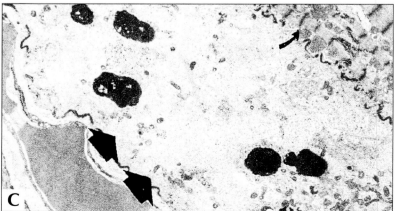

FIGURE 3-32. Anthracycline cardiomyopathy. Survivors of childhood malignancy represent one of the largest new groups of patients at risk for premature cardiovascular disease: 15% of patients in a pediatric cardiomyopathy registry had been treated for malignancy [59]. The anthracyclines doxorubicin and daunorubicin, widely used as chemotherapeutic agents, produce dose-related cardiotoxicity. It is likely that doxorubicin treatment impairs myocardial growth and leads to inadequate myocardial development. **A,** The cumulative probability of developing doxorubicin-induced congestive heart failure as a reflection of total cumulative dose in 3941 patients, 88 of whom experienced heart failure. **B,** Histologic changes characteristic of adriamycin cardiotoxicity. Light microscopic section showing characteristic myofibril loss and vacuolar degeneration (*arrow*). Hematoxylin and eosin, × 400. **C,** Electron microscopic image demonstrating extensive loss of myofilaments (*large arrows*). Normal, unaffected myocytes are also seen (*small arrows*). Original magnification, × 2800. (Parts B and C *from* Shan *et al.* [60]; with permission.)

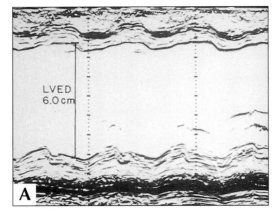

FIGURE 3-33. Left ventricular dysfunction secondary to hypocalcemia. M-mode echocardiograms from a patient with hypocalcemia before (**A**) and after (**B**) calcium repletion. Calcium exerts a fundamental regulatory role on cardiac contraction. Experimentally, the level of extracellular ionized calcium can be shown to correlate with the contractile state of the heart. Clinically, patients with persistent hypocalcemia may develop a reversible dilated cardiomyopathy. Shown is the echocardiogram of a patient with chronic renal insufficiency, previous subtotal parathyroidectomy, and persistent hypocalcemia. Chronic repletion of calcium with intravenous ionized calcium led to significant improvement of hemodynamics and partial resolution of cardiac dilatation over a 6-month period. LVED—left ventricular end-diastolic dimension. (*From* Feldman *et al.* [61]; with permission.)

INHERITED CAUSES

MYOCARDIAL DISEASE IN THE MAJOR HEREDOFAMILIAL NEUROMYOPATHIC DISORDERS

DISORDER	GENETICS	CARDIOMYOPATHY	CONDUCTION SYSTEM ARRHYTHMIA
Progressive muscular dystrophy			
Duchenne dystrophy; early-onset, rapidly progressive	X-linked	DCM	+
Becker dystrophy; late-onset, slowly progressive	X-linked	DCM	+
Limb-girdle dystrophy of Erb	Variable	-	-
Facioscapulohumeral (Landouzy-Dejerine)	AD	-	+
Emery-Dreifuss muscular dystrophy	X-linked	AP, DCM	+
Myotonic dystrophy (Steinert's disease)	AD	DCM	+
Friedreich's ataxia	AR	HCM, DCM	-
Kearns-Sayre syndrome	Mitochondrial	DCM	+

Minus sign indicates absent; *plus sign indicates* present.

FIGURE 3-34. Myocardial disease in the major heredofamilial neuromyopathic disorders [62]. Shown are the major heredofamilial neuromyopathic disorders and their mode of inheritance. Also shown are the types of cardiomyopathic processes associated with these disorders, and whether arrhythmias or conduction system disease contribute to cardiovascular morbidity. AD—autosomal dominant; AP—atrial paralysis; AR—autosomal recessive; DCM—dilated cardiomyopathy; HCM—hypertrophic cardiomyopathy.

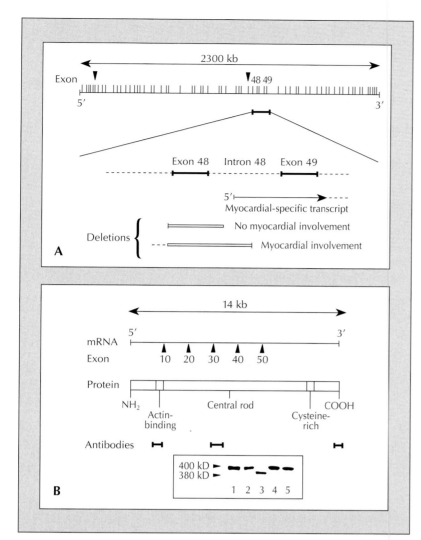

A

B

FIGURE 3-35. Neuromuscular disorders associated with cardiomyopathy and mutations in the dystrophin gene. The dystrophin gene, spanning more than 2.3 million base pairs, is the largest mammalian gene. It codes for a cytoskeletal protein found in both striated and cardiac myocytes. Mutations of this gene cause both Duchenne and Becker muscular dystrophy. The former is associated with the complete absence of dystrophin, which results from an out-of-frame intragenic deletion producing a stop codon in the downstream sequence. In contrast, Becker muscular dystrophy results from an in-frame deletion in which only a part of the coding sequence is absent. Cardiac involvement has been noted in more than 80% of patients with Duchenne dystrophy and in approximately 50% of patients with Becker dystrophy.

A, The dystrophin gene: exons are indicated by *vertical bars* and *arrowheads* mark the sites where deletion breakpoints occur most often in Duchenne and Becker dystrophy. Melacini *et al.* [63] have described an association between cardiac involvement and intragenic deletions that include exons 48 and 49 in patients with Becker dystrophy. The finding that patients with deletions only in exon 48 have no cardiac involvement has led to the hypothesis that a myocardium-specific transcript exists whose 5′ end is located within intron 48. Deletion of this sequence could be crucial in the development of cardiomyopathy in patients with muscular.

B, The 14-kb dystrophin mRNA with exon numbers indicated and its corresponding protein product. Several domains of the protein are indicated: NH_2 (amino-terminal) domain, actin-binding domain, central-rod domain, cysteinerich domain, and COOH (carboxy-terminal) domain. Using antibodies to various locations of the protein (*inset*), Western blotting can be used to demonstrate the abnormal lower molecular weight protein (lane 3380 kD) in a patient with Becker muscular dystrophy compared to the normal 400-kD dystrophin protein in lanes 1, 2, 4, and 5. (*Adapted from* Melacini *et al.* [63].)

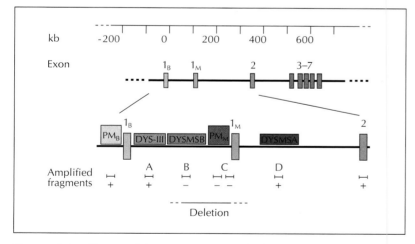

FIGURE 3-36. Dystrophin mutations in X-linked cardiomyopathies. Genetics may play a significant role in the etiology of idiopathic dilated cardiomyopathy (DCM) in the absence of neuromyopathic findings [64]. In 1987, Berko and Swift [65] reported a large kindred in which a progressive cardiomyopathy observed in teenage boys was inherited as an X-linked trait. Because both Duchenne and Becker muscular dystrophy have an X-linked pattern of inheritance, the intriguing possibility was raised that X-linked DCM was due to similar genetic abnormalities. Two studies in 1993 have now confirmed the association of X-linked DCM with mutations in the dystrophin gene [66] or its promoter region [67]. This figure shows the 5′ end of the dystrophin gene. Muntoni *et al.* [67] used the polymerase chain reaction (PCR) to detect the presence of three polymorphic microsatellite loci (DYS-III, DYSMSB, and DYSMSA) in a kindred of patients with X-linked DCM. The *bars* beneath these regions indicate the fragments subject to PCR analysis. The letters *A, B, C,* and *D* above the bars correspond to the regions for which the PCR amplification was performed. The *plus* and *minus* signs indicate the presence or absence of the region in affected individuals, respectively. The approximate extent of the deletion is indicated at the bottom of the figure. These data indicate that X-linked cardiomyopathy is associated with a deletion of the muscle promoter and the first exon of the dystrophin gene, and imply that expression of dystrophin must be driven by the brain promoter (PM_B). PM_M—muscle promoter; 1_B—first brain exon; 1_M—first muscle exon. (*Adapted from* Muntoni *et al.* [67].)

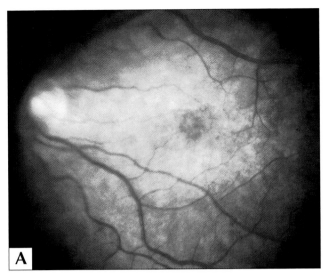

FIGURE 3-37. The Kearns-Sayre syndrome and mitochondrial cardiomyopathies. Dilated cardiomyopathy (DCM) is rarely associated with mitochondrial skeletal myopathies [68]. Kearns-Sayre syndrome is a rare mitochondrial myopathy characterized by ptosis, chronic progressive external ophthalmoplegia, abnormal retinal pigmentation, and conduction system abnormalities. Fewer than 20% of patients have cardiac involvement manifesting either as conduction system disease or cardiomyopathy. The genetics of mitochondrial cardiomyopathies have recently been elucidated; both mutations and deletions in the mitochondrial DNA have been associated with DCM [69,70]. **A,** The typical "salt and pepper" retinal pigmentation of Kearns-Sayre syndrome. **B,** Electron microscopic sections of normal and abnormal cardiac mitochondria from patients with Kearns-Sayre syndrome. *Panel I* demonstrates the appearance of normal mitochondria with closely packed cristae and granules. *Panels II* to *IV* depict mitochondrial abnormalities, with huge mitochondria with concentric cristae (*panel II*), enlarged mitochondria with transverse cristae (*panel III*), and small vacuolized mitochondria (*panel IV*). These abnormalities were found in seven of nine patients with Kearns-Sayre syndrome, demonstrating that a mitochondrial cardiomyopathy is part of this condition. (Part A *courtesy of* Tatsuo Hirose and Paul Arrigg; part B *from* Schwartzkopff *et al.* [71].)

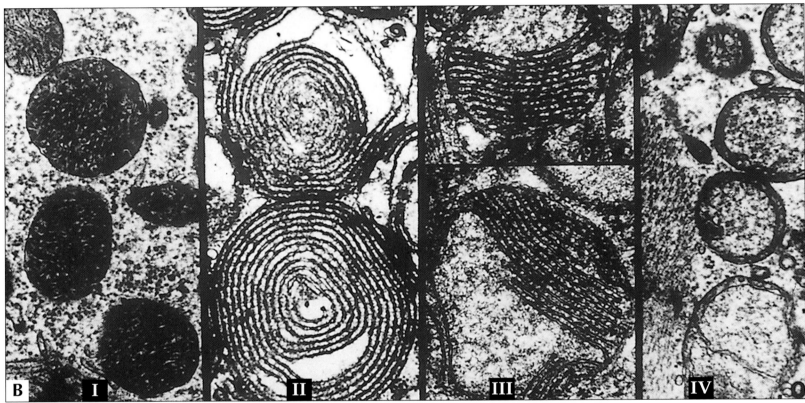

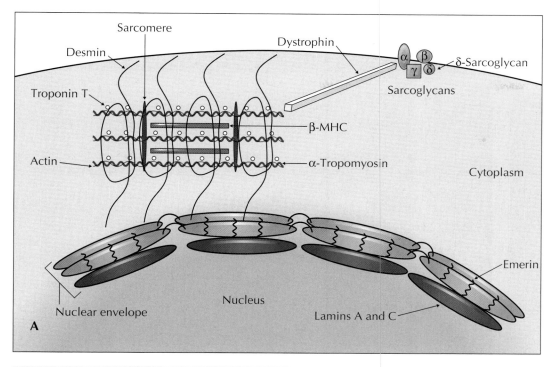

A

DOMINANT AND X-LINKED DILATED CARDIOMYOPATHY LOCI

LOCUS	DISEASE GENE	ADDITIONAL FEATURES	SYNDROME
1p1-q21	Lamin A/C	Conduction disease ≥ skeletal myopathy	CMD1A
1q32	?	None	CMD1D
1q32	Cardiac troponin T	None (mutations may also cause HCM)	CMD1D ?
2q14-q22	?	Conduction disease	CMD1H
2q31	?	None	CMD1G
2q35	Desmin	Skeletal myopathy	CMD1I
3p22-25	?	SVT, conduction disease	CMD1E
5q33	δ-Sarcoglycan	LGMD	LGMD2F
6q12-q16	?	None	None
6q23	?	Skeletal myopathy and conduction disease	CMD1F
6q23-24	?	Sensorineural hearing loss	CMD1J
9q13-q22	?	None	CMD1B
10q21-q23	?	MVP	CMD1C
14q11	Cardiac β MHC	None (mutations may also cause HCM)	None
15q14	Cardiac actin	None (mutations may also cause HCM)	None
15q22.1	α-Tropomyosin	None (mutations may also cause HCM)	None
19q13.2	?	Anemia, short stature	BDS
Xp21	Dystrophin	Skeletal myopathy	DMD, BMD
Xq28	Emerin	Skeletal myopathy	EDMD
Xq28	Tafazzin	Skeletal myopathy, endocardial fibroelastosis	Barth

FIGURE 3-38. The genetics of dilated cardiomyopathy. Familial inheritance has been implicated in 20% to 35% of cases of dilated cardiomyopathy [72]. This figure may underestimate the true prevalence of inherited disorders, as apparently spontaneous cases may arise from de novo mutations. Additionally, incomplete penetrance, age-dependent phenotype, and small families also limit recognition of genetically determined cardiomyopathy. **A,** Genes implicated in familial cardiomyopathy encode cellular structural proteins, contractile proteins, nuclear envelope proteins, and as-yet-unidentified products. Alterations in cytoskeletal elements may lead to ineffective force transmission whereas abnormal sarcomeric elements may disrupt force generation. Other structural proteins participate in organizing the contractile apparatus and maintaining myocyte structural integrity. For example, the actin cytoskeleton is linked to the extracellular matrix by dystrophin and the dystrophin-associated glycoprotein complex. Mutations in dystrophin and other members of the dystrophin-associated glycoprotein complex (the sarcoglycans) have been shown to produce dilated cardiomyopathy in humans. Other subcellular components that interact with these proteins are prime candidates for the responsible proteins whose genes are in linked genomic intervals. Mutations in the sarcomeric proteins depicted can also cause hypertrophic cardiomyopathy. The mechanism by which mutations in the nuclear envelope proteins cause DCM is unknown. **B,** Published genomic loci linked to familial dilated cardiomyopathy. The table lists the known genes and loci that are linked to this disorder with both autosomal dominant (most common) and X-linked patterns of inheritance. Phenotypic features other than ventricular enlargement and systolic dysfunction are also described if present. The syndromes are named according to their Online Mendelian Inheritance in Man (OMIM) designation. As shown, approximately one half of familial dilated cardiomyopathy gene loci have as yet unidentified gene-products [72]. With at least twenty described loci, it is estimated that additional loci will be discovered as the search continues. BDS—Blackfan-Diamond syndrome; BMD—Becker muscular dystrophy; CMD—cardiomyopathy, dilated; DMD—Duchenne muscular dystrophy; EDMD—Emery-Dreifuss muscular dystrophy; HCM—hypertrophic cardiomyopathy; LGMD—limb-girdle muscular dystrophy; MVP—mitral valve prolapse; SVT—supraventricular tachycardia. (*Courtesy of* Daniel Judge, Baltimore, MD.)

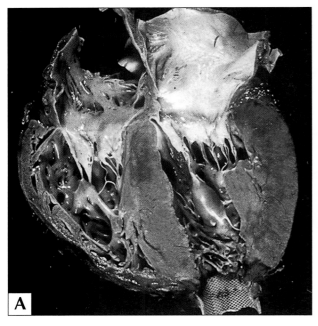

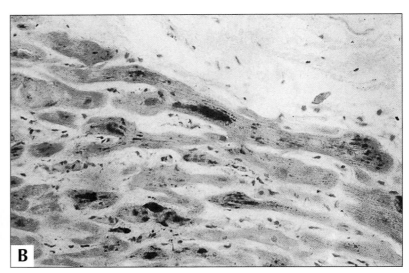

FIGURE 3-39. (*See* Color Plate.) Myocardial iron deposition from hemochromatosis. Hemochromatosis is an inherited HLA-linked disorder of iron metabolism that results in iron deposition within parenchymal cells of the heart, liver, pancreas, synovium, and various endocrine glands, including the thyroid, parathyroid, and anterior pituitary. Infiltration of the heart produces a classic dilated cardiomyopathy. Early diagnosis is essential, as periodic venesection can prevent or reduce iron deposition. Iron depletion from the heart may not reverse cardiac dysfunction after a certain threshold of myocyte damage has been reached [73]. Iron loading from repeated blood transfusions can also produce iron deposition in parenchymal disease; patients with anemias associated with erythroid marrow hyperplasia and ineffective erythropoiesis are predisposed to iron deposition with transfusion.

A, The heart of a patient with hemochromatosis, demonstrating four-chamber hypertrophy and dilatation (heart weight, 500 g). The patient had received left and right ventricular assist devices for advanced heart failure. Shown is the left ventricular apical insertion site of a left ventricular assist device.

B, Microscopic section of myocardium from a patient with hemochromatosis, stained for iron with Prussian blue. The extensive hemosiderin deposits within the myocytes stain blue. (Part A *courtesy of* Richard Mitchell, Boston, MA; part B *courtesy of* Ralph Hruben, Baltimore, MD.)

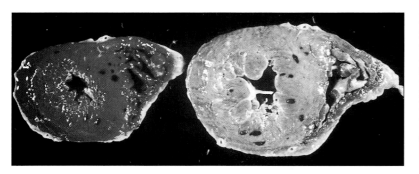

FIGURE 3-40. Neoplastic infiltration of the heart with metastatic melanoma. Tumor invasion of the heart is a rare cause of congestive heart failure. Flipse *et al.* [74] reported on a series of seven patients over a 7-year period in whom malignant neoplasms of the heart were diagnosed during life by endomyocardial biopsy. The important differential diagnosis to be considered in patients with known neoplasia is that of cardiac toxicity induced by treatment with anthracycline-based chemotherapy (*see* Fig. 3-32) or mediastinal radiation. (*Courtesy of* Richard Mitchell, Boston, MA.)

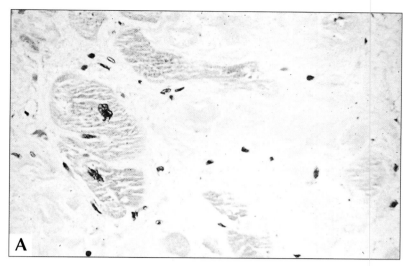

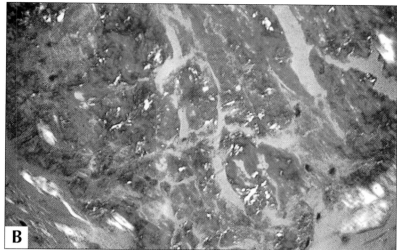

FIGURE 3-41. (*See* Color Plate.) Cardiac amyloidosis. Amyloidosis is a condition in which tissue atrophy and necrosis result from deposition of insoluble protein fibrils. Although different proteins have the potential to deposit as amyloid, their common feature is the ability to form a specific molecular configuration, that of the β sheet. Cardiac amyloidosis may develop from the deposition of 1) proteins of immunologic origin, usually variable (κ or λ) immunoglobulin light chains, also known as Bence-Jones proteins (associated with multiple myeloma and primary amyloidosis); 2) abnormal transthyretin protein (familial amyloidosis); or 3) pre-albumin (senile cardiac amyloidosis). Amyloid deposition may result in either dilated, restrictive, or hypertrophic-like cardiomy-

opathy. Survival of patients with familial amyloidosis is significantly better than that of patients with light chain amyloidosis, which warrants distinguishing these two etiologies by identifying the abnormal protein with immunohistochemistry or electrophoresis in the heart, bone-marrow, serum, or urine [75]. Digitalis, calcium channel blockers, and β-blocking drugs are contraindicated in amyloidosis. **A,** Histologic section from myocardium of a patient with senile amyloidosis, revealing scattered viable myocytes surrounded by a pale, hazy material, which represents the amyloid deposition (hematoxylin and eosin). **B,** Amyloid can be histologically identified by a characteristic green birefringence when viewed under polarized light (Sirius red).

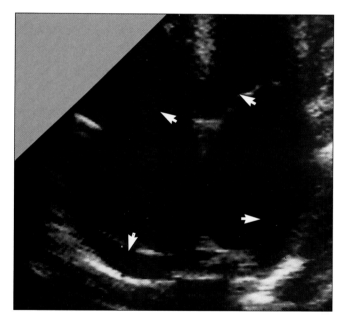

FIGURE 3-42. Echocardiographic features of restrictive cardiomyopathy. Apical four-chamber echocardiogram obtained from an 82-year-old man with progressive right heart failure. The notable features include thickened ventricular walls (*lower arrows*) with normal cavity sizes. There is biatrial enlargement (*upper arrows*), which develops to compensate for the restriction to filling. At cardiac catheterization the patient had equalization of the right atrial, right ventricular diastolic, pulmonary diastolic, and pulmonary arterial wedge pressures. Endomyocardial biopsy revealed cardiac amyloidosis.

HYPERTROPHIC CARDIOMYOPATHY

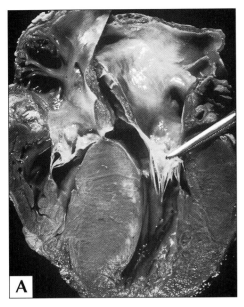

A

FIGURE 3-43. (*See* Color Plate.) Hypertrophic cardiomyopathy. Familial hypertrophic cardiomyopathy is inherited as an autosomal-dominant trait. It causes hypertrophy of the ventricular walls in association with myofiber disarray. The genetic etiology of this condition has been linked to mutations in the cardiac β-myosin heavy chain gene [76]. The two most important clinical manifestations of hypertrophic cardiomyopathy are heart failure and sudden death. The development of heart failure is a consequence of increased chamber stiffness and diastolic dysfunction.

A, Gross appearance of hypertrophic cardiomyopathy. Although several different distributions of left ventricular hypertrophy exist, the most common is that of asymmetric septal hypertrophy. A characteristic fibrous plaque can be seen at the base of the septum in proximity to the anterior mitral leaflet, which probably results from systolic contact between the mitral valve and the septum. This interaction manifests on echocardiography as systolic anterior motion. **B,** Myocardial histology in hypertrophic cardiomyopathy. The characteristic appearance is that of bizarre and disordered myocardial architecture (hematoxylin and eosin). **C,** Myocardial fibrosis in hypertrophic cardiomyopathy (Masson's trichrome). (*Courtesy of* Frederick J. Schoen, Boston, MA.)

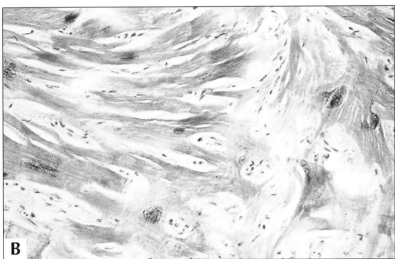

B

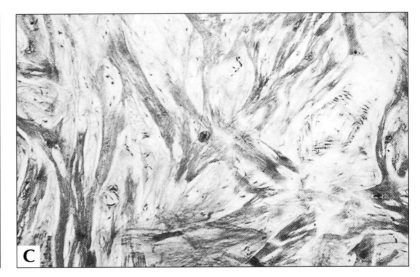

C

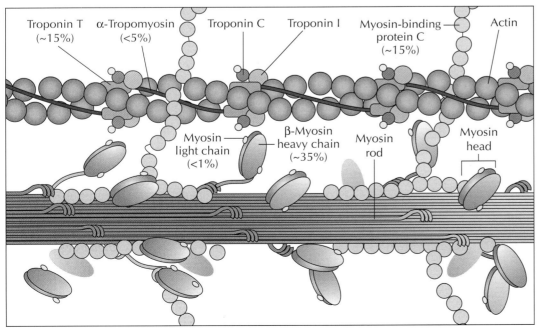

FIGURE 3-44. The genetics of hypertrophic cardiomyopathy. Hypertrophic cardiomyopathy may be caused by mutations affecting components of the myocardial contractile apparatus, thereby impairing myosin-actin interactions responsible for the generation of force. Mutations in four genes encoding proteins of the cardiac sarcomere have been implicated as causing hypertrophic cardiomyopathy. Mutations have been found in the genes for β-myosin heavy chain; cardiac troponin T, α-tropomyosin; and myosin-binding protein C genes. Percentages represent the estimated frequency with which a mutation on the corresponding gene causes hypertrophic cardiomyopathy. (*Adapted from* Spirito [76].)

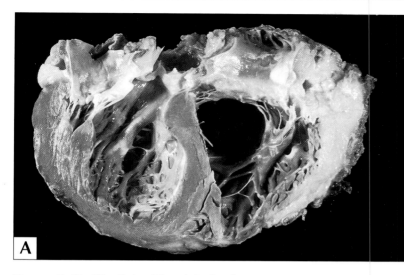

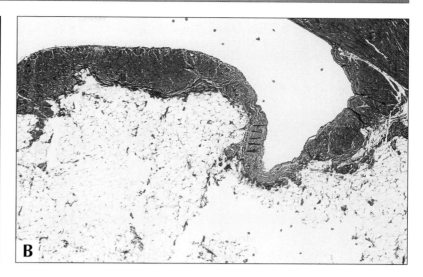

FIGURE 3-45. (*See* Color Plate.) Arrhythmogenic right ventricular dysplasia. Arrhythmogenic right ventricular dysplasia is an isolated right ventricular cardiomyopathy characterized by extensive fibrotic and adipose infiltration of the right ventricular free wall. Approximately one third of patients have an autosomal dominant inheritance. Clinically there is a male predominance, symptoms of palpitations and syncope, a risk of sudden death often associated with ventricular fibrillation, and right ventricular dyskinesis. **A,** Explanted heart of a patient with right ventricular dysplasia. The right ventricle is markedly dilated, infiltrated with adipose tissue, and has a very thin rim of myocardial tissue. **B,** Histologic section through the right ventricular apex, showing regions of fibrosis, adipose infiltration, and myocardial thinning (Mason's trichrome). (*Courtesy of* G. Winters, Boston, MA.)

REFERENCES

1. Manolio TA, Baughman KL, Rodeheffer R, *et al.*: Prevalence and etiology of idiopathic dilated cardiomyopathy (summary of a National Heart, Lung, and Blood Institute workshop). *Am J Cardiol* 1992, 69:1458–1466.

2. Felker GM, Thompson RE, Hare JM, *et al.*: Etiology and long-term survival in unexplained cardiomyopathy. *N Engl J Med* 2000, 342:1077–1084.

3. Lieberman EB, Hutchins GM, Herskowitz A, *et al.*: Clinicopathologic description of myocarditis. *J Am Coll Cardiol* 1991, 18:1617–1626.

4. Hrobon P, Kuntz KM, Hare JM: Should endomyocardial biopsy be performed for detection of myocarditis? A decision analytic approach. *J Heart Lung Transplant* 1998, 17:479–486.

5. Ho KKL, Pinsky JL, Kannel WB, *et al.*: The epidemiology of heart failure: the Framingham Study. *J Am Coll Cardiol* 1993, 22 (suppl A):6–13.

6. Teerlink JR, Goldhaber SZ, Pfeffer MA: An overview of contemporary etiologies of congestive heart failure. *Am J Cardiol* 1991, 121:1852–1853.

7. Bonow RO, Udelson JE: Left ventricular diastolic dysfunction as a cause of congestive heart failure: mechanisms and management. *Ann Intern Med* 1992, 117:502–510.

8. Gaasch WH, Levine HJ, Quinones NM, *et al.*: Left ventricular compliance: mechanisms and clinical implications. *Am J Cardiol* 1976, 38:645–653.

9. Weber KT, Anversa P, Armstrong PW, *et al.*: Remodeling and reparation of the cardiovascular system. *J Am Coll Cardiol* 1992, 20:3–16.

10. Hare JM, Walford GD, Hruban RH, *et al.*: Ischemic cardiomyopathy: endomyocardial biopsy and ventriculographic evaluation of patients with congestive heart failure, dilated cardiomyopathy and coronary artery disease. *J Am Coll Cardiol* 1992, 20:1318–1325.

11. Mangschau A, Forfang K, Rootwelt K, *et al.*: Improvement in cardiac performance and exercise tolerance after left ventricular aneurysm surgery: a prospective study. *Thorac Cardiovasc Surg* 1988, 36:320–325.

12. Kloner RA, Przyklenk K, Patel B: Altered myocardial states: the stunned and hibernating myocardium. *Am J Med* 1989, 86(suppl 1A):14–22.

13. Pagley PR, Beller GA, Watson DD, *et al.*: Improved outcome after coronary bypass surgery patients with ischemic cardiomyopathy and residual myocardial viability. *Circulation* 1997, 96:793–800.

14. Ross J Jr: Afterload mismatch in aortic and mitral valve disease: implications for surgical therapy. *J Am Coll Cardiol* 1985, 5:811–826.

15. Morgan DJR, Hall RJC: Occult aortic stenosis as cause of intractable heart failure. *Br Med J* 1979, 1:784–787.

16. Kontos GJ Jr, Schaff HV, Gersh BJ, *et al.*: Left ventricular function in subacute and chronic mitral regurgitation: effect of function early postoperatively. *J Thorac Cardiovasc Surg* 1989, 98:163–169.

17. Rozich JD, Carabello BA, Usher BW, *et al.*: Mitral valve replacement with and without chordal preservation in patients with chronic mitral regurgitation: mechanisms for differences in postoperative ejection performance. *Circulation* 1992, 86:1718–1726.

18. Liu CP, Ting CT, Yang TM, *et al.*: Reduced left ventricular compliance in human mitral stenosis: role of reversible internal constraint. *Circulation* 1992, 85:1447–1456.

19. Aretz HT, Bellingham ME, Edwards WD, *et al.*: Myocarditis: a histopathologic definition and classification. *Am J Cardiovasc Pathol* 1986, 1:3–14.

20. Jones SR, Herskowitz A, Hutchins GM, *et al.*: Effects of immunosuppressive therapy in biopsy-proved myocarditis and borderline myocarditis on left ventricular function. *Am J Cardiol* 1991, 68:370–376.

21. Chow LH, Radio SJ, Sears TD, *et al.*: Insensitivity of right ventricular endomyocardial biopsy in the diagnosis of myocarditis. *J Am Coll Cardiol* 1989, 14:915–920.

22. Deckers JW, Hare JM, Baughman KL: Complications of transvenous right ventricular endomyocardial biopsy in adult cardiomyopathy patients: a seven year survey of 546 consecutive diagnostic procedures in a tertiary referral center. *J Am Coll Cardiol* 1992, 19:43–47.

23. Starling RC, VanFossen DB, Hammer DF, *et al.*: Morbidity of endomyocardial biopsy in cardiomyopathy. *Am J Cardiol* 1991, 68:133–136.

24. Eck M, Greiner A, Kandolf R, *et al.*: Active fulminant myocarditis characterized by T-lymphocytes expressing the gamma-delta T-cell receptor: a new disease entity? *Am J Surg Patho* 1997, 21:1109–1112.

25. Mason JW, O'Connell JB, Herskowitz A, *et al.*: A clinical trial of immunosuppressive therapy for myocarditis. *N Engl J Med* 1995, 333:269–275.

26. Hare JM, Baughman KL: Myocarditis: current understanding of the etiology, pathophysiology, natural history and management of inflammatory diseases of the myocardium. *Cardiol Rev* 1994, 2:165–173.

27. Martin AB, Webber S, Fricker FJ, *et al.*: Acute myocarditis: rapid diagnosis by PCR in children. *Circulation* 1994, 90:330–339.

28. Jin O, Sole MJ, Butany JW, *et al.*: Detection of enterovirus RNA in myocardial biopsies from patients with myocarditis and cardiomyopathy using gene amplification by polymerase chain reaction. *Circulation* 1990, 82:8–16.

29. Kandolf R: The impact of recombinant DNA technology on the study of enterovirus heart disease. In *Coxsackieviruses: A General Update*. Edited by Bendinelli M, Friedman H. New York: Plenum Publishing; 1988:293–318.

30. Kandolf R: Molecular biology of viral heart disease. *Herz* 1993, 18:238–244.

31. McCarthy RE, Boehmer JP, Hruban RH, *et al.*: Long-term transplant-free survival of patient with fulminant and acute nonfulminant myocarditis. *N Engl J Med* 2000, 342:690–695.

32. Felker GM, Boehmer JP, Hruban RH, *et al.*: Echocardiographic findings in fulminant and acute myocarditis. *J Am Coll Cardiol* 2000, 36:227–232.

33. Dec GW, Palacios I, Yasuda T, *et al.*: Antimyosin antibody cardiac imaging: its role in the diagnosis of myocarditis. *J Am Coll Cardiol* 1990, 16:97–104.

34. Narula J, Khaw BA, Dec GW, *et al.*: Recognition of acute myocarditis masquerading as acute myocardial infarction. *N Engl J Med* 1993, 328:100–104.

35. Davidoff R, Palacios I, Southern J, *et al.*: Giant cell versus lymphocytic myocarditis: a comparison of their clinical features and long-term outcomes. *Circulation* 1991, 83:953–961.

36. Cooper LT, Berry GJ, Shabetai R: Idiopathic giant-cell myocarditis: natural history and treatment. *N Engl J Med* 1997, 336:1861–1866.

37. Johns CJ, Paz H, Kasper EK, *et al.*: Myocardial sarcoidosis: course and management. *Sarcoidosis* 1992, 9(suppl 1):231–236.

38. Kounis NG, Zavras GM, Soufras GD, *et al.*: Hypersensitivity myocarditis. *Ann Allergy* 1989, 62:71–73.

39. Getz MA, Subramanian R, Logemann T, *et al.*: Acute necrotizing eosinophilic myocarditis as a manifestation of severe hypersensitivity myocarditis: antemortem diagnosis and successful treatment. *Ann Intern Med* 1991, 115:201–202.

40. Herskowitz A, Campbell S, Deckers J, *et al.*: Demographic features and prevalence of idiopathic myocarditis in patients undergoing endomyocardial biopsy. *Am J Cardiol* 1993, 71:982–986.

41. Felker GM, Jaeger CJ, Klodas E, *et al.*: Myocarditis and long-term survival in peripartum cardiomyopathy. *Am Heart J* 2000, 140:785–791

42. Stevens MB: Lupus carditis. *N Engl J Med* 1988, 319:861–862.

43. Doherty HE, Siegel RJ: Cardiovascular manifestations of systemic lupus erythematosus. *Am Heart J* 1985, 110:1257–1265.

44. Stanek G, Klein J, Bittner R, *et al.*: Isolation of *Borrelia burgdorferi* from the myocardium of a patient with longstanding cardiomyopathy. *N Engl J Med* 1990, 322:249–252.

45. Kirchhoff LV: American trypanosomiasis (Chagas' disease): a tropical disease now in the United States. *N Engl J Med* 1993, 329:639–644.

46. Morris SA, Tanowitz HB, Wittner M, *et al.*: Pathophysiologic insights into the cardiomyopathy of Chagas' disease. *Circulation* 1990, 82:1900–1909.

47. Bestetti RB, Muccillo G: Clinical course of Chagas' heart disease: a comparison with dilated cardiomyopathy. *Int J Cardiol* 1997, 60:187–193.

48. Ladenson PW, Sherman SI, Baughman KL, *et al.*: Reversible alterations in myocardial gene expression in a young man with dilated cardiomyopathy and hypothyroidism. *Proc Natl Acad Sci U S A* 1992, 89:5251–5255.

49. Woeber KA: Thyrotoxicosis and the heart. *N Engl J Med* 1992, 327:94–98.

50. Lam JB, Shub C, Sheps SG: Reversible dilatation of hypertrophied left ventricle in pheochromocytoma: serial two-dimensional echocardiographic observations. *Am Heart J* 1985, 109:613–615.

51. Imperato-McGinley J, Gautier T, Ehlers K, *et al.*: Reversibility of catecholamine-induced dilated cardiomyopathy in a child with pheochromocytoma. *N Engl J Med* 1987, 316:793–797.

52. Case records of the Massachusetts General Hospita:Case 15-1988. *N Engl J Med* 1988, 318:970–998.

53. Sugihara N, Genda A, Shimizu M, *et al.*: Intramural coronary angiitis of periarteritis nodosa proved by endomyocardial biopsy. *Am Heart J* 1990, 119:1414–1416.

54. Follansbee WP, Miller TR, Curtiss EI, *et al.*: A controlled clinico-pathologic study of myocardial fibrosis in systemic sclerosis (scleroderma). *J Rheumatol* 1990, 17:656–662.

55. Alexander EL, Firestein GS, Weiss JL, *et al.*: Reversible cold-induced abnormalities in myocardial perfusion and function in systemic sclerosis. *Ann Intern Med* 1986, 105:661–668.

56. Kahan A, Nitenberg A, Foult JM, *et al.*: Decreased coronary reserve in primary scleroderma myocardial disease. *Arthritis Rheum* 1985, 28:637–646.

57. Urbano-Marquez A, Estruch R, Navarro-Lopez F, *et al.*: The effects of alcoholism on skeletal and cardiac muscle. *N Engl J Med* 1989, 320:409–415.

58. Kloner RA, Hale S, Alker K, *et al.*: The effects of acute and chronic cocaine use on the heart. *Circulation* 1992, 408:407–419.

59. Lipshultz SE, Sallan SE: Cardiovascular abnormalities in long-term survivors of childhood malignancy. *J Clin Oncol* 1993, 11:1199–1203.

60. Shan K, Lincoff AM, Young JB: Anthracycline-induced cardiotoxicity. *Ann Intern Med* 1996, 125:47–58.

61. Feldman AM, Fivush B, Zahka K, *et al.*: Congestive cardiomyopathy in patients on continuous ambulatory peritoneal dialysis. *Am J Kidney Dis* 1988, 11:76–79.

62. Perloff JK: Neurologic disorders and heart disease. In *Heart Disease, A Textbook of Cardiovascular Medicine*, edn 5. Edited by Braunwald E. Philadelphia: WB Saunders; 1997:1865–1886.

63. Melacini P, Fanin M, Danieli GA, *et al.*: Cardiac involvement in Becker muscular dystrophy. *J Am Coll Cardiol* 1993, 22:1927–1934.

64. Michels VV, Moll PP, Miller FA, *et al.*: The frequency of familial dilated cardiomyopathy in a series of patients with idiopathic dilated czardiomyopathy. *N Engl J Med* 1992, 326:77–82.

65. Berko BA, Swift M: X-linked dilated cardiomyopathy. *N Engl J Med* 1987, 316:1186–1191.

66. Towbin JA, Hejtmancik JF, Brink P, *et al.*: X-linked cardio-myopathy: molecular evidence of linkage to the Duchenne muscular dystrophy (dystrophin) gene at the Xp21 locus. *Circulation* 1993, 87:1854–1865.

67. Muntoni F, Cau M, Ganua A, *et al.*: Deletion of the dystrophin muscle-promoter region associated with X-linked dilated cardiomyopathy. *N Engl J Med* 1993, 329:921–925.

68. Channer KS, Channer JL, Campbell MJ, *et al.*: Cardiomyopathy in the Kearns-Sayre syndrome. *Br Heart J* 1988, 59:486–490.

69. Zeviani M, Gellara C, Antozzi C, *et al.*: Maternally inherited myopathy and cardiomyopathy: association with mutation in mitochondrial DNA tRNA Leu(UUR). *Lancet* 1991, 338:143–147.

70. Suomalainen A, Paetau A, Leinonen H, *et al.*: Inherited idiopathic dilated cardiomyopathy with multiple deletions of mitochondrial DNA. *Lancet* 1992, 340:1319–1320.

71. Schwartzkopff B, Frenzel H, Breithardt G, *et al.*: Ultrastructural findings in endomyocardial biopsy of patients with Kearns-Sayre syndrome. *J Am Coll Cardiol* 1988, 12:1522–1528.

72. Bowles KR, Gajarski R, Porter P, *et al.*: Gene mapping of familial autosomal dominant dilated cardiomyopathy to chromosome 10q21-23. *J Clin Invest* 1996 98:1355–60.

73. Westra WH, Hruban RH, Baughman KL, *et al.*: Progressive hemo-chromatotic cardiomyopathy despite reversal of iron deposition after liver transplantation. *Am J Clin Pathol* 1993, 99:39–44.

74. Flipse TR, Tazelaar HD, Holmes DR Jr: Diagnosis of malignant cardiac disease by endomyocardial biopsy. *Mayo Clin Proc* 1990, 65:1415–1422.

75. Dubrey SW, Cha K, Skinner, *et al.*: Familial and primary (AL) cardiac amyloidosis: echocardiographically similar diseases with distinctly different clinical outcomes. *Heart* 1997, 78:74–82.

76. Spirito P, Seidman CE, McKenna WJ, *et al.*: The management of hypertrophic cardiomyopathy. *N Engl J Med* 1997, 336:775.

MOLECULAR AND CELLULAR EVENTS IN MYOCARDIAL HYPERTROPHY AND FAILURE

CHAPTER 4

Douglas B. Sawyer and Wilson S. Colucci

Whereas cardiac failure was once thought to be a static condition reflecting a damaged myocardium, it is now apparent that it reflects a dynamic process involving the continuous structural and functional reorganization, or remodeling, of the heart in response to environmental stresses and stimuli. The fundamental events that lead to cardiac remodeling occur at the molecular and cellular level in both the myocytes and the nonmyocyte cells of the heart. Observations made in failing human myocardium and in myocardium from animals with hypertrophy or failure suggest that there are multiple molecular and cellular alterations involving the excitation-contraction process, contractile and regulatory proteins, growth factors, and signaling pathways. A variety of stimuli that may be responsible for these alterations have been identified, including mechanical wall stresses, hormones, neurotransmitters, and peptide growth factors. Genetic manipulations in small animal models are refining our understanding of the stimuli and molecular events that lead to progression of heart failure. Although much remains to be learned about how these stimuli interact with signaling pathways to regulate the remodeling of the myocardium, it is now apparent that these events have an important impact on the clinical course of the patient and may offer new approaches to the prevention and treatment of myocardial failure.

As our understanding of the basic molecular and cellular biology of myocardial hypertrophy and failure advances, it is likely that additional new diagnostic and therapeutic approaches will emerge. For example, the ability to assess the "molecular status" of the myocardium may allow better tracking of disease progression, earlier detection of asymptomatic patients, improved prognostication, and the design of therapeutic regimens tailored at the molecular level. New classes of therapeutic agents will emerge. Drugs that block cytokine or growth factor receptors already exist, and these offer exciting prospects that may be evaluated in the near future. Finally, it is already reasonable to speculate that progress in our understanding of the regulation of cardiac gene expression will lead to the development of molecular therapies (*eg*, utilizing the transfer of genes or antisense oligonucleotides) aimed at preventing or reversing fundamental abnormalities that occur at the molecular and cellular level.

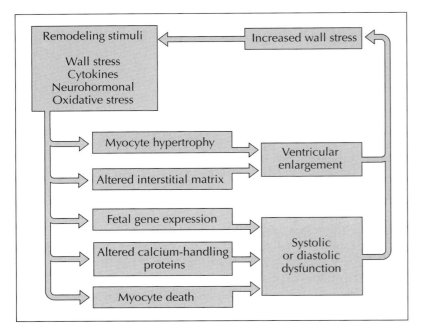

FIGURE 4-1. Remodeling stimuli. Chronic hemodynamic stimuli such as pressure and volume overload lead to ventricular remodeling through increases in myocardial wall stress, cytokines, signaling peptides, neuroendocrine signals, and perhaps, oxidative stress. The myocardium responds with adaptive as well as maladaptive changes. Myocyte hypertrophy and changes in interstitial matrix might at first normalize the wall stress but these occur at the expense of ventricular compliance. Re-expression of fetal contractile proteins and calcium handling proteins may contribute to impaired contraction and relaxation. Myocytes unable to adapt might be triggered to undergo programmed cell death (apoptosis). The net result of these changes is further impairment in pump function and increased wall stress, thus completing a vicious cycle that leads to further progression of the myocardial dysfunction.

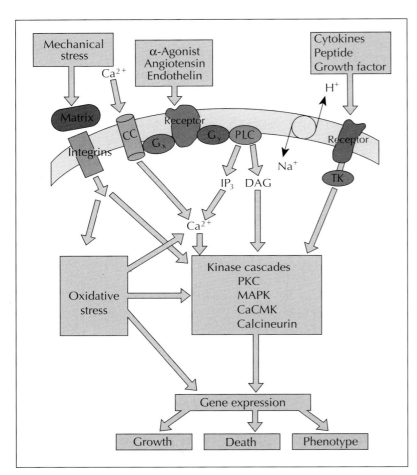

FIGURE 4-2. Signaling pathways in myocardial remodeling. Many signaling pathways have the potential to regulate the growth of cardiac cells acting through an increasingly complex network of intracellular signaling cascades. Agonists for α-adrenergic, angiotensin, and endothelin receptors couple to phospholipase C (PLC) and calcium influx channels (CC) by way of G-proteins (Gx and Gy). Activation of PLC results in the generation of two second messengers, inositol triphosphate (IP_3) and diacylglycerol (DAG). IP_3 causes the release of calcium from intracellular stores, and DAG activates protein kinase C (PKC). Changes in intracellular calcium stores can activate calcium-calmodulin–dependent kinases (Ca-CMK), as well as calcineurin, which can affect gene expression in multiple ways. PKC can affect gene expression directly or indirectly by its effects on Na^+-H^+ exchange (to regulate cellular pH) or by activating mitogen-activated protein kinase (MAPK) cascades.

Cytokines and peptide growth factors can be elaborated by various cells within the heart and may act in an autocrine or paracrine manner. These growth factors activate cellular receptors that usually possess tyrosine kinase (TK) activity and are coupled to a cascade of protein kinases (ras, Raf, MAPKK, MAPK). Mechanical deformation of cardiac myocytes through matrix–integrin interactions can lead to activation or modulation of several signaling pathways, at least in part through autocrine action of released agonists such as angiotensin. Both nitric oxide and oxidative stress may be induced after stimulation of signaling pathways and modulate the activity of kinase cascades and transcription factors leading to alterations in contractile phenotype, growth, and death in myocytes.

MYOCYTE HYPERTROPHY

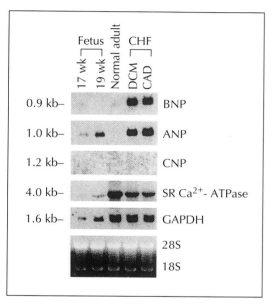

FIGURE 4-3. Isolated cardiac myocytes obtained from mice, showing cellular hypertrophy. **A,** Myocyte from the left ventricle of the normal mouse heart. **B,** Hypertrophied myocyte from the left ventricle of a mouse 6 months after myocardial infarction, viewed at the same magnification as in A. In the myocyte from the failing heart, there has been series addition of sarcomeres, which are otherwise organized in a normal pattern. The resulting myocyte elongation, a form of hypertrophy, likely contributes to ventricular dilatation that occurs during myocardial remodeling.

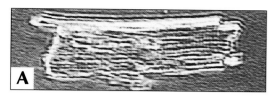

FIGURE 4-4. Although the sarcomeres in remodeled myocardium retain a normal gross morphologic appearance, the expression of several functionally important proteins is altered. Characteristics of the ventricular remodeling response to hemodynamic overload include reexpression of fetal genes that are not normally present in adult myocardium and reduced expression of several muscle-specific adult genes. Shown is a Northern blot illustrating mRNA levels for several proteins in human ventricular myocardium from a normal adult (*center lane*), fetal tissue (Fetus) and from two patients with heart failure (CHF), one due to dilated cardiomyopathy (DCM) and the other due to coronary artery disease (CAD).

Atrial natriuretic peptide (ANP) and brain natriuretic peptide (BNP), which are normally expressed in fetal tissue but are not present in normal adult ventricular tissue, are reexpressed in patients with heart failure. The quantity of cardiac sarcoplasmic reticulum Ca^{2+}-ATPase (Sr Ca^{2+}-ATPase), a protein important for excitation-contraction coupling and normally expressed in abundance in normal adult myocardium, is reduced in the myocardium from the patients with CHF. The amounts of glyceraldehyde-3-phosphate dehydrogenase (GAPDH) mRNA and ribosomal (28S and 18S) RNAs are shown as internal controls. CNPNC—C-type natriuretic peptide. (*Adapted from* Takahashi *et al.* [3].)

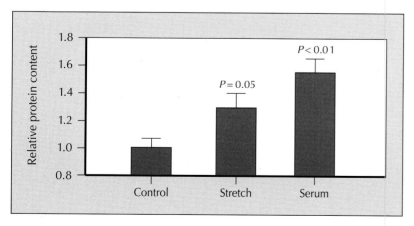

FIGURE 4-5. An increase in the mechanical stresses on cardiac myocytes is a potential growth stimulus common to many forms of hypertrophy. To examine this mechanism experimentally, cardiac myocytes cultured from neonatal rat hearts were grown on a deformable membrane that could be stretched. Compared with control cells that were not stretched, cells that were stretched to increase their length by 20% for 48 hours showed an approximately 30% increase in cellular protein content, indicative of hypertrophy. Serum, which is rich in growth factors, was used for comparison purposes. Because under the conditions of these experiments no other cell types or extrinsic growth factors are present, these observations suggest that mechanical deformation of the myocyte can in itself cause hypertrophy. *P* values are versus control cells. (*Adapted from* Sadoshima *et al.* [4].)

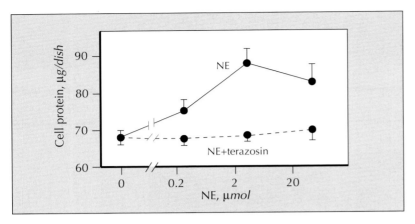

FIGURE 4-6. Another regulator of cell growth and differentiation is sympathetic innervation. Norepinephrine (NE), the primary sympathetic neurotransmitter, can affect the growth of cardiac myocytes. Neonatal rat cardiac myocytes in culture dishes were exposed to NE in various concentrations for 24 hours, after which cellular protein was measured. NE caused cellular hypertrophy (*ie*, increased protein), which was inhibited by terazosin, an α_1-selective antagonist. These findings indicate that the hypertrophic effect of NE is mediated by an α_1-adrenergic receptor located on the cardiac myocyte. (*Adapted from* Simpson and McGrath [5].)

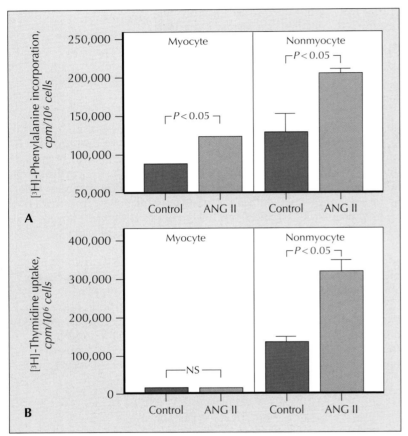

FIGURE 4-7. The levels of both circulating and tissue angiotensin are increased in many conditions associated with myocardial hypertrophy, and this peptide has therefore been implicated as a causative factor in myocardial hypertrophy. To examine whether angiotensin exerts direct effects on protein synthesis in cardiac cells, 10 nmol angiotensin (ANG II) was applied for 24 to 48 hours to either myocytes or nonmyocytes (the latter consisting primarily of fibroblasts) cultured from neonatal rat hearts. **A,** In both cardiac myocytes and nonmyocytes, angiotensin increased [3H]-phenylalanine incorporation, indicating a hypertrophic effect. **B,** Interestingly, angiotensin increased [3H]-thymidine incorporation, an index of DNA synthesis, only in the nonmyocytes. This observation suggests that, in addition to causing myocyte hypertrophy, angiotensin may play a role in the proliferation of fibroblasts and the development of interstitial fibrosis, important components of cardiac remodeling. NS—not significant. (*Adapted from* Sadoshima and Izumo [6].)

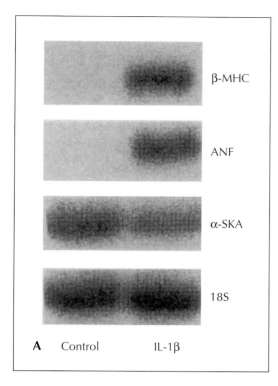

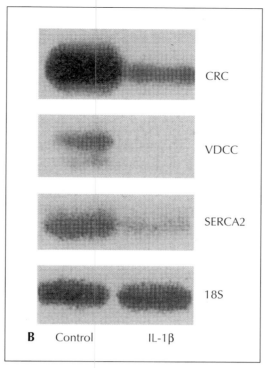

FIGURE 4-8. Cytokines alter myocardial phenotype. Circulating or myocardial levels of cytokines including interleukin-1β, tumor necrosis-α and interleukin-6 are increased in some patients with heart failure. **A** and **B**, In isolated ventricular myocytes, Thaik *et al.* [7] showed that interleukin-1 β induces cell growth, as evidenced by increases in protein synthesis, the reexpression of the fetal genes for β-myosin heavy chain (β-MHC) and atrial natriuretic factor (ANF), and the decreased expression of several adult genes, including those for sarcoplasmic reticulum calcium adenosine triphosphatase (ATPase) (*ie*, SERCA2) and the calcium release channel (*ie*, CRC). Other investigators have shown that some inflammatory cytokines such as tumor necrosis factor-α can stimulate apoptosis in cardiac myocytes. These data suggest that the local production of inflammatory cytokines in the myocardium in response to hemodynamic overload or inflammatory conditions can, among other things, regulate the growth and death of cardiomyocytes and may thus play an important role in the process of myocardial remodeling. (*From* Thaik *et al.* [7].)

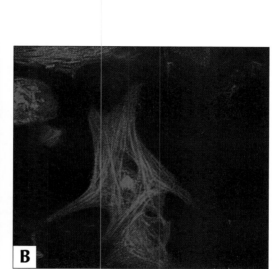

FIGURE 4-9. Peptide growth factors for heart failure. Some peptide growth factors may exert a survival effect on the myocardium. For example, neuregulins are a family of peptide growth factors that function in several organ systems, including the heart, to control normal tissue architecture. Mice genetically engineered to lack neuregulins or their receptors have growth arrest and die in utero with a poorly developed left ventricle. Neuregulins are expressed on nonmyocytes, including the micro-vascular endothelium of the heart in adulthood, and induce a growth response in isolated cardiac myocytes. Neuregulins also prevent the programmed cell death of isolated myocytes, suggesting that their stimulation may have survival value. **A**, Control myocytes. **B**, Myocytes treated with neuregulin. Neuregulin-treated myocytes show a spreading of myofilaments typical of myocytes undergoing a growth response in tissue culture.

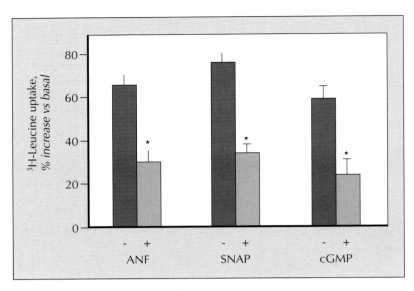

FIGURE 4-10. Counter-regulatory pathways. Myocyte hypertrophy is balanced in the cell by counter-regulatory pathways. Norepinephrine (NE) and adrenergic stimuli cause myocyte hypertrophy, as evidenced by an increased rate of protein synthesis, in this case tritiated leucine incorporation. The addition of atrial natriuretic factor (ANF), or the nitric oxide (NO) donor SNAP (S-nitroso-*N*-acetyl-D,L-penicillamine), inhibits the norepinephrine (NE)-induced increase in protein synthesis. Myocyte hypertrophy is associated with the reexpression of ANF. Thus, ANF in turn may act on the myocyte in an autocrine manner to limit the growth response. ANF increases intracellular levels of cGMP, and cGMP alone has similar effects. SNAP also increases myocyte levels of cGMP, suggesting that this pathway may play a role in the control of sympathetically stimulated myocyte hypertrophy by the parasympathetic system, which is known to regulate the activity of nitric oxide synthase. (*Adapted from* Calderone *et al.* [8].)

CALCIUM HANDLING AND CONTRACTILE PROTEIN EXPRESSION

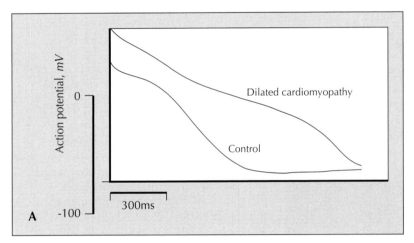

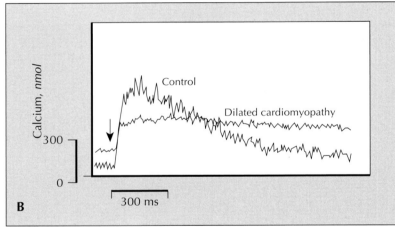

FIGURE 4-11. There is evidence that calcium handling is deranged in the myocardium of patients with end-stage heart failure. **A,** The action potentials in single human cardiac myocytes obtained from patients with normal ventricular function (control) or dilated cardiomyopathy. The action potential is substantially prolonged in the cell from the patient with dilated cardiomyopathy. **B,** The intracellular calcium transients in single cells, as assessed by the fura-2 technique. In the cell from a patient with dilated cardiomyopathy, the intracellular calcium fails to increase normally after stimulation and remains elevated for a prolonged time. Such abnormalities in calcium transients probably contribute to both systolic and diastolic ventricular dysfunction. (*Adapted from* Beuckelmann *et al.* [9].)

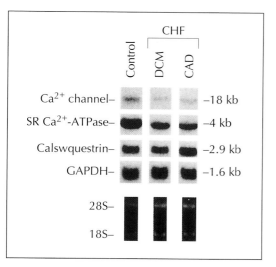

FIGURE 4-12. Abnormal calcium handling in failing myocardium appears to reflect altered expression of one or more important proteins. Shown is a Northern blot demonstrating typical decreases in the mRNA levels for both voltage-dependent Ca^{2+} channels and sarcoplasmic reticulum Ca^{2+}-ATPase (SR Ca^{2+}-ATPase) in myocardium from patients with idiopathic dilated cardiomyopathy (DCM) or ischemic cardiomyopathy (CAD). The mRNA level for calsequestrin, a protein that binds calcium within the sarcoplasmic reticulum, is normal in the myopathic myocardium. The levels of glyceraldehyde-3-phosphate dehydrogenase (GAPDH) and ribosomal RNA (18S and 28S) are shown as internal controls. kb—kilobases. (*Adapted from* Takahashi *et al.* [10].)

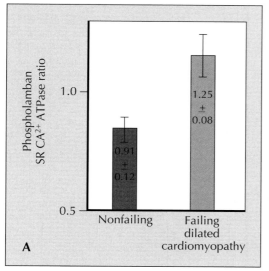

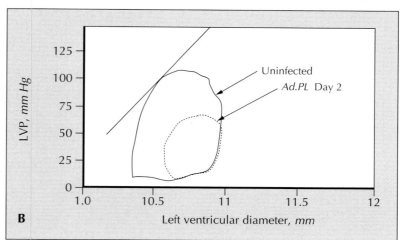

FIGURE 4-13. Phospholamban in heart failure. Phospholamban regulates the activity of SERCA2 in the cardiac myocyte and thereby alters the cytosolic concentrations of calcium (Ca^{2+}). Whereas both phospholamban and SERCA2 expression are decreased in failing myocardium, phospholamban is not as reduced as SERCA2, so that the ratio of phospholamban to SERCA2 is increased (A). When the phospholamban/SERCA2 ratio was increased in rat heart by means of viral-mediated transfer of the phospholamban gene (Ad.PL), there was a downward shift in the left ventricular end-systolic pressure/volume relationship consistent with worsening systolic function (B). Thus, abnormal expression of calcium-regulating proteins could contribute to myocardial dysfunction in remodeled hearts. (Part A *adapted from* Hasenfuss *et al.* [11]; part B *adapted from* Hajjar *et al.* [12].)

CALCIUM HOMEOSTASIS IN FAILING HUMAN MYOCARDIUM

INTRACELLULAR CALCIUM CONCENTRATION	CALCIUM-HANDLING PROTEINS (mRNA LEVELS)
Basal (diastolic) ↑	Voltage-dependent Ca^{2+} channels ↓
Peak (systolic) ↓	Na^+/Ca^{2+} exchanger ↑
Rate of fall ↓	SR Ca^{2+}-ATPase ↓
	Phospholamban ↓
	Phospholamban/SR Ca^{2+} ATPase ↑
	Ca^{2+} release channel ↓
	Calsequestrin ↔

FIGURE 4-14. The observed alterations in calcium handling and the levels of mRNA expression for several key calcium-handling proteins in myocardium from patients with cardiomyopathy. In failing myocardium there is elevation of the basal concentration of intracellular calcium and attenuation of the peak rise with depolarization. These functional abnormalities are associated with alterations in the mRNA levels for proteins involved in myocyte excitation-contraction coupling, suggesting that at least some of the functional abnormalities in failing myocardium are caused by alterations in gene expression. SR—sarcoplasmic reticulum.

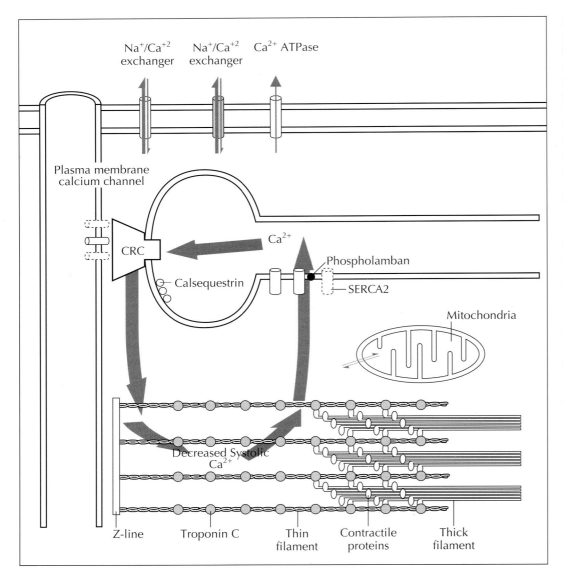

FIGURE 4-15. Myocyte contraction and relaxation in heart failure. As discussed in Chapter 1 (see Fig. 1-9), normal myocyte contraction and relaxation are dependent on the interaction of several calcium regulatory proteins. Changes in expression and activity of several of these have been observed in failing myocardium (see Fig. 4-16), as illustrated here. Increased expression is represented by *shaded proteins.* Decreased expression is represented by *dotted proteins.* Increases in the ratio of phospholamban to SERCA2 and the sodium/calcium exchanger reduces the amount of calcium in the sarcoplasmic reticulum that is available for release during systole, thereby diminishing the amplitude of the calcium transient, as shown in Figure 4-11. Decreases in the calcium release channel (CRC) and L-type calcium channels likewise diminish the calcium transient. As discussed in the next section, other alterations in the expression and calcium sensitivity of the contractile proteins may also contribute to the abnormal contractile phenotype of the failing heart. (*Adapted from* Katz [13].)

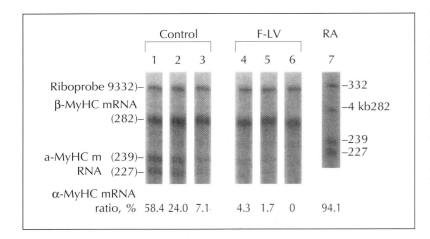

FIGURE 4-16. The myosin heavy chains (MHCs). The MHCs are the molecular motors of muscle that convert the calcium transients into muscle contraction. The α and β isoforms of MHC differ in their relative adenosine triphosphatase (ATPase) activity and velocity of shortening. Whereas α-MHC has relatively more ATPase activity and an increased velocity of shortening, β-MHC shortens more slowly and with greater economy of energy stores. The adult human heart has approximately 90% β-MHC and 10% α-MHC. In myocardium from patients with left ventricular failure (F-LV), Nakao *et al.* [14] have shown that there is decreased expression of α-MHC, which would be expected to result in a reduced velocity of shortening. (*Adapted from* Nakao *et al.* [14].)

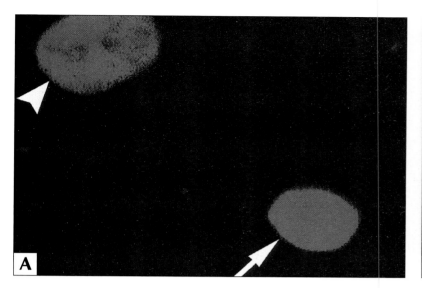

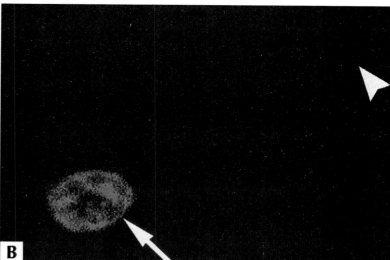

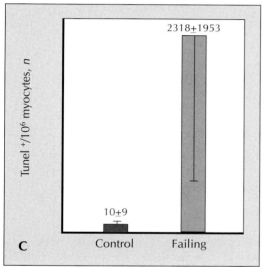

FIGURE 4-17. Loss of myocytes in heart failure. The slow loss of myocytes may contribute to the progressive decline in systolic function in heart failure. All cells have the ability to undergo programmed cell death, or apoptosis, in the presence of stimuli that activate the necessary signaling cascades. Cardiac apoptosis appears to play an important role in embryonic life as the heart "remodels" during development. Thus, apoptosis may be part of a fetal gene program. Apoptosis also occurs as a defense mechanism to rid an organ of infected or damaged cells without activation of inflammatory systems as would occur with necrosis. Olivetti *et al.* [16] demonstrated that apoptosis occurs in myocardium obtained from patients with heart failure by staining for fragmented DNA, a hallmark of the apoptotic process. **A,** Confocal microscopy of myocardial nuclei stained with propridium iodide. **B,** DNA fragments labeled with deoxyuridine triphosphate (Tunel) in apoptotic nucleus (*arrow*) but not normal nucleus (*arrowhead*). **C,** Counting of stained cells shows a large number of apoptotic cells (Tunel[+]) in failing, but not normal, myocardium. (Parts A and B *from* Olivetti *et al.* [16]; with permission. Part C *adapted from* Olivetti *et al.* [16].).

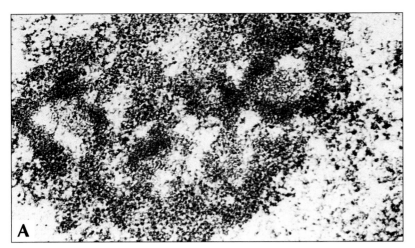

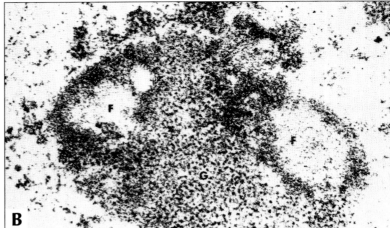

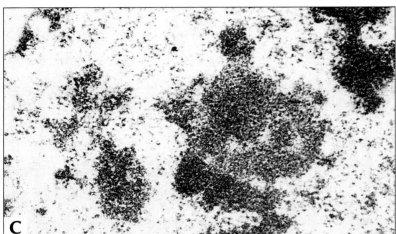

FIGURE 4-18. Electron micrographs of apoptotic cells show condensed chromatin due to the activity of specific endonucleases that cleave DNA between nucleosomes. Unverferth *et al.* [17] demonstrated this finding in the myocardium of patients 24 hours after a single dose of adriamycin, suggesting that myocyte apoptosis may play a role in the cardiotoxicity of anthracylines. **A,** Normal nucleus. **B,** Myocardial nucleus from a patient 4 hours after a single dose of adriamycin, showing some chromatin condensation. **C,** Nucleus from a patient 24 hours after adriamycin dose, showing chromatin condensation typical of apoptosis. (*From* Unverferth *et al.* [17].)

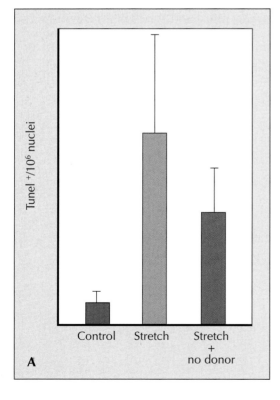

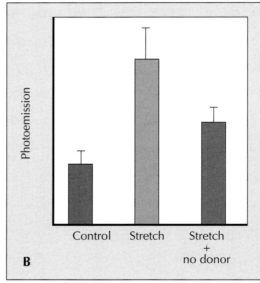

FIGURE 4-19. Mechanical stress–induced myocyte apoptosis. Increased wall stress as occurs in the dilated failing heart is sufficient to induce myocyte apoptosis. When Cheng *et al.* [18] applied gentle mechanical strain to rat myocardium in vitro, the stretched myocardium exhibited an increase in the number of myocytes with DNA fragmentation characteristic of apoptosis (**A**). They further showed that mechanical stretch increased the production of reactive oxygen (*eg*, superoxide anion), and that the addition of a nitric oxide donor that can reduce the availability of superoxide anion reduced the extent of stretch-induced apoptosis (**B**) as detected using the Tunel method. Other studies have suggested that the release of angiotensin from the myocardium in response to mechanical stretch may be a signal for apoptosis and that stretch-mediated apoptosis can be inhibited by the angiotensin receptor antagonist losartan. (*Adapted from* Cheng *et al.* [18].)

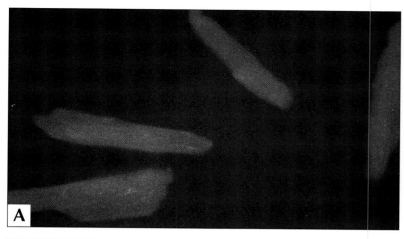

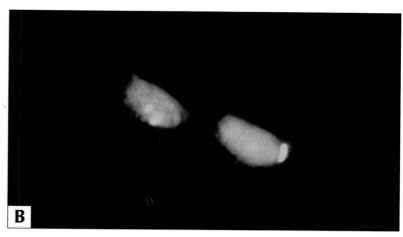

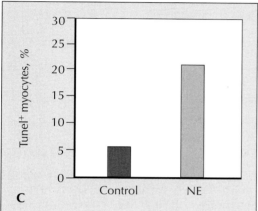

FIGURE 4-20. Neurohormonal systems, including the sympathetic nervous system, have been implicated in the induction of apoptosis. Norepinephrine (NE) can stimulate apoptosis in isolated rat ventricular myocytes as demonstrated here by an increase in the number of cells staining positive for fragmented DNA using the Tunel method. **A,** Control myocytes. **B,** Apoptotic myocytes after 24 hours' treatment with 10 mm NE. **C,** The percent of apoptotic cells increases approximately four-fold. This effect is mediated by β-adrenergic receptors since it is blocked by the β-adrenergic antagonist propranolol but not the α-adrenergic antagonist prazosin. These observations suggest that increased sympathetic tone could contribute to progressive myocyte loss and provide a possible mechanism by which β-adrenergic antagonists might exert beneficial effects in patients with heart failure. (Part A and B *from* Communal *et al.* [19], with permission; part C *adapted from* Communal *et al.* [19].)

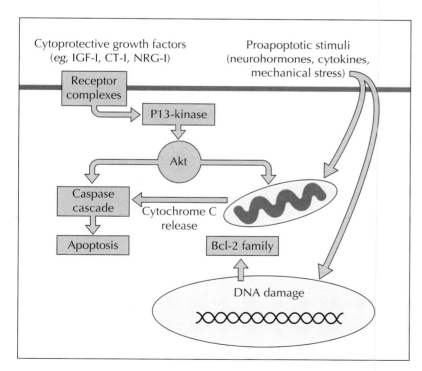

FIGURE 4-21. Regulation of myocyte survival in heart failure. The proapoptotic effect of chronic neurohormonal, inflammatory cytokine, mechanical stress, and other stimuli are counterbalanced by prosurvival pathways. The fate of any single myocyte is a function of the *net* effect of these influences. Antiapoptotic influences in the myocardium are mediated in part by cyto-protective growth factors including insulin-like growth factor-1 (IGF-1), cardiotrophin-1 (CT-1), and neuregulin-1 (NRG-1) that suppress the apoptotic cascade at multiple levels at least in part through the activation of PI-3kinase and Akt as depicted.

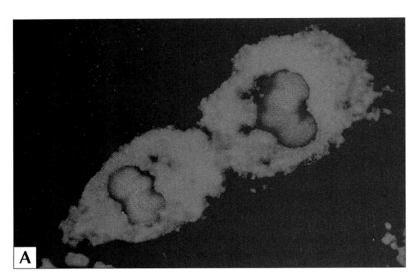

A

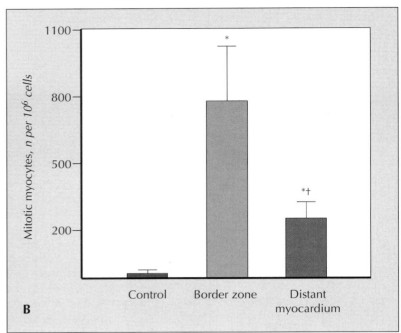

B

FIGURE 4-22. (*See* Color Plate.) Myocyte cell division in the failing heart. The long-held belief that the adult myocyte is a postmitotic cell unable to divide after birth has recently been challenged by studies showing evidence of myocyte division in the adult heart. Autopsy specimens from patients who died 4 to 12 days after myocardial infarction were examined for evidence of myocyte division including mitotic spindles, contractile rings, karyokinesis, and cytokinesis. **A,** A cardiac myocyte undergoing cytokinesis. *Red stain* is for α-sarcomeric actin, whereas green is propidium iodide staining of the nuclei. **B,** The number of dividing myocytes was markedly increased in hearts with recent myocardial infarction. The mediators and mechanisms for division of the adult myocyte are not known. (*From* Beltrami *et al.* [20]; with permission.)

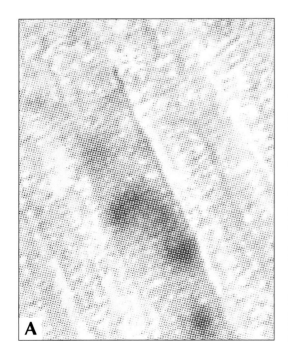

A

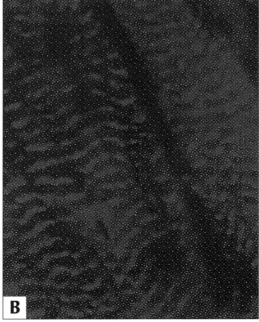

B

FIGURE 4-23. Myocyte differentiation from progenitor stem cells. There is also evidence that myocytes continue to differentiate after birth from pluripotent stem cells derived from the adult bone marrow, and potentially other organs, and this process might offset the cell loss that occurs in the remodeling heart. Jackson *et al.* [21] showed that hematopoietic stem cells incorporate into the hearts of mice after myocardial infarction. Similarly, Malouf *et al.* [22] were able to show that a liver-derived stem cell line was able to differentiate into cardiac myocytes when placed into the normal heart. In both studies, investigators used prelabeling of the stem cells with bacterial β-galactosidase gene to allow identification. **A,** Bright-field microscopy of a galactosidase positive (*darker areas*) myocyte differentiated from a hematopoietic stem cell. **B,** α-actinin staining of the same section confirming this cell has fully differentiated. *Continued*

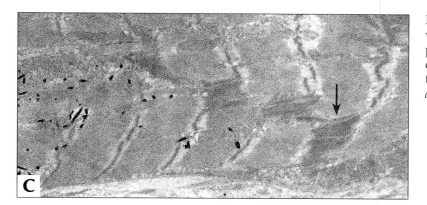

FIGURE 4-23. (*Continued*) **C,** Electron micrograph from heart tissue 6 weeks after injection of liver stem cells shows a β-galactosidase positive myocyte (with electron-dense crystalloid precipitate in cytoplasm) connected by intercalated disk and gap junction (*arrow*) to an unlabeled myocyte from the recipient heart. (Parts A and B *adapted from* Jackson [21]; part C *from* Malouf [22].

EXTRACELLULAR MATRIX

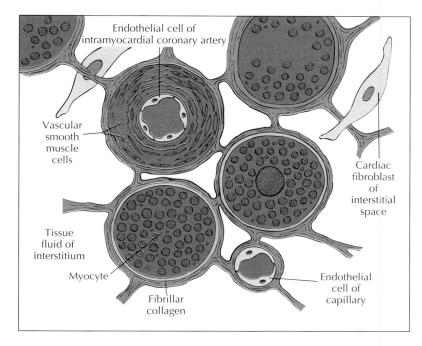

FIGURE 4-24. Although myocytes are the major components of the heart on the basis of mass, they represent only a minority of the cells on the basis of number. Nonmyocyte cellular constituents of the myocardium include fibroblasts, smooth muscle cells, and endothelial cells. Myocytes and nonmyocytes are interconnected by a complex of connective tissue and extracellular matrix. Components of the extracellular matrix include collagens, proteoglycans, glycoproteins (such as fibronectin), several peptide growth factors, and proteases (such as plasminogen activators). There is increasing appreciation that by regulating the nature and quantity of the extracellular matrix, nonmyocytes in the heart play an important role in determining the response of the myocardium to pathologic stimuli, such as hemodynamic overload. (*Adapted from* Weber and Brilla [23].)

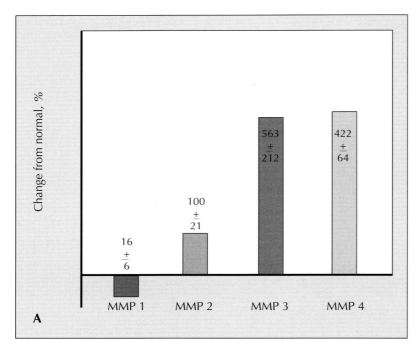
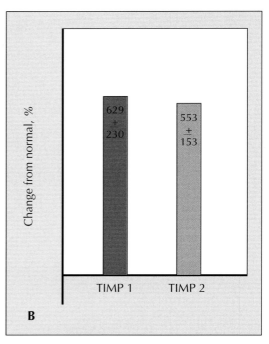

FIGURE 4-25. Metalloproteinases (MMPs) in remodeling of the extracellular matrix. The extracellular matrix that mechanically couples the myocytes must also "remodel" as the ventricle dilates. The extracellular matrix of the heart is constantly being broken down and reformed. This occurs in part through the activity of a group of enzymes called MMPs that degrade the extracellular matrix. **A,** The expression of at least two MMPs, MMP 3 and MMP 9, is increased in myocardium obtained from patients with heart failure. **B,** At the same time there appears to be increased expression of counter-regulatory inhibitors of MMPs referred to as tissue inhibitors of metalloproteinase (TIMP). Although the structural and functional consequences of these changes in matrix regulatory proteins is not yet known, it is possible that they play a role in myocardial remodeling by facilitating slippage of myocytes and thereby leading to chamber dilation. (*Adapted from* Thomas *et al.* [24].)

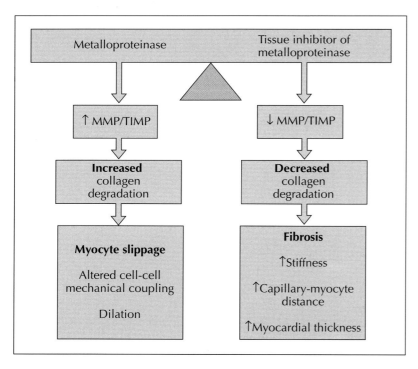

FIGURE 4-26. The balance between metalloproteinase (MMP) and tissue inhibitors of metalloproteinase (TIMP) activity. This balance determines the rate of matrix degradation and turnover. Increased MMP activity theoretically favors myocyte slippage, with reduced myocyte-to-myocyte mechanical coupling and dilation. Increased TIMP activity results in a net decrease in MMP activity and therefore theoretically favors matrix deposition. This perhaps leads to interstitial fibrosis, which may lead to increased stiffness and impaired supply of nutrients to myocytes because of an increased capillary-to-myocyte distance.

β-ADRENERGIC PATHWAY

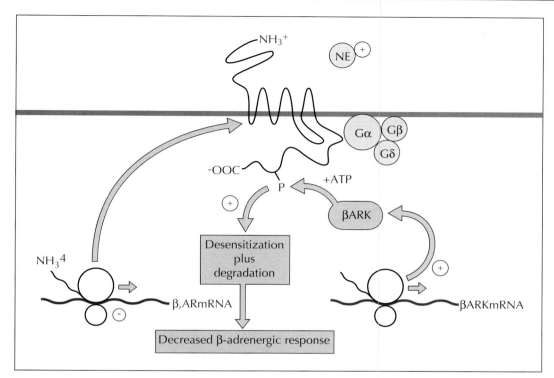

FIGURE 4-27. Alterations in β-adrenergic pathways in the failing heart. A characteristic physiologic abnormality in patients with heart failure is a reduction in the inotropic and chronotropic responses to exercise and other types of sympathetic stimulation. The molecular basis for this appears to involve multiple changes in the β_1-adrenergic receptor coupling that are a response to the chronic increase in adrenergic stimulation. In myocardium from patients with end-stage heart failure, compared with control tissue from patients without failure, the level of β-adrenergic receptor kinase (βARK) mRNA is increased and the level of β_1-adrenergic receptor mRNA is reduced [24]. This leads not only to reduction in transcription of new β_1-adrenergic receptors, but increased phosphorylation of receptors leading to desensitization and degradation of receptors.

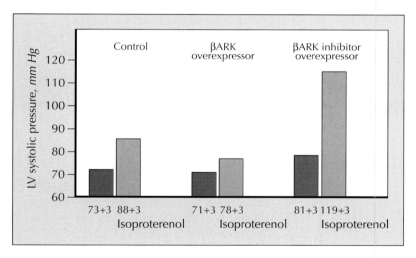

FIGURE 4-28. The functional importance of the increased expression of β-adrenergic receptor kinase (β ARK) in failing myocardium. In transgenic mice with overexpression of β ARK, there is a decreased ionotropic response to administration of the β-adrenergic agonist isoproterenol. Conversely, in mice with overexpression of the β ARK inhibitor has the opposite effect is seen with augmentation of the inotropic response to isoproterenol. LV—left ventricle. (*Adapted from* Koch *et al.* [25].)

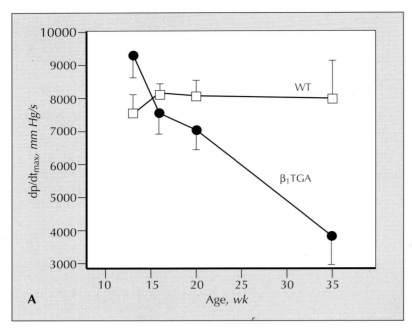

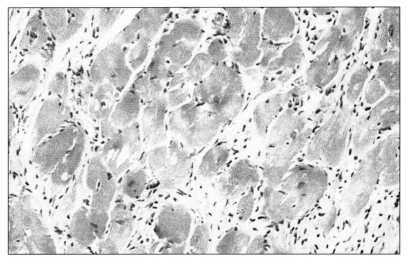

FIGURE 4-29. Adverse effects of chronic β-adrenergic receptor (β-AR) activation. Overwhelming clinical and scientific evidence now support the thesis that while desensitization of β-AR impairs myocardial contractility, this response protects against the effects of chronic β-AR on myocardial remodeling. Lohse *et al.* demonstrated the deleterious effects of β-AR stimulation by generating transgenic mice that overexpressed the β_1-AR in the heart. **A,** Using in vivo measurements of dp/dt, they found that while mice expressing approximately 15-fold the normal level of β_1-AR had evidence of increased cardiac function at 12 weeks of age, the mice went on to develop systolic dysfunction and evidence of heart failure with premature death. **B,** Histopathologic examination of these hearts at the late timepoint showed findings consistent with chronic remodeling including myocyte hypertrophy and replacement fibrosis. (*Adapted from* Engelhardt *et al.* [26]).

RENIN-ANGIOTENSIN SYSTEM, ENDOTHELIN, AND INFLAMMATORY CYTOKINES

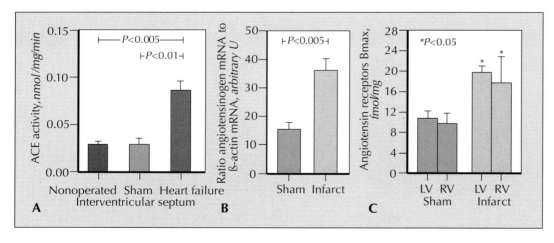

FIGURE 4-30. There is upregulation of several components of the renin-angiotensin system (RAS) in the noninfarcted myocardium of rats after myocardial infarction. There are significant increases in ACE activity (**A**), the level of angiotensinogen mRNA (**B,**), and the density of angiotensin-II receptors (**C**). The increase in angiotensin-II receptor density suggests that in addition to increased activity of the tissue RAS, the responsiveness of the tissue to angiotensin may be increased. LV—left ventricle; RV—right ventricle. (*Adapted from* Hirsch *et al.* [27]; Lindpaintner *et al.* [28]; Meggs *et al.* [29].)

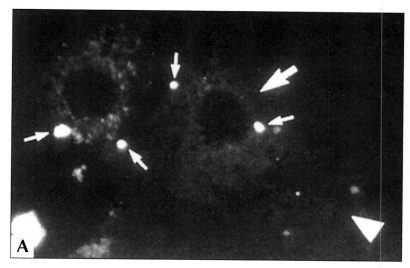

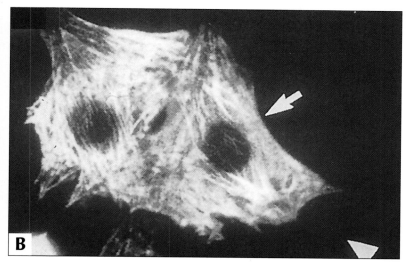

FIGURE 4-31. The cardiac myocyte may be a source of tissue angiotensin II. **A,** Fluorescence staining of a rat ventricular myocyte with an antibody directed against angiotensin II is shown. The focal areas of staining (*small arrows*) within the cell indicate the presence of angiotensin II. **B,** The same cell (note location of large arrow) stains avidly with an antisarcomeric myosin antibody, indicating that it is a myocyte. The *arrowhead* indicates a nonmyocyte. Stretching of cultured neonatal rat cardiac myocytes on a silicone membrane induced the expression of fetal genes and increased protein synthesis, and these effects were blocked by the angiotensin-receptor antagonist losartan. These observations suggest that angiotensin II released from cardiac myocytes plays an autocrine role in regulating the cardiac myocyte growth response to hemodynamic overload. (*Adapted from* Sadoshima *et al.* [30]; with permission.)

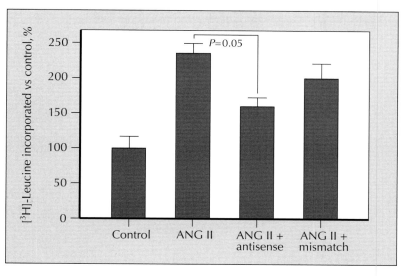

FIGURE 4-32. There is evidence that endothelin-1 (ET-1) may serve as an autocrine or paracrine regulator of the molecular and cellular effects of angiotensin II (ANG II) on cardiac myocyte growth. In cultured neonatal rat cardiac myocytes, ANG II induces the expression of ET-1. By using an antisense oligonucleotide directed against preproendothelin-1 mRNA (ppET-1, the precursor of ET-1), it was shown that cells treated with antisense to ppET-1 to block ET-1 synthesis have a significantly reduced growth response to ANG II, as reflected by leucine incorporation into protein. In other experiments, an antagonist for ET-1 receptors was similarly shown to inhibit the growth effects of ANG II. These observations raise the intriguing possibility that in cardiac myocytes, ET-1 plays a critical autocrine role in the cellular response to ANG II. Data are mean $\pm$ SD. (*Adapted from* Ito *et al.* [31].)

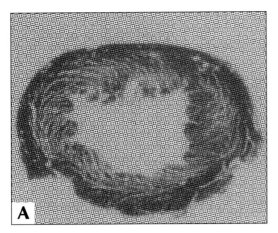

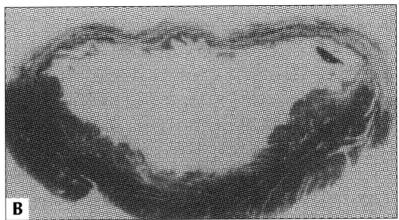

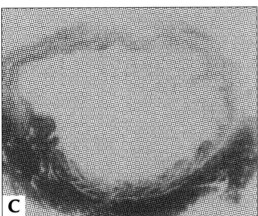

FIGURE 4-33. Role of endothelin in heart failure. Because endothelin can stimulate myocyte growth and regulate extracellular matrix turnover in vitro and is increased in the plasma of patients with heart failure, it has been suggested that it might play a pathophysiologic role in myocardial failure. Sakai *et al.* [32] examined this thesis by treating rats with BQ-123, an endothelin receptor antagonist, or placebo after myocardial infarction. Rats treated with BQ-123 had improved left ventricular (LV) function and better survival than placebo-treated animals. Masson trichrome–stained sections of LV from sham-operated rat (**A**), infarcted rat (**B**), and infarcted rat treated with BQ-123 (**C**) show less LV dilation in the treated animals. These effects are similar to those observed by other investigators with angiotensin-converting enzyme inhibitors. At this time it is unclear whether endothelin and angiotensin exert independent effects on ventricular remodeling or whether they act in series, as suggested by Figure 4-35. (*From* Sakai *et al.* [32]; with permission.)

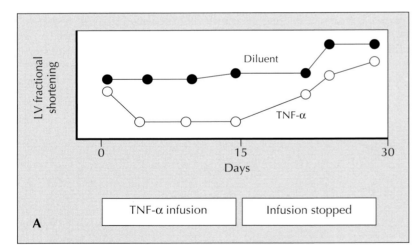

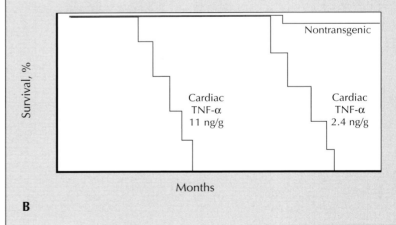

FIGURE 4-34. Tumor necrosis factor (TNF)-α in heart failure. Circulating levels of cytokines including TNF-α are elevated in patients with heart failure. There is now reason to believe that these levels play a role in the pathogenesis of heart failure, although the mechanism by which this occurs remains unclear. Bozkurt *et al.* [33] were able to demonstrate a decrease in left ventricular (LV) fractional shortening as assessed by serial echocardiograms in rats subjected to a continuous infusion with TNF-α (**A**). Interestingly, this decrease in LV function was completely reversed 30 days after the infusion was stopped. When Bryant *et al.* [34] caused overexpression of TNF-α in transgenic mice, there was ventricular dilation and impaired survival of mice that was related to the intensity of TNF-α expression (**B**). (*Adapted from* Bozkurt *et al.* [33] and Bryant *et al.* [34].

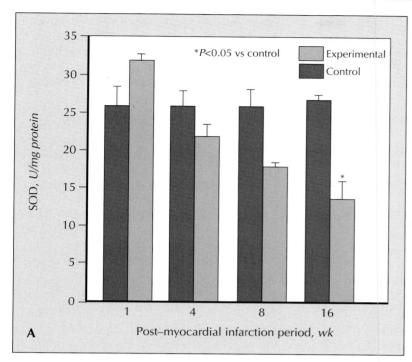

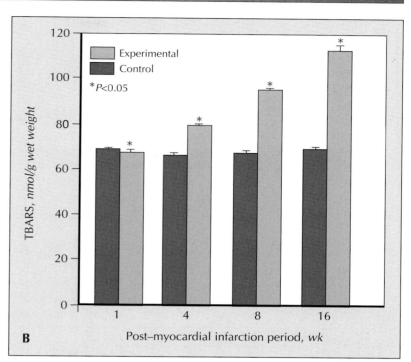

FIGURE 4-35. Role of oxidative stress in progression of myocardial failure. There is evidence that oxidative stress is increased in heart failure and may play a role in progression of the underlying myocardial failure. **A,** In the rat myocardial infarction model, Hill and Singal [35] found that increased oxidative stress in the myocardium was associated with decreased activity of antioxidant enzymes such as superoxide dismutase (SOD). **B,** In the same animals, the myocardial level of thiobarbituric acid reactive substances (TBARS), an index of oxidative stress, was elevated. In guinea pigs with pressure overload–induced myocardial failure, these same investigators were able to prevent the transition from hypertrophy to failure by supplementation of the diet with vitamin E, a lipid-soluble antioxidant. (*Adapted from* Hill and Singal [35].)

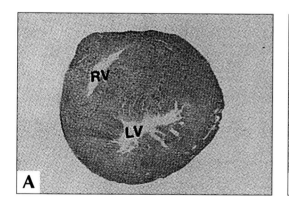

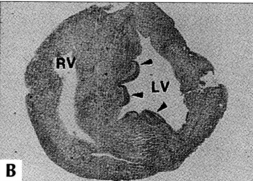

FIGURE 4-36. **A** and **B,** Transgenic animals offer further evidence for the importance of antioxidant enzymes in the control of cardiac function and remodeling. Removal of a functional copy of the enzyme manganese superoxide dismutase (MnSOD), the main form of superoxide dismutase (SOD) in the mitochondria, results in death of mice at a young age. These mice have anatomic evidence of heart failure, with dilated ventricles and thrombus formation on the ventricular wall (*arrowheads*), consistent with poor systolic function. LV— left ventricle; RV—right ventricle. (*From* Li *et al.* [36]; with permission.)

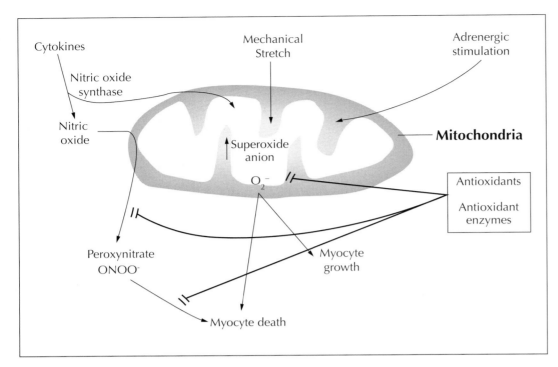

FIGURE 4-37. Oxidative stress as a mediator of the failure phenotype. Oxidative stress resulting from superoxide anion, nitric oxide (NO), and their reaction product, peroxynitrite, may act as important intracellular mediators for remodeling stimuli such as mechanical overload, inflammatory cytokines, and catecholamines. Mitochondria are the major source of superoxide anion in ventricular myocytes, although there are other potentially important oxidase systems in the cytoplasm. Superoxide anions that are unquenched by superoxide dismutase (SOD) or soluble antioxidants result in formation of hydrogen peroxide and hydroxyl radicals. In the presence of nitric oxide, peroxynitrite is also formed. Nitric oxide synthase under some circumstances can also become a significant source of superoxide anion. These reactive oxygen species may cause sublethal cell injury that can activate apoptotic pathways, as well as activate growth pathways through oxidative stress–responsive transcription factors.

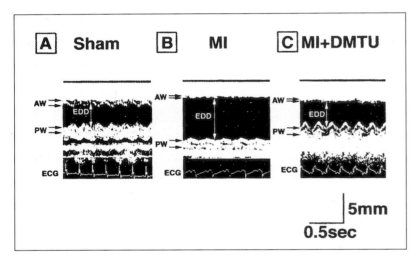

FIGURE 4-38. Oxidative stress contributes to myocardial remodeling. Studies with pharmacologic delivery of antioxidants in animal models of myocardial remodeling have shown beneficial effects that may be occurring through multiple mechanisms. Echocardiograms of mice 28 days after myocardial infarction (MI) show evidence of dilation and dysfunction that was prevented by treatment with the antioxidant dimethylthiourea (DMTU). Histopathologic examination of the hearts from these animals showed that DMTU prevented the increase in myocyte diameter, increase in collagen content, and increased activity of MMP-2, suggesting that both oxidative stress was mediating myocyte as well as matrix remodeling. (*Adapted from* Kinugawa *et al.*[37]).

REFERENCES

1. Swynghedauw B, Moalic JM, Delcayre C: The origins of cardiac hypertrophy. In *Research in Cardiac Hypertrophy and Failure*. Edited by Swynghedauw B. London: INSERM/John Libbey Eurotext; 1990:23–50.

2. Gerdes AM, Kellerman SE, Moore JA, *et al.*: Structural remodeling of cardiac myocytes in patients with ischemic cardiomyopathy. *Circulation* 1992, 86:426–430.

3. Takahashi T, Allen PD, Izumo S: Expression of A-, B-, and C-type natriuretic peptide genes in failing and developing human ventricles. *Circ Res* 1992, 71:9–17.

4. Sadoshima J-I, Jahn L, Takahashi T, *et al.*: Molecular characterizations of the stretch-induced adaptation of cultured cardiac cells: an in vitro model of load-induced cardiac hypertrophy. *J Biol Chem* 1992, 267:10551–10560.

5. Simpson P, McGrath A: Norepinephrine-stimulated hypertrophy of cultured rat myocardial cells is an a1 adrenergic response. *J Clin Invest* 1983, 72:732–738.

6. Sadoshima J-I, Izumo S: Molecular characterization of angiotensin II-induced hypertrophy of cardiac myocytes and hyperplasia of cardiac fibroblasts: critical role of the AT1 receptor subtype. *Circ Res* 1993, 73:413–423.

7. Thaik CM, Calderone A, Takahashi N, Colucci WS: Interleukin-1b modulates the growth and phenotype of neonatal rat cardiac myocytes. *J Clin Invest* 1995, 96:1093–1099.

8. Calderone A, Thaik CM, Takahashi N, *et al.*: Nitric oxide, atrial natriuretic peptide, and cGMP inhibit the growth-promoting effects of norepinephrine in cardiac myocytes and fibroblasts. *J Clin Invest* 1998, 101:812–818.

9. Beuckelmann DJ, Nabauer M, Erdmann E: Intracellular calcium handling in isolated ventricular myocytes from patients with terminal heart failure. *Circulation* 1992, 85:1046–1055.

10. Takahashi T, Allen PD, Lacro RV, *et al.*: Expression of dihydropyridine receptor (Ca^{2+} channel) and calsequestrin genes in the myocardium of patients with end-stage heart failure. *J Clin Invest* 1992, 90:927–935.

11. Hasenfuss G, Meyer M, Schillinger W, *et al.*: Calcium handling proteins in the failing human heart. *Basic Res Cardiol* 1997, 92 (suppl 1):87–93.

12. Hajjar RJ, Schmidt U, Matsui T, *et al.*: Modulation of ventricular function through gene transfer in vivo. *Proc Natl Acad Sci U S A* 1998, 95:5251–5256.

13. Katz AM: *Physiology of the Heart*, edn 2. New York: Raven Press; 1992.

14. Nakao K, Minobe W, Roden R, *et al.*: Myosin heavy chain gene expression in human heart failure. *J Clin Invest* 1997, 100:2362–2370.

15. Anderson PAW, Malouf NN, Oakeley AE, *et al.*: Troponin T isoform expression in the normal and failing human left ventricle: a correlation with myofibrillar ATPase activity. *Basic Res Cardiol* 1992, 87:175–185.

16. Olivetti G, Abbi R, Quaini F, *et al.*: Apoptosis in the failing human heart. *N Engl J Med* 1997, 336:1131–1141.

17. Unverferth DV, Magorien RD, Unverferth BP, *et al.*: Human myocardial morphologic and functional changes in the first 24 hours after doxorubicin administration. *Cancer Treat Reports* 1981, 65:1093–1097.

18. Cheng W, Li B, Kajistura J, *et al.*: Stretch-induced programmed myocyte cell death. *J Clin Invest* 1995, 96:2247–2259.

19. Communal C, Singh K, Pimentel DR, Colucci WS: Norepinephrine stimulates apoptosis in adult rat ventricular myocytes by activation of the β-adrenergic pathway. *Circ Res* 1998, 98: 1329–1334.

20. Beltrami AP, Urbanek K, Kajstura J, *et al.*: Evidence that human cardiac myocytes divide after myocardial infarction. *N Engl J Med* 2001, 344:1750–1757.

21. Jackson KA, Majka SM, Wang H, *et al.*: Regeneration of ischemic cardiac muscle and vascular endothelium by adult stem cells. *J Clin Invest* 2001, 107:1395–1402.

22. Malouf NN, Coleman WB, Grisham JW, *et al.*: Adult-derived stem cells from the liver become myocytes in the heart in vivo. *Am J Pathol* 2001, 158:1929–1935.

23. Weber KT, Brilla CG: Pathological hypertrophy and cardiac interstitium: fibrosis and renin-angiotensin-aldosterone system. Circulation 1991, 83:1849_1865.

24. Thomas CV, Coker ML, Zellner JL, *et al.*: Increased matrix metalloproteinase activity and selective upregulation in LV myocardium from patients with end-stage dilated cardiomyopathy. *Circulation* 1998, 97:1708–1715.

25. Koch WJ, Rockman HA, Samama P, *et al.*: Cardiac function in mice overexpressing the beta-adrenergic receptor kinase or a bARK inhibitor. *Science* 1995, 268:1350–1353.

26. Engelhardt S, Hein L, Wiesmann F, Lohse MJ: Progressive hypertrophy and heart failure in beta 1 - adrenergic receptor transgenic mice. Proc Natl Acad Sci U S A 1999, 96: 7059–7064.

27. Hirsch AT, Talsness CE, Schunkert H, *et al.*: Tissue-specific activation of cardiac angiotensin converting enzyme in experimental heart failure. *Circ Res* 1991, 69:475–482.

28. Lindpaintner K, Lu W, Niedermajer N, *et al.*: Selective activation of cardiac angiotensinogen gene expression in post-infarction ventricular remodeling in the rat. *J Mol Cell Cardiol* 1993, 25:133–143.

29. Meggs LG, Coupet J, Huang H, *et al.*: Regulation of angiotensin II receptors on ventricular myocytes after myocardial infarction in rats. *Circ Res* 1993, 72:1149–1162.

30. Sadoshima J-I, Xu Y, Slayter HS, Izumo S: Autocrine release of angiotensin II mediates stretch-induced hypertrophy of cardiac myocytes in vitro. *Cell* 1993, 75:977–984.

31. Ito H, Hirata Y, Adachi S, *et al.*: Endothelin-1 is an autocrine/paracrine factor in the mechanism of angiotensin II-induced hypertrophy in cultured rat cardiomyocytes. *J Clin Invest* 1993, 92:398–403.

32. Sakai S, Miyauchi T, Kobayashi M, *et al.*: Inhibition of myocardial endothelin pathway improves long-term survival in heart failure. *Nature* 1996, 384:353–355.

33. Bozkurt B, Kribbs SB, Clubb FJ, *et al.*: Pathophysiologically relevant concentrations of tumor necrosis factor-a promote progressive left ventricular dysfunction and remodeling in rats. *Circulation* 1998, 97:1382–1391.

34. Bryant D, Becker L, Richardson J, *et al.*: Cardiac failure in transgenic mice with myocardial expression of tumor necrosis factor-a. *Circulation* 1998, 97:1375–1381.

35. Hill MF, Singal PK: Antioxidant and oxidative stress changes during heart failure subsequent to myocardial infarction in rats. *Am J Pathol* 1996, 148:291–300.

36. Li Y, Huang T-T, Carlson EJ, *et al.*: Dilated cardiomyopathy and neonatal lethality in mutant mice lacking manganese superoxide dismutase. *Nat Genet* 1995, 11:376–381.

37. Kinugawa S, Tsutsui H, Hayashidani S, *et al.*: Treatment with dimethyliourea prevents left ventricular remodeling and failure after experimental myocardial infarction in mice: role of oxidative stress. *Circ Res* 2000, 87:392–398.

CARDIAC REMODELING AND ITS PREVENTION

5

CHAPTER

Marc A. Pfeffer

Cardiac chambers have the capacity to alter (remodel) their size and configuration in response to a chronic change in their hemodynamic load. Whether across or within species, the mass and volume of the ventricular chambers maintain a close relationship with the required external work. The changes in chamber volume and mass that accompany normal growth provide the most striking example of the heart's intrinsic capacity to remodel in response to the insidious alterations in demand that take place as a consequence of body growth. Under pathologic conditions of chronic pressure or volume overload, the chamber remodels in direct relation to the imposed hemodynamic burden. The mass increase is attributable to fiber hypertrophy. However, the manner of rearrangement of these additional contractile tissues can lead to either an eccentric (chamber volume > mass) or a concentric (chamber mass > volume) pattern of ventricular growth. Although remodeling in response to a pathologic condition can in one sense be considered adaptive because it permits the restoration of pump function in the face of an imposed hyperfunctional condition, the extent of ventricular remodeling is nevertheless an important marker for a less than optimal prognosis.

A specific type of chamber remodeling can occur as the result of myocardial infarction (MI). In this situation the left ventricle (LV) can undergo an immediate contour change as a result of thinning and elongation of the region affected by myocardial necrosis. This topographic alteration in the infarcted region, termed *infarct expansion*, is a consequence of slippage between muscle fiber bundles, resulting in a reduction across the ventricular wall of the number of myocytes in the noncontractile region. This regional stretching and thinning can continue until connective tissue elements within the infarcted region provide sufficient resistance to oppose further deformation. Both the initial loss of contractile tissues and this subsequent distortion combine to augment the effect of workload and wall stress on the remaining viable myocardium. These events, which occur relatively early during acute MI, provide the substrate for the more insidious global process of subsequent progressive ventricular enlargement.

As with other forms of systolic dysfunction, the greater the degree of ventricular enlargement, the more guarded the prognosis. This is particularly true for survivors of MI in whom a small quantitative augmentation of ventricular volume is associated with a great increase in the relative risk for death. Current methods of noninvasive imaging enable serial assessments of ventricular size and shape to be obtained and have thus delineated the progressive nature of the remodeling that occurs in the impaired LV. Remodeling after MI is a multifactorial process that can be influenced by infarct size and transmurality, the degree of histologic healing in the infarcted region, and ventricular wall stress. Prompt restoration of myocardial flow by thrombolytic therapy or primary coronary angioplasty reduces infarct size and transmurality and diminishes the risk for postinfarction ventricular remodeling. Therapy with anti-inflammatory agents during the early phase of MI can prolong the phase during which the ventricle is vulnerable to infarct expansion. Therefore, avoidance of these agents may reduce the extent of local distortion. Infarct expansion and the more insidious process of global ventricular enlargement have been successfully attenuated by chronic therapy with angiotensin-converting enzyme (ACE) inhibitors. These factors that influence ventricular remodeling after MI have practical value because they can be modified, and favorable alterations in ventricular size and shape have been shown to result in improved clinical outcome. Indeed, limiting the extent of ventricular remodeling in asymptomatic patients after MI can be considered as preventive therapy for symptomatic congestive heart failure.

CARDIAC GROWTH AND REMODELING

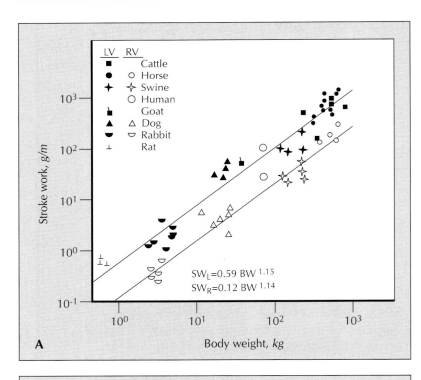

A

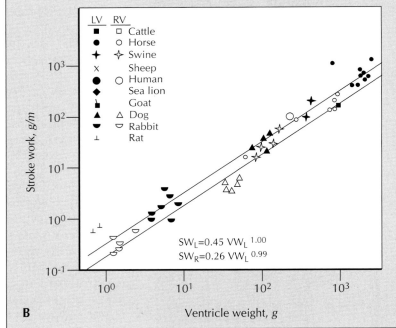

B

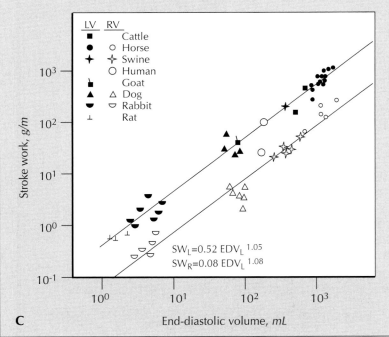

C

FIGURE 5-1. The logarithmic relationship between ventricular stroke work (SW) and body weight (BW; *panel A*), stroke work and ventricular weight (VW; *panel B*), and stroke work and end-diastolic volume (EDV; *panel C*) [1]. These relationships between external work, ventricular chamber weight, and volume were developed across 10 mammalian species ranging in size from rats to cattle and provide an excellent example of the close association between workload and structure. LV—left ventricle; RV—right ventricle. (*Adapted from* Holt *et al.* [1].)

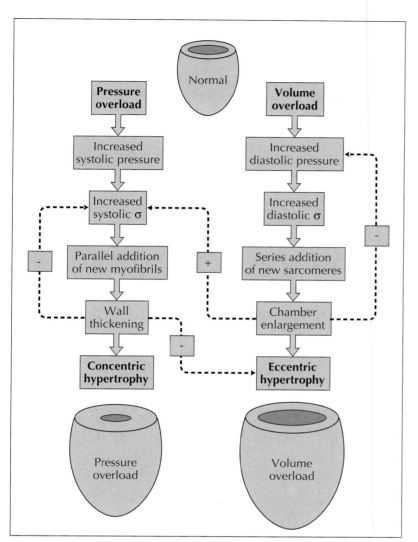

FIGURE 5-2. Patterns of ventricular hypertrophy. Specific patterns of ventricular remodeling occur in response to the imposed augmentation in workload. A pattern of hypertrophic growth characterized as concentric, in which increased mass is out of proportion to chamber volume, is particularly effective in reducing systolic wall stress (σ) under conditions of heightened pressure load. In contrast, in volume overload conditions, in which the major stimulus is diastolic loading, a predominant finding is a great increase in the cavity size or volume. Although there can be extensive increases in mass, the relationship between mass and volume is either preserved or, in severe cases, reduced. The fundamental response is generated by cellular hypertrophy. However, the configuration of the new contractile tissue is specific and offsets the major mechanical stimulus. (*Adapted from* Grossman *et al.* [2].)

VENTRICULAR REMODELING: ALTERATION IN CONTOUR OR VOLUME OF VENTRICULAR CAVITY THAT IS NOT ATTRIBUTED TO ACUTE CHANGES IN DISTENDING PRESSURE

Remodeling with preservation of mass/volume ratio
Remodeling with alteration in mass/volume ratio
  Alteration in mass/volume relationship
    ↑ Concentric hypertrophy
  Mass/volume
    ← ↓ Eccentric hypertrophy
    ↓ Failure

FIGURE 5-3. Definition of ventricular remodeling. In a definition of ventricular remodeling, it is important to note that these alterations in size and volume or shape are not related to acute changes in distension [3]. Although alterations in filling pressure change chamber volume, these acute changes do not reflect a true structural modification. Systolic dysfunction impairs ventricular emptying and initially leads to a predominant condition of volume overload. With chamber enlargement, systolic load is also increased. With left ventricular dysfunction and enlargement, the chamber volume may increase out of proportion to mass. This sets up a pathophysiologic condition in which, at any comparable intraventricular pressure, the wall stress is increased compared with that of a ventricle with a preserved mass-to-volume ratio. Although ventricular mass is increased in all three situations, the relationship between the augmented mass and volume differs.

EARLY REMODELING AFTER MYOCARDIAL INFARCTION AND INFARCT EXPANSION

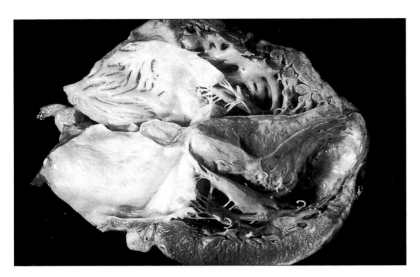

FIGURE 5-4. Pathologic specimen of a human heart that experienced a prior infarction leading to marked apical infarct expansion. Thinning and elongation of the involved apical region have resulted in distortion and enlargement of the ventricular cavity. The scarred apex not only would be unable to contract but would lead to a distortion of the ventricular cavity, resulting in hypertrophy of the remaining viable myocardium. (*Courtesy of* Frederick Schoen, MD, PhD, Boston, MA.)

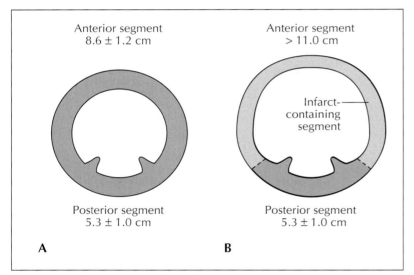

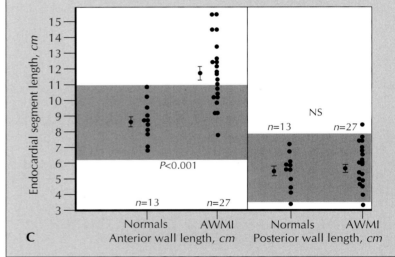

FIGURE 5-5. *In vivo* echocardiographic diagnosis of remodeling. The echocardiographic diagnosis of remodeling was made from the short-axis plane at the level of the papillary muscle. Using the internal landmarks provided by the papillary muscle, the ventricle was divided into two segments, anterior and posterior. **A,** Whereas the normal anterior segment length is 8.6±1.2 cm, the posterior segment is 5.3±1 cm. **B,** In patients with first myocardial infarcts, the segment with the noncontractile region is the obvious infarct-containing segment. Patients who experience infarct expansion develop elongation of this segment within the first week of the infarction. **C,** Actual data points from 27 patients with acute anterior wall myocardial infarction (AWMI) demonstrate that almost 60% of patients with an anterior infarct developed an elongation of the anterior segment that was greater than 2 SD from normal. In these patients, the posterior wall length was not increased 3 days after the infarction. Conversely, in patients with posterior infarcts, one can anticipate that the anterior segment would be normal and that a proportion would have elongation of the posterior segment. *Shaded areas* indicate normal ranges ± SD. (*Adapted from* Erlebacher *et al.* [4].)

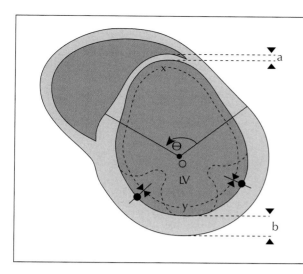

Θ Angular extent of asynergy

x   Endocardial length of asynergy-containing segment

y   Endocardial length of segment without asynergy

a   Average thickness of asynergic zone

b   Average thickness of non-asynergic zone

FIGURE 5-6. A more extensive method of quantitating infarct expansion developed by Jugdutt and Michorowski [5]. The length of the infarct-containing segment is, of course, determined. However, in this method, which also utilizes two-dimensional short-axis echocardiography, at the mid-papillary muscle level the thickness of the infarcted segment is related to the wall thickness of the noninfarcted region to provide a thinning ratio, the other major component of infarct expansion. Expansion index is calculated by dividing the length of the asynergy-containing segment by the length of the segment without asynergy (x/y). Thinning ratio is determined by dividing average thickness of the asynergic zone by average thickness of the non-asynergic zone (a/b). LV—left ventricle. (*Adapted from* Jugdutt and Michorowski [5].)

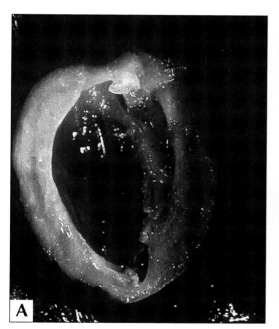

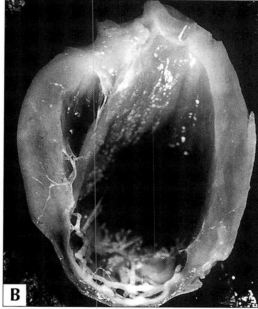

FIGURE 5-7. Predilection of the left ventricular apex for expansion. The left ventricular apex is particularly vulnerable to infarct expansion and initiation of global enlargement. **A,** A normal apex has the greatest radius (r) of curvature and therefore, by the Law of Laplace, has the lowest wall tension (T). **B,** When this region undergoes expansion and thinning, the elongation produces a marked distortion and greatly increases the radius of curvature. Because this area usually has the least wall thickness (h), it is the most vulnerable to any increase in the radius. P—pressure.

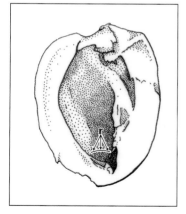

Law of Laplace
$$T = \frac{P \times r}{2}$$

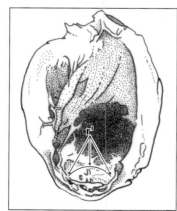

Wall stress (σ)
$$\sigma = \frac{T}{h} = \frac{P \times r}{2h}$$

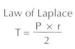

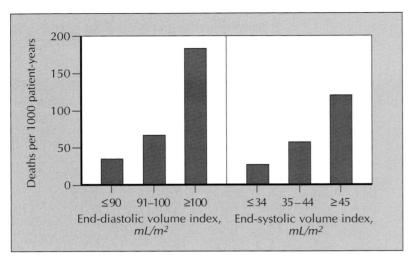

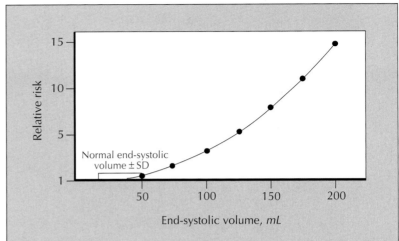

FIGURE 5-8. Mortality rate as related to left ventricular size. In an extensive database that included clinical demographics, catheterization data, and exercise capacity of 733 patients with coronary artery disease, the most powerful predictor of long-term outcome was left ventricular size as measured by volume biplane left ventriculography. The relationship between deaths per thousand patient- years and left ventricular size in either end-diastole or end-systole illustrates the major increase in risk for death that occurs with relatively small changes in left ventricular volume. (*Adapted from* Hammermeister *et al.* [6].)

FIGURE 5-9. Relative risk for death in survivors of myocardial infarction. End-systolic volume has been found to be a most important prognostic factor for determinations of long-term survival after myocardial infarction. For each 25-mL increment in end-systolic volume, the risk for death increased exponentially over that of other survivors of myocardial infarction with preserved left ventricular volume. (*Adapted from* White *et al.* [7].)

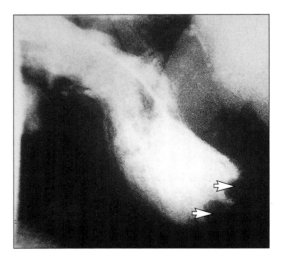

FIGURE 5-10. Morphologic classification of early change in shape of left ventricle (LV). A myocardial infarction (MI) can alter left ventricular LV shape as well as volume. Although much more difficult to quantitate, this scheme has been developed to characterize the distortion that occurs after an MI. LV shape is an important determinant of outcome. Meizlish *et al.* [8] developed a classification for LV shape changes based on radionuclide angiograms and found that greater degrees of distortion were associated with a higher likelihood of death even when adjustment was made for comparable LV ejection fractions. In the above grading system, shape abnormalities of grades 1 and 2 are confined to the diastolic contour. Grades 3 through 5 involve overt alterations in the LV contour that are present in diastole as well as systole. In patients with a first anterior MI, the greater the shape distortion, the higher the likelihood of ventricular thrombus. (*Adapted from* Meizlish *et al.* [8] and Lamas *et al.* [9].)

FIGURE 5-11. Contrast left ventriculogram of a patient with a first anterior infarct. This frame in end-systole shows enlargement and distortion of the cavity, with apical expansion. Intraluminal thrombi (*arrows*) are detected as filling defects. (*From* Lamas *et al.* [9]; with permission.)

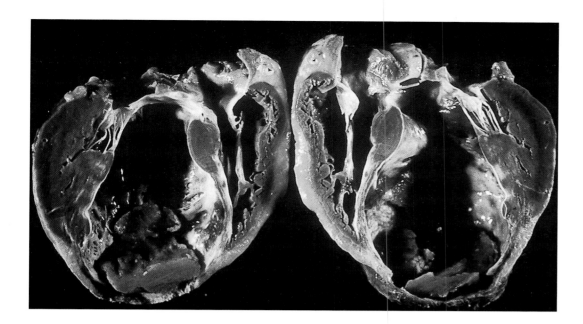

FIGURE 5-12. A heart removed from a cardiac transplant recipient. This specimen, from a survivor of one large anterior septal apical infarction, demonstrates the thinning and elongation of the infarcted region, the cavity enlargement, and hypertrophy of the remaining segment, as well as a large apical thrombus. (*Courtesy of* Lynda Biedrzycki, MD, Boston, MA.)

PROGRESSIVE ENLARGEMENT AFTER MYOCARDIAL INFARCTION

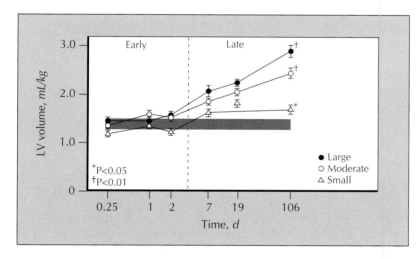

FIGURE 5-13. Progressive ventricular remodeling in a rat model of myocardial infarction. Left ventricular (LV) volumes in rats with various degrees of histologic damage were studied in the acute to chronic period after coronary ligation. The *shaded area* represents mean values ± 2 SEM from normal (not infarcted) animals. Volumes were obtained from the pressure/volume relationship and are compared at the common distending pressure of 20 mm Hg. Therefore, under these conditions, a change in volume is caused by true remodeling rather than altered distention. The extent of this remodeling is a function of both the duration and the degree of histologic damage. Although infarct expansion has been noted as an early process, when filling pressure is taken into account it becomes apparent that the bulk of the global enlargement occurs in the weeks to months after an infarction, when fibrous connective tissue has been established in the infarcted region. (*Adapted from* Pfeffer *et al.* [10].)

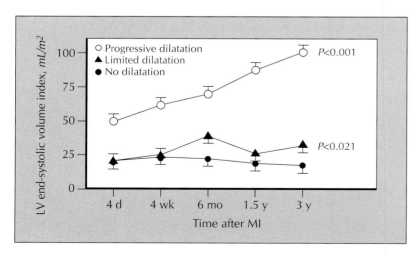

FIGURE 5-14. Progressive ventricular enlargement after myocardial infarction (MI) in humans. In a sequential study of left ventricular (LV) volumes of 99 patients from 4 days to 3 years after acute MI, Gaudron *et al.* [11] demonstrated that progressive enlargement continued in about 25%. Those who experienced progressive and marked changes in ventricular size were more likely to have had large anterior infarctions with limited collateral flow. Recurrent infarction was excluded in this patient population as a potential explanation for this late enlargement. (*Adapted from* Gaudron *et al.* [11].)

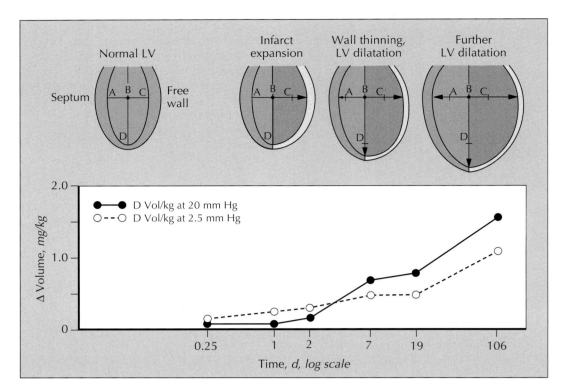

FIGURE 5-15. Time course and components of remodeling after experimental infarction. Changes in volume per kilogram of body weight at common distending pressures indicate a true structural change. *Numerical values* represent actual experimental data. *Upper diagrams*, although not drawn to scale, illustrate the various components of remodeling after infarction. Lengths BA and BC represent the minor radius at the midpoint of the left ventricle (LV), and length BD represents the major radius. In the initial period there is thinning and elongation of the infarcted region, and axis B to C increases. The change in the shape of the perimeter leads to a net increase in ventricular volume. During the early healing period there is further thinning and elongation. However, there is an additional component of chamber enlargement that now involves the viable myocardium, as axes B to A and B to D are also increased. This more global process of enlargement continues long after histologic resolution. (*Adapted from* Pfeffer [12].)

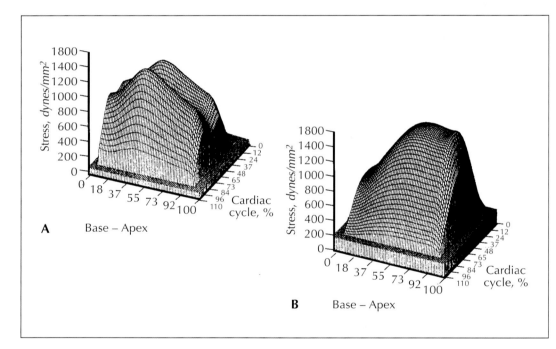

FIGURE 5-16. Regional midwall circumferential wall stress from base to apex calculated during the cardiac cycle in a rat model of myocardial infarction (MI), showing the regionality and complexity of wall stress over the entire cardiac cycle. **A,** Wall stress declines during the early ejection phase in a normal ventricle, despite the increased pressure caused by both systolic wall thickening and a marked decrease in chamber radius. **B,** The infarcted (dilated) ventricle starts from a greater diastolic radius or volume and wall stress. During ejection, there is a much lesser reduction in the radius of the enlarged ventricle (even for the same stroke volume) so that wall stress is actually exacerbated rather than relieved with the development of systolic pressure during early ejection. Also shown is the regionality of abnormal wall stress, consistent with the clinical observation that the base is least affected. (*Adapted from* Capasso *et al.* [13].)

MODIFICATION OF REMODELING AFTER MYOCARDIAL INFARCTION

MODIFIABLE FACTORS FOR INTERVENTIONS TO LIMIT ENLARGEMENT AFTER MYOCARDIAL INFARCTION

INTERDEPENDENT FACTORS	INTERVENTIONS
Infarct	Restoration of infarct vessel patency
Size	Thrombolytic therapy + aspirin
Transmurality	Mechanical PTCA
Location	Avoid NSAIDs, steroids
Scar formation	Nitroglycerin
Ventricular wall stress	ACE inhibition

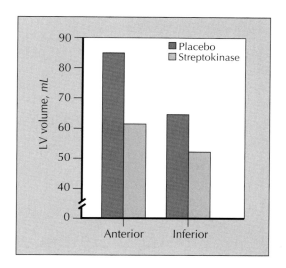

FIGURE 5-17. Modifiable factors for limitation of postinfarction ventricular remodeling. The extent of the infarction, in terms of both the amount of wall motion abnormality and the degree of transmurality, plays a major role in determining the risk for progressive ventricular enlargement. Primary prevention measures should be considered as the major key to reducing the initial risk for myocardial infarction (MI) and subsequent distortion of the left ventricle. During an acute MI, prompt attention to the supply-and-demand balance, with restoration of coronary artery flow, preserves myocardium and reduces infarct size and transmurality. Infarct vessel patency is an independent factor that reduces the risk for late enlargement. Interference with the connective fibers that buttress the infarct region can prolong the vulnerable period for infarct expansion and worsen this condition. Nonsteroidal anti-inflammatory drugs (NSAIDs) and steroids should be avoided. Aspirin does not appear to have this same detrimental effect on infarct expansion. Heightened ventricular wall stress should be viewed as a long-term inciting stimulus for progressive remodeling in both the infarcted and the noninfarcted regions. Although several studies have demonstrated beneficial effects of nitroglycerin on infarct expansion, there is consistent information that angiotensin-converting enzyme (ACE) inhibition therapy favorably alters this process and is associated with improved clinical outcome. PTCA—percutaneous transluminal coronary angioplasty.

FIGURE 5-18. Effects of thrombolytic therapy (streptokinase) on left ventricular (LV) volumes in survivors of acute myocardial infarction (MI). Thrombolytic therapy is associated with less LV enlargement, as assessed in this randomized, double-blind trial that used biplanar left ventriculography 3 weeks after the MI. This study also illustrates that patients with anterior MI are at greater risk for enlargement than patients with inferior infarctions. However, in both instances, the use of thrombolytic therapy led to a reduction in ventricular enlargement. (*Adapted from* White *et al.* [14].)

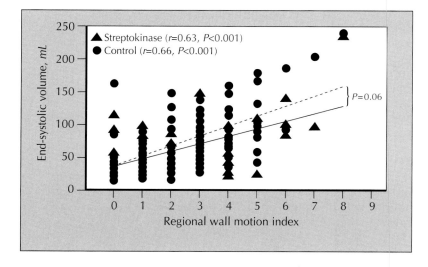

FIGURE 5-19. Echocardiographic substudy from the GISSI (Gruppo Italiano per lo Studio della Streptochinasi nell'Infarto Miocardico) trial. This study demonstrated that left ventricular enlargement 6 months after myocardial infarction is a function of the extent of the wall motion abnormality and that thrombolytic therapy resulted in a strong trend toward smaller ventricular volumes for every degree of abnormality. (*Adapted from* Marino *et al.* [15].)

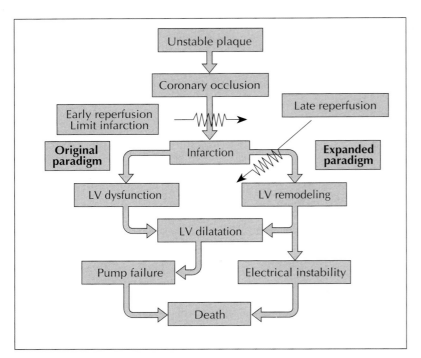

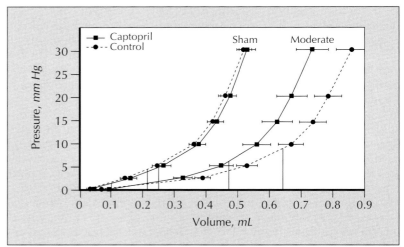

FIGURE 5-20. Expansion of the paradigm of the beneficial actions of early reperfusion therapy. The original paradigm appears on the *left* and the expanded paradigm is on the *right*. Restoration of coronary flow during the early (salvage) phase of acute myocardial infarction (MI) is administered to reduce MI size and transmurality. This preservation of myocardium was anticipated to reduce the wall motion abnormality, improve the ejection fraction, and ultimately lead to a reduction in mortality. Although these observations are accurate, the reduction in death appears to be out of proportion to the improvement in ejection fraction observed in the large placebo-controlled trials [16]. However, recent observations of the influence of infarct vessel patency on left ventricular (LV) remodeling and electrical stability led to an expansion of the original paradigm. The favorable effects of reperfusion therapy in reducing LV dilatation have a prominent role in the more current hypothesis explaining the beneficial actions of reperfusion therapy. (*Adapted from* Kim and Braunwald [17].)

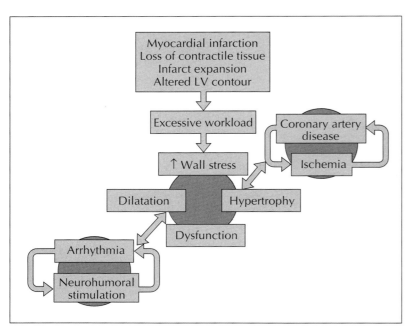

FIGURE 5-21. Algorithm for wall stress. This algorithm for wall stress underscores the central importance of excessive workload and wall stress in the progressive structural alterations in a positive-feedback cycle whereby the structural alterations of left ventricular (LV) dilatation lead to further augmentations in wall stress, reinforcing the progression of the cycle. This scheme is central to understanding the progressive nature of dysfunction, with and without symptoms. This construct provided the rationale for the use of an angiotensin-converting enzyme inhibitor in asymptomatic patients with LV dilatation to prevent further structural changes and reduce the risk for development of congestive heart failure.

FIGURE 5-22. Pressure-volume relationship in rats with moderate-sized infarctions, demonstrating the effects of captopril therapy. Rats with chronic infarctions have a passive pressure-volume relationship, which is shifted to the right of normal. Such a shift defines a larger ventricle at any common filling pressure (*ie*, postinfarction remodeling). Chronic therapy with captopril, an angiotensin-converting enzyme (ACE) inhibitor, resulted in less enlargement, even when compared for the same amount of histologic damage. The captopril-treated animals also had a lower filling pressure than untreated controls, and therefore the operating volume (*circles*) was reduced with ACE inhibition therapy because of the structural change (*ie*, attenuation of remodeling) and the reduced distending pressure. *Sham* rats were operated and noninfarcted; *moderate* rats had histologic infarct sizes ranging from greater than 20% to less than 40% surface area. (*Adapted from* Pfeffer *et al.* [18].)

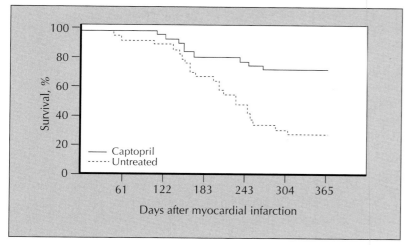

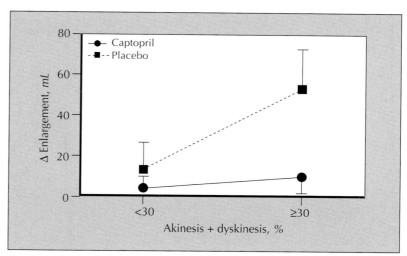

FIGURE 5-23. Influence of angiotensin-converting enzyme (ACE) inhibition therapy (captopril) on survival in the rat myocardial infarction model. Long-term improvement in survival with ACE inhibition was seen in rats with moderate (<40%, >20% surface area) infarctions. In infarcts within this size range, therapy was most effective in prolonging survival. Of interest is that the benefits of ACE inhibition therapy increased with the duration of administration. (*Adapted from* Pfeffer *et al.* [19].)

FIGURE 5-24. Late volume enlargement after first anterior infarction. In asymptomatic patients with left ventricular (LV) dysfunction, late (*ie*, from 3 weeks to 1 year) volume enlargement occurred with administration of conventional therapy. The magnitude of this increase in LV end-diastolic volume was greatest in patients with an occluded infarct-related vessel and a higher degree of wall motion abnormality, as assessed by percent akinesis plus dyskinesis of the baseline left ventriculogram. In a randomized, placebo-controlled study, administration of the angiotensin-converting enzyme (ACE) inhibitor captopril was effective in attenuating the late LV enlargement observed in these selected survivors of myocardial infarction. (*Adapted from* Pfeffer *et al.* [20].)

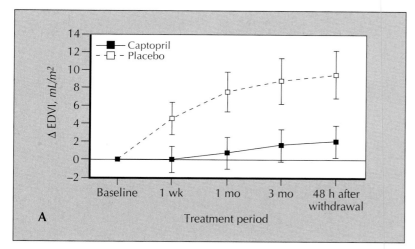

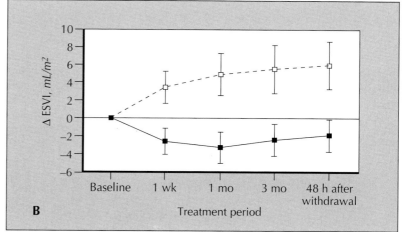

FIGURE 5-25. Change in end-diastolic volume index (EDVI; *panel A*) and end-systolic volume index (ESVI; *panel B*) in patients with Q-wave infarctions as assessed by serial echocardiography. A study by Sharpe [21] has extended prior observations to an earlier time period and has expanded the patient group to include both inferior and anterior Q-wave infarctions. Once again, progressive enlargement is seen with conventional therapy, and this alteration in left ventricular (LV) volume was significantly reduced by the addition of the angiotensin-converting enzyme (ACE) inhibitor captopril. This study also measured LV volume after withdrawal of the ACE inhibitor, demonstrating that the observed differences are not merely a consequence of acute unloading. (*Adapted from* Sharpe [21].)

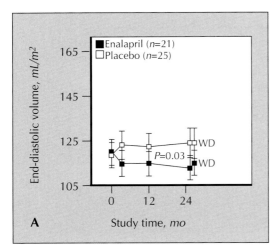

	3 wk	1 y
End-diastolic volume, *mL*	302	377
End-systolic volume, *mL*	186	271
Circumference, *cm*	59.5	62.8
Contractile segment, *cm*	30.5	33.8
Noncontractile segment, *cm*	23.7	23.5
Diastolic sphericity index	0.70	0.74
Systolic sphericity index	0.60	0.77

FIGURE 5-26. Components of late enlargement. Late (*ie,* 3 weeks to 1 year) ventricular enlargement in patients with first anterior myocardial infarction is shown. Although major changes in the noncontractile region characterized the early process of infarct expansion, the increase in volume during the later phase is a consequence of lengthening of the contractile portion and a further shape change, resulting in a more spherical contour. (*Adapted from* Mitchell *et al.* [22].)

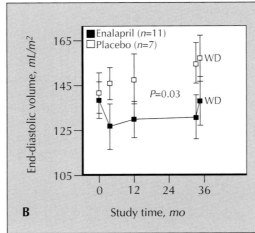

FIGURE 5-27. Serial left ventricular (LV) end-diastolic volume changes in SOLVD (Studies of Left Ventricular Dysfunction) study participants. In an ancillary trial of the SOLVD study, both the prevention (*panel A*) and the treatment (*panel B*) arms

demonstrated significant reductions in LV volume in the patients randomized to receive long-term angiotensin-converting enzyme (ACE) inhibitor therapy with enalapril. In general, the asymptomatic patients in the prevention arm experienced less LV enlargement than the symptomatic patients in the treatment arm. In both study groups, enalapril therapy was effective in attenuating progressive LV enlargement. An interesting component of this study was withdrawal data (WD). The ACE inhibitor was withheld for a minimum of 5 days, and the difference in LV end-diastolic volume was sustained, indicating that this therapy was influencing structural enlargement rather than merely an acute unloading effect. (*Adapted from* Konstam *et al.* [23].)

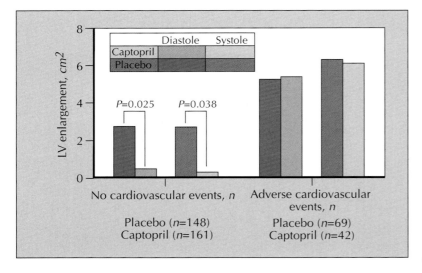

FIGURE 5-28. Changes in left ventricular (LV) area related to adverse cardiovascular events and therapy with captopril. The echocardiographic substudy of the Survival and Ventricular Enlargement trial did indeed confirm that chronic angiotensin-converting enzyme (ACE) inhibition therapy was associated with less ventricular enlargement 1 year after myocardial infarction. Importantly, this study extended previous observations to indicate that patients who had experienced an adverse cardiovascular event were much more likely to demonstrate progressive LV enlargement. Although ACE inhibitor therapy reduced the number of patients who experienced adverse cardiovascular events by approximately 20%, those who experienced either cardiovascular death, heart failure, or MI despite therapy were as likely as patients receiving placebo to demonstrate LV enlargement. These observations point to an important link between LV enlargement and adverse clinical outcome. (*Adapted from* St. John Sutton *et al.* [24].)

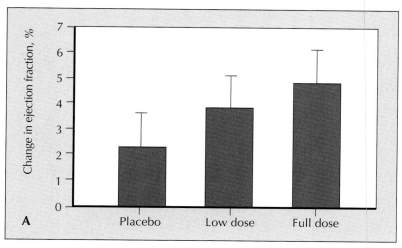

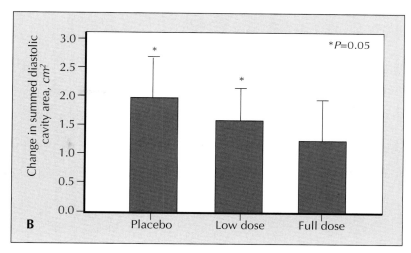

FIGURE 5-29. Change in ejection fraction in the first 14 days after an anterior myocardial infarction. In the cohort of 299 patients with paired studies on day 1 and day 0, there was an overall improvement in ejection fraction. **A,** Those who received an angiotensin-converting enzyme (ACE) inhibitor had a greater benefit, particularly those who were randomized to a full dose of the ACE inhibitor ramipril. **B,** Despite the general improvement in ejection fraction, there was evidence of left ventricular enlargement, which was most prominent in the patients who were not treated with an ACE inhibitor during the first 14 days of an infarction. These data indicate a relative dissociation between a measure of ventricular performance (*ie,* ejection fraction) and the assessment of remodeling (*ie,* diastolic cavity area). (*Adapted from* Pfeffer *et al.* [25].)

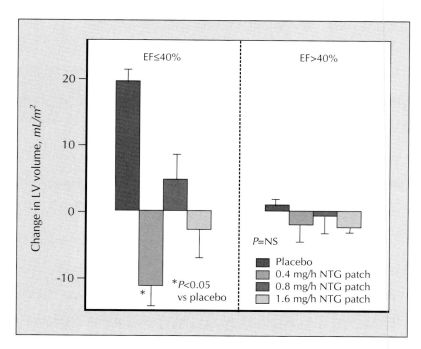

FIGURE 5-30. Changes in left ventricular (LV) end-systolic volume from the early phase (first 3 days to 6 months) after myocardial infarction and the influence of randomization to a transdermal nitroglycerin (NTG) patch. Chronic therapy with nitroglycerin reduced ventricular enlargement. In this randomized study, it is of interest that, consistent with prior studies, most of the ventricular enlargement occurred in placebo-treated patients who had an LV ejection fraction (LVEF) of 40% or less than in those with an LVEF greater than 40%. The favorable influence of nitro-glycerin was demonstrated in the group with LVEF of 40% or less. The authors are careful to indicate that their study was designed to address the LV remodeling influence of nitrates and was not powered to address the issue of clinical outcomes. The observations do support the notion that remodeling is mainly a problem for larger infarcts and that factors that favorably influence filling pressures, such as angiotensin-converting enzyme inhibitors and nitroglycerin, can have long-term benefits on structure. (*Adapted from* Mahmarian *et al.* [26].)

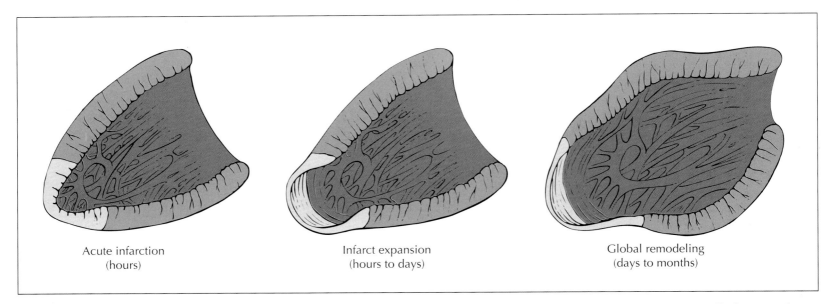

| Acute infarction (hours) | Infarct expansion (hours to days) | Global remodeling (days to months) |

FIGURE 5-31. Left ventricular remodeling after myocardial infarction (MI). During the critical initial hours of MI when acute ischemia progresses to true necrosis, regional systolic dysfunction is already present. However, in this particularly crucial period, measures to restore the balance between O_2 demand and delivery can lead to salvage of contractile tissue. Once cell death has occurred, and particularly if there is a transmural infarction involving the ventricular apex, there is a high likelihood that this initially functional distortion of ventricular contour will become structural for infarct expansion. The distorted ventricle undergoes further remodeling as a consequence of heightened wall stress on the remaining viable myocardium, which leads to further cavity enlargement and shape distortion. The latter insidious process is associated with a greater likelihood of cardiovascular morbidity and mortality.

REFERENCES

1. Holt J, Rhode E, Kines H: Ventricular volumes and body weight in mammals. *Am J Physiol* 1968, 215:704–715.

2. Grossman W, Carabello BA, Gunther S, *et al.*: Ventricular wall stress and the development of cardiac hypertrophy and failure. In *Perspectives in Cardiovascular Research. Myocardial Hypertrophy and Failure*, vol 7. Edited by Alpert NR. New York: Raven Press; 1993:1–15.

3. Hutchins GM, Bulkley BH: Infarct expansion versus extension: two different complications of acute myocardial infarction. *Am J Cardiol* 1978, 41:1127–1132.

4. Erlebacher JA, Weiss JL, Weisfeldt ML, *et al.*: Early dilation of the infarcted segment in acute transmural myocardial infarction: role of infarct expansion in acute left ventricular enlargement. *J Am Coll Cardiol* 1984, 4:201–208.

5. Jugdutt BI, Michorowski BL: Role of infarct expansion in rupture of the ventricular septum after acute myocardial infarction: a two-dimensional echocardiographic study. *Clin Cardiol* 1987, 10:641–652.

6. Hammermeister KE, DeRouen TA, Dodge HT: Variables predictive of survival in patients with coronary disease: selection by univariate and multivariate analyses from the clinical, electrocardiographic, exercise, arteriographic, and quantitative angiographic evaluations. *Circulation* 1979, 59:421–430.

7. White HD, Norris RM, Brown MA, *et al.*: Left ventricular end-systolic volume as the major determinant of survival after recovery from myocardial infarction. *Circulation* 1987, 76:44–51.

8. Meizlish JL, Berger HJ, Plankey M, *et al.*: Functional left ventricular aneurysm formation after acute anterior transmural myocardial infarction: incidence, natural history, and prognostic implications. *N Engl J Med* 1984, 311:1001–1006.

9. Lamas GA, Vaughan DE, Pfeffer MA: Left ventricular thrombus formation after first anterior wall acute myocardial infarction. *Am J Cardiol* 1988, 62:31–35.

10. Pfeffer JM, Pfeffer MA, Fletcher PJ, *et al.*: Progressive ventricular remodeling in rat with myocardial infarction. *Am J Physiol* 1991, 29 (suppl H):1406–1414.

11. Gaudron P, Eilles C, Kugler I, *et al.*: Progressive left ventricular dysfunction and remodeling after myocardial infarction: potential mechanisms and early predictors. *Circulation* 1993, 87:755–763.

12. Pfeffer JM: Progressive ventricular dilatation in experimental myocardial infarction and its attenuation by angiotensin converting enzyme inhibition. *Am J Cardiol* 1991, 68:17D–25D.

13. Capasso J, Zhang P, Anversa P: Heterogeneity of ventricular remodeling after acute myocardial infarction in rats. *Am J Physiol* 1992, 262(suppl H):486–495.

14. White HD, Norris RM, Brown MA, *et al.*: Effect of intravenous streptokinase on left ventricular function and early survival after acute myocardial infarction. *N Engl J Med* 1987, 317:850–855.

15. Marino P, Zanolla L, Zardini P: Effect of streptokinase on left ventricular modeling and function after myocardial infarction: the GISSI (Gruppo Italiano per lo Studio della Streptochinasi nell'Infarto Miocardico) Trial. *J Am Coll Cardiol* 1989, 14:1149–1158.

16. Braunwald E: Myocardial reperfusion, limitation of infarct size, reduction of left ventricular dysfunction, and improved survival: should the paradigm by expanded? *Circulation* 1989, 79:441–444.

17. Kim C, Braunwald E: Potential benefits of late reperfusion of infarcted myocardium: the open artery hypothesis. *Circulation* 1993, 88:2426–2436.

18. Pfeffer JM, Pfeffer MA, Braunwald E: Influence of chronic captopril therapy on the infarcted left ventricle of the rat. *Circ Res* 1985, 57:84–95.

19. Pfeffer MA, Pfeffer JM, Steinberg C, Finn P: Survival after an experimental myocardial infarction: beneficial effects of long-term captopril therapy. *Circulation* 1985, 72:406–412.

20. Pfeffer MA, Lamas GA, Vaughan DE, *et al.*: Effect of captopril on progressive ventricular dilatation after anterior myocardial infarction. *N Engl J Med* 1988, 319:80–86.

21. Sharpe N: Early preventive treatment of left ventricular dysfunction following myocardial infarction: optimal timing and patient selection. *Am J Cardiol* 1991, 68(suppl D):64–69.

22. Mitchell GF, Lamas GA, Vaughan DE, *et al.*: Left ventricular remodeling in the year following first anterior myocardial infarction: a quantitative analysis of contractile segment lengths and ventricular shape. *J Am Coll Cardiol* 1992, 19:1136–1144.

23. Konstam M, Kronenberg M, Rousseau M, *et al.*: Effects of the angiotensin converting enzyme inhibitor enalapril on the long-term progression of left ventricular dilatation in patients with asymptomatic systolic dysfunction. *Circulation* 1993, 88:2277–2283.

24. St. John Sutton M, Pfeffer M, Plappert T, *et al.*: Quantitative two dimensional echocardiographic measurements are major predictors of adverse cardiovascular events following acute myocardial infarction: the protective effects of captopril. *Circulation* 1994, 89:68–75.

25. Pfeffer MA, Greaves SC, Arnold JMO, *et al.*: Early versus delayed angiotensin-converting enzyme inhibition therapy in acute myocardial infarction: the Healing and Early Afterload Reducing Therapy Trial. *Circulation* 1997, 95:2643–2651.

26. Mahmarian JJ, Moyé LA, Chinoy DA, *et al.*: Transdermal nitro-glycerin patch therapy improves left ventricular function and prevents remodeling after acute myocardial infarction: results of a multicenter prospective randomized, double-blind, placebo-controlled trial. *Circulation* 1998, 97:2017–2024.

Neurohumoral, Renal, and Vascular Adjustments in Heart Failure

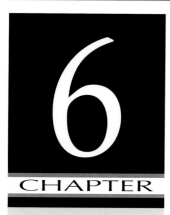

6

CHAPTER

Anju Nohria, Jorge A. Cusco, and Mark A. Creager

Congestive heart failure resulting from left ventricular dysfunction is accompanied by peripheral circulatory changes that influence cardiac function and contribute to the clinical manifestations of heart failure. Neurohumoral systems that modulate both vascular tone and the retention of salt and water are activated. These include the sympathetic nervous system, the renin-angiotensin-aldosterone system, arginine vasopressin, and the natriuretic peptides. In addition, the peripheral circulation undergoes local changes in response to heart failure that are fundamental to the pathophysiology of this disease state. Such changes include an increased release of endothelin and prostaglandins, as well as a possible decrease in the activity of nitric oxide. In addition, there may be enhanced local production of angiotensin II.

Taken together, these systemic and local vasoactive systems modulate vascular resistance and determine the regional distribution of the cardiac output. Whereas blood flow to the limb, kidneys, and splanchnic bed may decrease, blood flow to the heart and brain is usually preserved. Diminished exercise capacity in patients with congestive heart failure may be due in part to chronically diminished limb blood flow and failure to increase blood flow normally with metabolic stimulation. Renal hypoperfusion alters intrarenal hemodynamics and may contribute to sodium and water retention.

This chapter reviews the mechanisms in congestive heart failure that underlie systemic activation of the sympathetic nervous system, the renin-angiotensin system, and circulatory neurohormones such as arginine vasopressin and natriuretic peptides. It also focuses on local vasodilator and vasoconstrictor mechanisms that are mediated by the endothelium and the vascular smooth muscle.

Mechanisms in Heart Failure

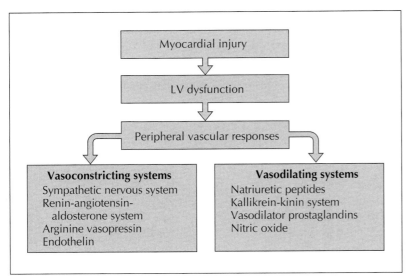

FIGURE 6-1. Myocardial injury causes left ventricular (LV) dysfunction. This activates or alters a variety of peripheral vasomotor mechanisms that are both beneficial (compensatory) and deleterious. Vasoconstrictor systems such as the sympathetic nervous system, the renin-angiotensin-aldosterone system, arginine vasopressin, and endothelin increase afterload and contribute to salt and water retention. Vasodilating systems such as the natriuretic peptides, the kallikrein-kinin system, nitric oxide, and prostaglandins unload the left ventricle and may facilitate natriuresis.

Sympathetic Nervous System

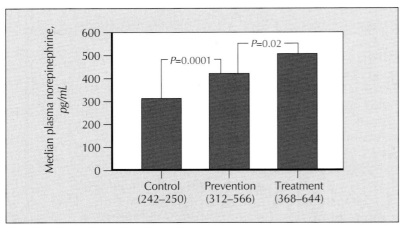

FIGURE 6-2. Sympathetic nervous system activity is increased in patients with congestive heart failure (CHF). In a substudy of the SOLVD (Studies of Left Ventricular Dysfunction) trial, plasma norepinephrine was measured in 54 control subjects, 151 patients with left ventricular dysfunction but no evidence of CHF (prevention group), and 81 patients with left ventricular dysfunction and mild to moderate CHF (treatment group). The median plasma norepinephrine levels for these groups were 317 pg/mL, 422 pg/mL, and 507 pg/mL, respectively (interquartile ranges are shown in parentheses). Mean values for plasma norepinephrine were significantly higher in patients with left ventricular dysfunction compared with those in normal subjects ($P=0.0001$). Levels were significantly higher in patients with overt heart failure compared with those in asymptomatic patients with left ventricular dysfunction ($P=0.02$). This study demonstrates that sympathetic nervous system activation occurs in the early stages of CHF. (*Adapted from* Francis *et al.* [1].)

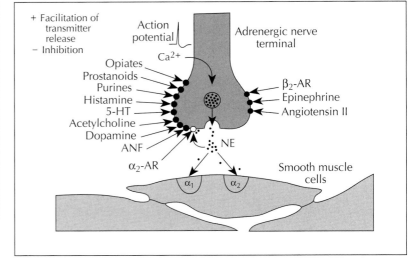

FIGURE 6-3. Sympathetic nerve terminal. Sympathetic nerve activity can be measured directly by measuring the electrical activity in the peripheral nerves and indirectly by measuring the plasma norepinephrine (NE) concentration. Plasma NE is derived from sympathetic nerves, but the amount that reaches the circulation depends on several processes. Plasma NE can be increased by increased nerve release, decreased local uptake, or reduced systemic clearance. Neurotransmitter release at the sympathetic neuroeffector junction is also modulated locally by a variety of hormones and other substances that act on specific receptors located on the presynaptic nerve ending. Several α_2-receptor agonists, including NE itself (via α_2-adrenergic receptors [α_2-AR]), opioids, prostanoids, purines, histamine, 5-hydroxytryptamine (5-HT), atrial natriuretic factor (ANF), dopamine, and acetylcholine, *inhibit* NE release. In contrast, epinephrine (via β_2-adrenergic receptors [β_2-AR]) and angiotensin II *increase* NE release from the neuroeffector junction. (*Adapted from* Vanhoutte and Luscher [2].)

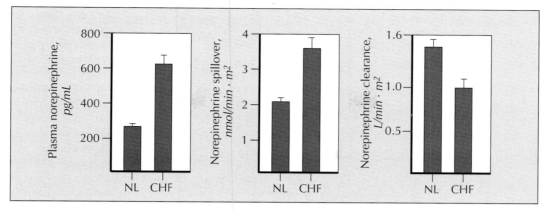

FIGURE 6-4. To determine whether elevated plasma norepinephrine levels in heart failure are secondary to increased neural release of norepinephrine, decreased clearance, or both, Davis *et al.* [3] used a radiotracer technique to measure plasma norepinephrine levels, spillover, and clearance in 18 normal subjects (NL) and 19 patients with severe New York Heart Association functional class III to IV congestive heart failure (CHF). Patients with CHF had significantly higher baseline plasma norepinephrine levels (249±20 pg/mL vs 628±68 pg/mL; *P*<0.001). A 73% greater spillover of norepinephrine and a 33% reduction in clearance were found in the CHF group. These studies of norepinephrine kinetics demonstrated that both increased spillover and decreased clearance contribute to the higher norepinephrine levels observed in CHF patients. (*Adapted from* Davis *et al.* [3].)

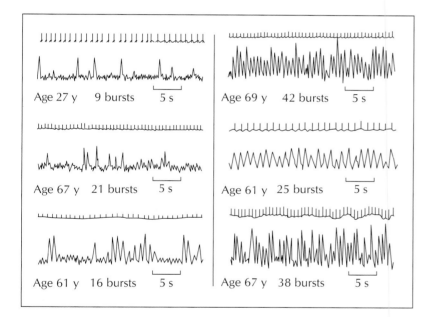

FIGURE 6-5. Microneurography. Sympathetic neural activity can be measured directly in humans by microneurography. Leimbach *et al.* [4] used microneurography for direct recording of intraneural sympathetic nerve activity from the peroneal nerve in normal subjects and patients with congestive heart failure (CHF). This figure illustrates microneurographic recordings from three normal subjects (*left*) and three patients with congestive heart failure (*right*). A burst represents a summation of nerve action potentials from multiple fibers. Note the increased sympathetic burst frequency in patients with CHF. These data provide further evidence that sympathetic nerve activity is increased in patients with CHF and that elevated plasma norepinephrine levels occur as a consequence of increased sympathetic neural activity. (*Adapted from* Leimbach *et al.* [4].)

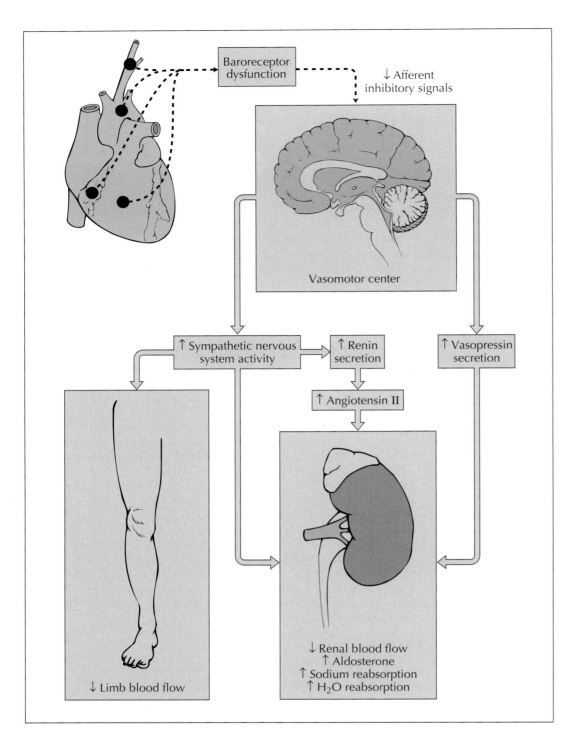

FIGURE 6-6. Baroreceptor dysfunction may account for increased sympathetic and reduced parasympathetic nervous system activity in most patients with congestive heart failure. Normally, autonomic balance is regulated by afferent input from multiple peripheral receptors, including baroreceptors in the heart, lungs, and great vessels, chemoreceptors in the carotid bodies, metaboreceptors in skeletal muscle, sensory receptors in skin, a variety of visceral receptors, and from signals originating in the central nervous system. Of these, the baroreceptors are the principal modulators of sympathetic and parasympathetic activity during changes in intravascular volume or pressure. Mechanoreceptors in the heart and pulmonary vasculature (cardiopulmonary baroreceptors) and in the aortic arch and carotid sinus (arterial baroreceptors) respond to stretch by relaying afferent neural signals to the central system via branches of the vagus and glossopharyngeal nerves. These signals *inhibit* sympathetic and *augment* parasympathetic efferent activity. In plasma volume depletion or hypotension, decreased receptor stretch reduces the afferent stimuli, thus decreasing parasympathetic activity and increasing sympathetic activity. Because baroreceptor function is impaired in heart failure, inhibitory input from arterial and cardiopulmonary baroreceptors is decreased, thereby leading to excessive sympathetic and reduced parasympathetic activity. Abnormal baroreceptor function may also facilitate vasopressin release from the neurohypophysis and stimulate renal release of renin. (*Adapted from* Paganelli *et al.* [5].)

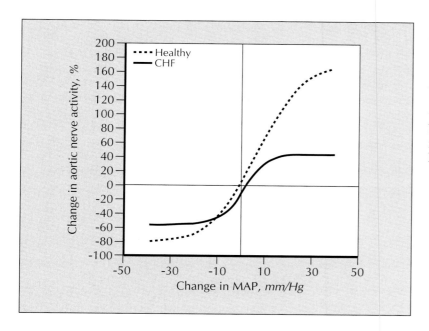

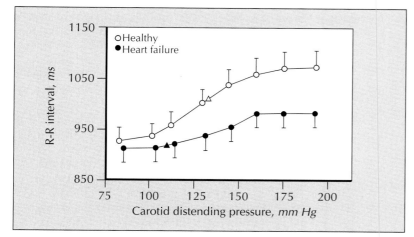

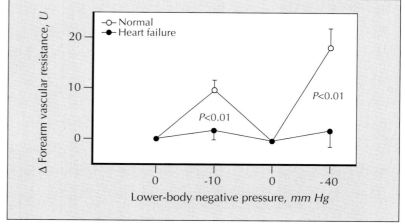

FIGURE 6-7. Abnormalities of arterial baroreceptor function have been demonstrated in animal models of heart failure. Dibner-Dunlap and Thames [6] measured the effect of changes in mean arterial pressure (MAP) on aortic nerve activity (nerve signals from aortic baroreceptors) in healthy dogs and in dogs with congestive heart failure (CHF) secondary to rapid ventricular pacing. Baroreceptor dysfunction is indicated by the observation that, for comparable increases in blood pressure induced by phenylephrine, there was a lesser increase in aortic nerve activity in dogs with CHF compared with that in healthy dogs. (*Adapted from* Dibner-Dunlap and Thames [6].)

FIGURE 6-8. Abnormalities in arterial baroreceptor reflex function have also been demonstrated in humans. Using a custom-designed neck chamber, Sopher *et al.* [7] applied progressive suction to the carotid sinus of healthy subjects and patients with congestive heart failure (CHF). Neck suction increases transmural pressure across the carotid sinus and simulates an increase in blood pressure, thereby stimulating the carotid sinus baroreceptors. The heart rate (R-R interval) was measured to assess the reflex response to carotid sinus baroreceptor stimulation. The heart rate slowed to a greater extent with increasing carotid distending pressure in healthy subjects compared with patients with CHF. The operational point (*triangle*), also known as the set point, is the starting or resting point of each group on the stimulus response curve. In patients with CHF, the operational point was shifted to the left. The shift in the baroreflex response curve defines an abnormality in the receptor firing function. These findings indicate that in patients with CHF, as shown in animal models, carotid sinus baroreceptor reflex function is impaired. (*Adapted from* Sopher *et al.* [7].)

FIGURE 6-9. Cardiopulmonary baroreceptor reflex function in humans can be assessed by encasing the lower part of the body in a rigid cylinder and subjecting the individual to negative pressure. Normally, increasing levels of lower-body negative pressure reduce cardiac filling pressures, inhibit cardiopulmonary baroreceptors, and increase sympathetic efferent nervous activity, thereby causing vasoconstriction. Whereas low levels of lower-body negative pressure (-10 mm Hg) selectively unload cardiopulmonary baroreceptors, high levels (-40 mm Hg) unload both cardiopulmonary and arterial baroreceptors (by reducing stroke volume and blood pressure). Forearm vasoconstriction occurs during lower-body negative pressure in normal subjects but not in patients with congestive heart failure. These data indicate that cardiopulmonary baroreceptor function is abnormal in patients with congestive heart failure, providing additional evidence for a mechanism that causes sympathetic activation in these individuals. (*Adapted from* Creager [8].)

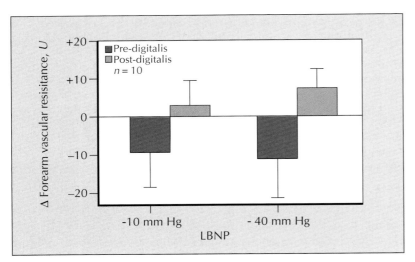

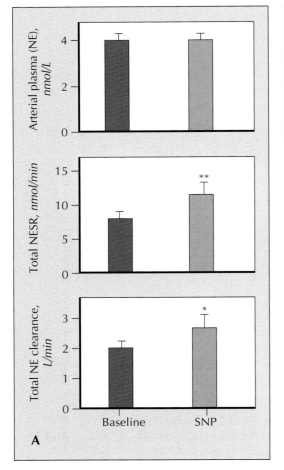

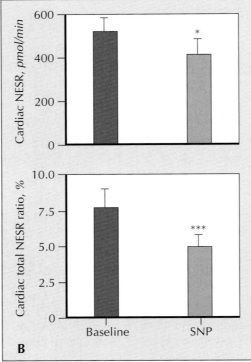

FIGURE 6-10. Some forms of therapy for patients with congestive heart failure favorably affect baroreceptor function. Ferguson *et al.* [9] administered a digitalis glycoside, lanatoside C, to patients with congestive heart failure and subjected them to lower-body negative pressure (LBNP). Before administration of digitalis, LBNP at -10 mm Hg and -40 mm Hg caused paradoxical forearm vasodilatation, indicating impaired baroreceptor function. After administration of digitalis, LBNP at -10 mm Hg and -40 mm Hg caused a more normal forearm vasoconstrictor response. These data suggest that part of the beneficial effect of digitalis in patients with congestive heart failure may be secondary to improvement in baroreceptor function, leading to withdrawal of sympathetic activity. (*Adapted from* Ferguson *et al.* [9].)

FIGURE 6-11. Baroreceptor unloading may affect sympathetic nervous system function in patients with congestive heart failure (CHF). Kaye *et al.* [10] used sodium nitroprusside (SNP) in doses sufficient to reduce both cardiac filling pressures and arterial pressure in patients with CHF. Nitroprusside infusion increased total body norepinephrine (NE) spillover rate (NESR) as well as total norepinephrine clearance (**A**). In contrast, nitroprusside decreased cardiac NESR (**B**). These findings indicate a differential effect of acute baroreceptor unloading on systemic and cardiac sympathetic activity in patients with heart failure, increasing the former but decreasing the latter. The clinical implication of these observations is that therapeutic interventions that reduce cardiac filling pressures would potentially impart a beneficial effect on survival by reducing cardiac sympathetic efferent activity. (*Adapted from* Kaye *et al.* [10].)

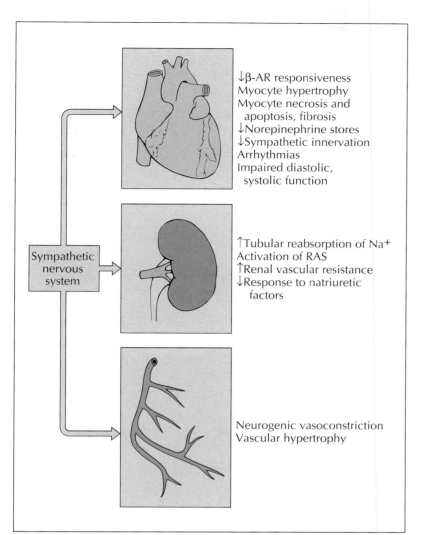

FIGURE 6-12. Increased sympathetic nervous system activity may contribute to the pathophysiology of congestive heart failure by multiple mechanisms involving cardiac, renal, and vascular function [11]. In the heart, increased sympathetic nervous system outflow may lead to desensitization of postsynaptic β-adrenergic receptors (β-AR), nonuniform depletion of norepinephrine stores, nonuniform destruction of sympathetic innervation, arrhythmias, and impairment of diastolic and systolic function, and act directly on myocardial cells, causing myocyte hypertrophy, necrosis, apoptosis, and fibrosis. In the kidneys, increased sympathetic activation induces arterial and venous vasoconstriction, activation of the renin-angiotensin system (RAS), increase in salt and water retention, and an attenuated response to natriuretic factors. In the peripheral vessels, neurogenic vasoconstriction and vascular hypertrophy are induced by increased sympathetic nervous activity. (*Adapted from* Floras [11].)

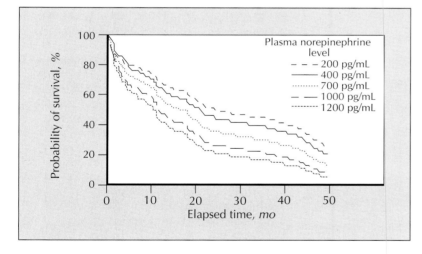

FIGURE 6-13. Activation of sympathetic nervous system activity, as reflected by elevated plasma norepinephrine levels, has been associated with a poor prognosis in patients with congestive heart failure. Cohn *et al.* [12] measured supine plasma norepinephrine levels in 106 patients with moderate to severe congestive heart failure. A multivariate analysis found that resting plasma norepinephrine levels were a significant independent predictor of mortality among these patients ($P<0.002$). In addition, the norepinephrine level was higher in patients who died from progressive heart failure (1014±699 pg/mL) than in those who died suddenly (619±238 pg/mL). The figure illustrates predicted survival curves for groups of patients with different baseline plasma norepinephrine levels. (*Adapted from* Cohn *et al.* [12].)

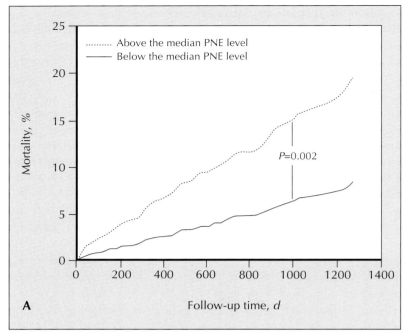

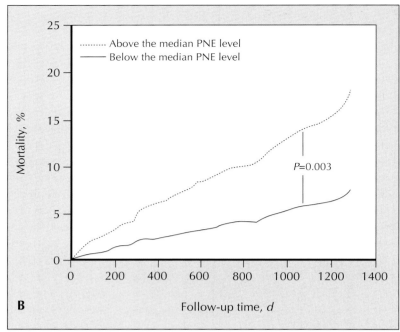

FIGURE 6-14. Plasma norepinephrine (PNE) levels also predict all cause and cardiovascular mortality in patients with asymptomatic left ventricular dysfunction. An analysis [13] from the Studies of Left Ventricular Dysfunction (SOLVD) trial found that PNE was the strongest predictor of clinical events in patients with asymptomatic left ventricular dysfunction. Adjusted all-cause mortality (**A**) and adjusted cardiovascular mortality (**B**) were significantly higher in patients with prerandomization

(*ie,* prior to placebo vs enalapril therapy) norepinephrine concentrations above or below the median value of 393 pg/mL. Plasma norepinephrine levels greater than 393 pg/mL were associated with a relative risk of 2.59 for all-cause mortality, 2.55 for cardiovascular mortality, 2.55 for hospitalization for heart failure, 1.88 for development of heart failure, 1.92 for ischemic events, and 2.59 for myocardial infarction. (*Adapted from* Benedict *et al.* [13].)

THE RENIN-ANGIOTENSIN-ALDOSTERONE SYSTEM

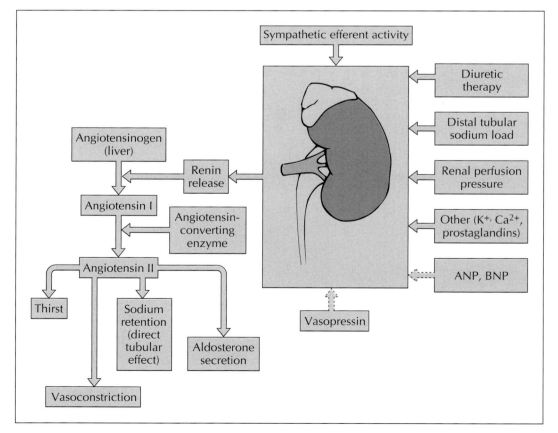

FIGURE 6-15. The renin-angiotensin system is activated in patients with congestive heart failure. The major site of release of circulating renin is the juxtaglomerular apparatus of the kidney, where multiple stimuli may contribute to renal release of renin into the systemic circulation, including increased renal sympathetic efferent activity, decreased distal tubular sodium delivery, reduced renal perfusion pressure, and diuretic therapy. Natriuretic peptides (ANP, BNP), and vasopressin (*dashed arrows*) may inhibit the release of renin. Renin enzymatically cleaves angiotensinogen, a tetrapeptide produced in the liver, to form the inactive decapeptide angiotensin I. Angiotensin I is converted to the octapeptide angiotensin II by the angiotensin-converting enzyme. Angiotensin II is a potent vasoconstrictor; it promotes sodium reabsorption by increasing aldosterone secretion and by a direct effect on the tubules, and it stimulates water intake by acting on the thirst center. Angiotensin II causes vasoconstriction directly and may also facilitate the release of norepinephrine by acting on sympathetic nerve endings. (*Adapted from* Paganelli *et al.* [5].)

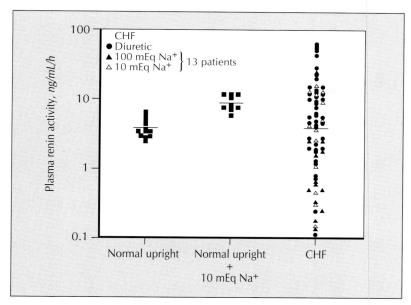

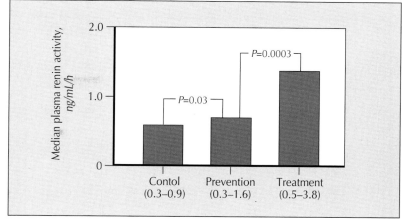

FIGURE 6-16. Cody and Laragh [14] evaluated the role of the renin-angiotensin system in patients with congestive heart failure (CHF). They studied 17 normal subjects in the upright position receiving an unrestricted sodium diet; 12 normal upright subjects receiving a low-sodium diet (10 mEq); and 52 patients with CHF receiving a low-sodium diet (10 mEq), a normal-sodium diet (100 mEq), or diuretics. The mean plasma renin activity in CHF did not differ significantly from that of normal subjects whose plasma renin activity was stimulated by upright position and a low-sodium diet. Nevertheless, many of the patients with CHF had marked elevation of plasma renin activity, as suggested by this logarithmic scale. (*Adapted from* Cody and Laragh [14].)

FIGURE 6-17. In the Studies of Left Ventricular Dysfunction (SOLVD), activation of the renin-angiotensin system was evaluated in patients with asymptomatic left ventricular dysfunction or mild congestive heart failure. Plasma renin activity was measured in 56 control subjects, 151 patients with left ventricular dysfunction but no evidence of congestive heart failure (prevention group), and 80 patients with left ventricular dysfunction with mild to moderate congestive heart failure (treatment group). The median plasma renin activity was 0.60 ng/mL/h in the prevention group and 1.4 ng/mL/h in the treatment group (interquartile ranges are shown in parentheses). Mean values for plasma renin activity were marginally increased in the prevention group compared with those in normal subjects. When the data were reanalyzed according to diuretic use, plasma renin activity was normal in patients in both the prevention and the treatment groups not taking diuretics. Therefore, there was no increase in the plasma renin activity in patients with asymptomatic left ventricular dysfunction or mild congestive heart failure who were not receiving diuretics. (*Adapted from* Francis *et al.* [1].)

FIGURE 6-18. Tissue renin-angiotensin systems. In addition to the hormonal effects of circulating angiotensin, many or all components of the renin-angiotensin system are present in several organs, including the heart, blood vessels, kidney, brain, and adrenal glands. Angiotensin produced within these tissues may act in a paracrine or autocrine manner to regulate cellular function, independent of the circulating hormone.

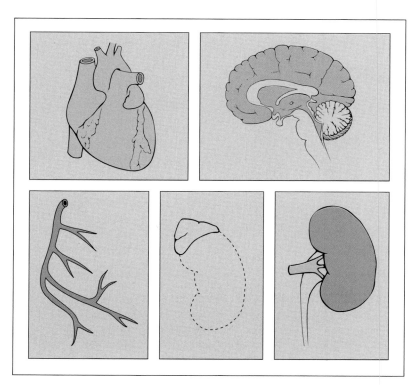

POTENTIAL CONTRIBUTIONS OF THE CARDIAC RENIN-ANGIOTENSIN SYSTEM TO THE PATHOPHYSIOLOGY OF HEART FAILURE

POTENTIAL TISSUE EFFECT	PATHOPHYSIOLOGIC CONSEQUENCES
Direct cellular angiotensin II effects	Positive inotropic effect
	Diastolic dysfunction
Facilitates adrenergic state	Positive inotropic effect
	Dysrhythmia induction
Coronary vasoconstriction	Subendocardial ischemia
Proto-oncogene expression	Cardiac hypertrophy and remodeling

FIGURE 6-19. Potential effects of the cardiac renin-angiotensin system on the pathophysiology of heart failure. The direct effects of angiotensin II on cardiac tissue include increased inotropy, decreased lusitropy, and coronary artery vasoconstriction. These effects may secondarily promote dysrhythmias and cause subendocardial ischemia. There is also evidence (*see* Chapter 4) that angiotensin contributes to myocardial hypertrophy and remodeling by acting directly on cardiac myocytes and fibroblasts. (*Adapted from* Hirsch *et al.* [15].)

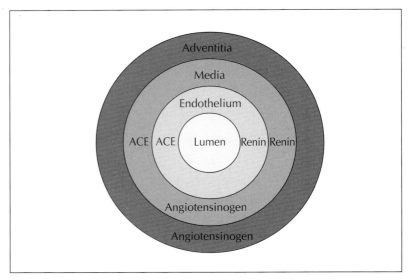

FIGURE 6-20. Distribution of the renin-angiotensin system components within the blood vessel wall. Angiotensinogen can be found in the adventitia and media. Renin, either synthesized locally or taken up from the circulation, has been found in the media and endothelium. Angiotensin-converting enzyme (ACE) has been localized in the media and endothelium. Thus, all of the components necessary for the generation of angiotensin are present in the vessel wall [16].

POTENTIAL CONTRIBUTIONS OF THE VASCULAR RENIN-ANGIOTENSIN SYSTEM TO THE PATHOPHYSIOLOGY OF HEART FAILURE

POTENTIAL TISSUE EFFECT	PATHOPHYSIOLOGIC CONSEQUENCES
Decreased conduit vessel compliance and increased arteriolar resistance	Increased afterload
Venoconstriction	Increased preload
Renal and splanchnic vasoconstriction	Regional blood flow redistribution

FIGURE 6-21. Potential contributions of the vascular renin-angiotensin system to the pathophysiology of heart failure. These contributions include decreased compliance, increased regional and systemic vascular resistance, and venoconstriction. Decreased compliance and increased resistance are due to both vasoconstriction and structural remodeling. (*Adapted from* Hirsch *et al.* [15].)

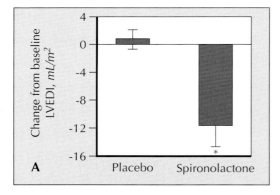

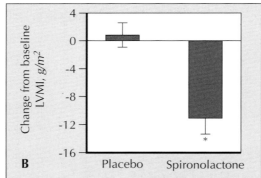

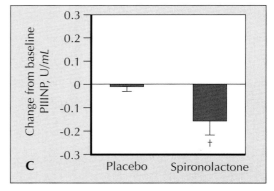

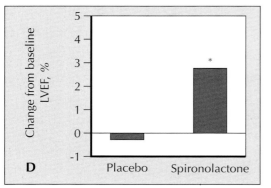

FIGURE 6-22. Aldosterone contributes significantly to structural remodeling in congestive heart failure. Despite angiotensin-converting enzyme inhibitor therapy, aldosterone levels remain elevated in patients with heart failure. This "escape" phenomenon is mediated by potassium-dependent aldosterone secretion that is independent of angiotensin concentration. Sustained elevations in circulating aldosterone result in proliferation of fibroblasts, and subsequent vascular remodeling of atria, ventricles, the great vessels, and other organs. Thirty-seven patients with mild-to-moderate congestive heart failure were randomly assigned to receive 4 weeks of spironolactone (*n*=20) or placebo (*n*=17). Plasma procollagen type III aminoterminal peptide (PIIINP), a marker of myocardial fibrosis, and left ventricular volume (LVEDI) and mass (LVMI) indices decreased with spironolactone treatment. Left ventricular ejection fraction (LVEF) increased in the spironolactone group. *Asterisk* indicates *P*<0.05. *Daggers* indicate *P*<0.01. (*Adapted from* Tsutamoto *et al.* [17].)

COMPONENTS OF THE INTRARENAL RENIN-ANGIOTENSIN SYSTEM

LOCALIZATION	COMPONENTS	POSSIBLE FUNCTION
Blood vessels (including vasa recta)	Renin	Intrarenal hemodynamics
	Angiotensinogen	Sodium-water homeostasis
	ACE	
	Angiotensin II receptors	
Glomerulus	Renin	Glomerular hemodynamics
	Angiotensin II receptors	
Proximal tubules	Renin (reabsorbed, interstitium)	Sodium reabsorption
	Angiotensinogen (synthesized)	
	ACE	
	Angiotensin II receptors	

FIGURE 6-23. Components of the intrarenal renin-angiotensin system. These components contribute to the regulation of renal hemodynamic function and sodium reabsorption. Angiotensinogen, renin, angiotensin-converting enzyme (ACE), and angiotensin II receptors are found in many portions of the kidney, including blood vessels, the glomerulus, and the proximal tubules. (*Adapted from* Dzau [18].)

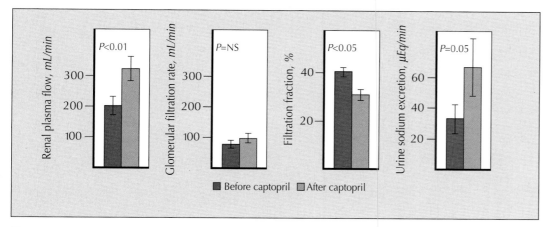

FIGURE 6-24. The contribution of the renin-angiotensin system to abnormal renal hemodynamics and sodium excretion in patients with congestive heart failure. The angiotensin-converting enzyme inhibitor captopril was administered to 12 patients with congestive heart failure. Captopril increased renal plasma flow but had no effect on glomerular filtration rate. Therefore, the filtration fraction, representing the ratio of glomerular filtration rate to renal plasma flow, decreased. In heart failure, renal sodium avidity is associated with a high filtration fraction, which has been postulated to increase peritubular oncotic pressure. After use of captopril, a decrease in filtration fraction, as well as a decrease in the plasma concentration of aldosterone, contributes to the increase in urine sodium excretion. These findings indicate that the renin-angiotensin system contributes importantly to renal vasoconstriction and sodium retention in patients with heart failure. (*Adapted from* Creager *et al.* [19].)

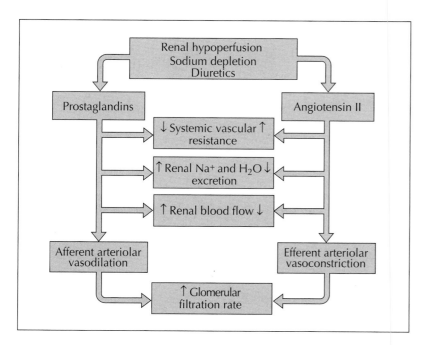

FIGURE 6-25. Stimuli to the release of prostaglandins and renin. Renal hypoperfusion, sodium depletion, and diuretics are potent stimuli for the release of both renin and prostaglandins from the kidney. The release of renal prostaglandins constitutes an adaptive response that counteracts the deleterious effects of the renin-angiotensin system in patients with congestive heart failure. The opposing effects on systemic vascular resistance and sodium and water excretion are also shown. (*Adapted from* Packer [20].)

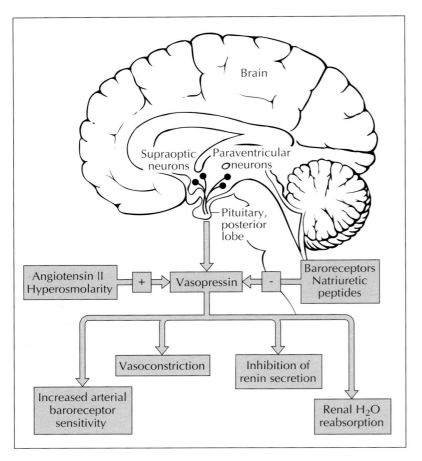

FIGURE 6-26. Arginine vasopressin is a peptide synthesized by the hypothalamic magnocellular neurons of the supraoptic and paraventricular nuclei, and is released into the circulation by axon terminals of the posterior pituitary gland. Osmotic and nonosmotic stimuli modulate vasopressin release. Whereas stimulation of hypothalamic osmoreceptors and elevated concentrations of angiotensin II stimulate vasopressin release, baroreceptor activation and natriuretic peptides (ANP, BNP) inhibit vasopressin secretion. Vasopressin acts at the tissue level by binding to specific receptors. It causes vasoconstriction via vasopressin 1 receptors and renal reabsorption of water, renal secretion of renin, and synthesis of renal prostaglandins via vasopressin 2 receptors. In addition, vasopressin may mediate vasodilatation via vasopressin 2 receptors by increasing the release and synthesis of nitric oxide and vasodilator prostaglandins. Vasopressin also sensitizes baroreceptors, and thus may cause vasodilatation by withdrawing sympathetic activity.

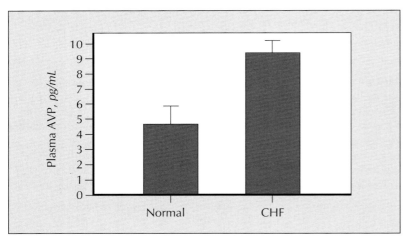

FIGURE 6-27. Plasma vasopressin in patients with heart failure. Francis *et al.* [21] measured basal levels of arginine vasopressin (AVP) in 31 patients with advanced congestive heart failure (CHF) and 11 age-matched normal control subjects. The mean vasopressin level was 9.5±0.89 pg/mL in the CHF group compared with 4.7±0.66 pg/mL in the control group (*P*<0.001). (*Adapted from* Francis *et al.* [21].)

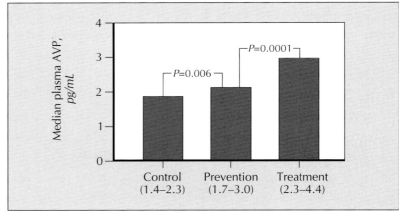

FIGURE 6-28. In a substudy of the Studies of Left Ventricular Dysfunction (SOLVD), arginine-vasopressin (AVP) levels were measured in patients with asymptomatic left ventricular dysfunction (ALVD) or mild congestive heart failure. Plasma AVP levels were measured in 54 control subjects, 147 patients with ALVD (prevention group), and 80 patients with left ventricular dysfunction and mild congestive heart failure (treatment group). The median plasma AVP was 1.9 pg/mL in the control group, 2.2 pg/mL in the prevention group, and 3.0 pg/mL in the treatment group (interquartile ranges are shown in parentheses). Mean values for plasma AVP were significantly higher in patients with left ventricular dysfunction compared with normal control subjects and significantly higher in patients with overt heart failure compared with patients with ALVD. (*Adapted from* Francis *et al.* [1].)

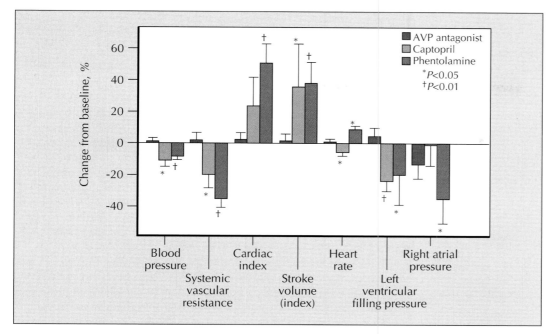

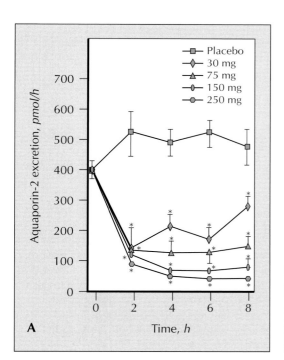
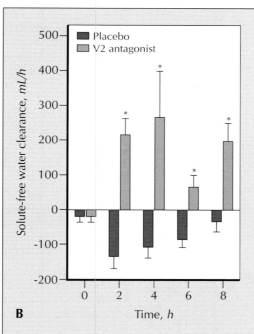

of each system. The hemodynamic responses to a V1 AVP antagonist, an angiotensin-converting enzyme inhibitor (captopril), and an α-receptor antagonist (phentolamine) in 10 patients with CHF are shown. The AVP antagonist had relatively little effect on systemic vascular resistance and cardiac function. In contrast, both phentolamine and captopril caused significant decreases in systemic vascular resistance and, consequently, increases in stroke volume and cardiac output. The effect of phentolamine was more profound than that of captopril. These findings suggest that of these three neurohormonal systems, the sympathetic nervous system activity contributes the greatest amount to vasoconstriction in patients with CHF. Whereas the renin-angiotensin system is also important, vasopressin probably contributes little to vasoconstriction in most patients with CHF. Vasopressin may contribute to vasoconstriction in heart failure only when the levels are extremely high. (*Adapted from* Creager *et al.* [22].)

FIGURE 6-29. The relative contributions of the sympathetic nervous system, renin-angiotensin system, and arginine-vasopressin (AVP) system to systemic vascular resistance in patients with congestive heart failure (CHF) was studied by administering an antagonist

osmotic gradient generated by the urinary countercurrent mechanism. In congestive heart failure (CHF), elevated levels of AVP lead to increased aquaporin-2 synthesis and translocation leading to inappropriate urinary concentration even in the setting of hyponatremia. Aquaporin-2 urinary excretion reflects increased aquaporin-2 translocation and is elevated in CHF. Martin *et al.* [23] assessed the effect of an oral, non-peptide V2 receptor antagonist on aquaporin-2 excretion (**A**) and free water clearance (B) in 21 patients with CHF. The V2 receptor antagonist (*n*=15) decreased aquaporin-2 excretion in a dose dependent manner compared to placebo (*n*=6, A). Solute-free water excretion was negative at baseline confirming the water retentive state of CHF. Although, free water excretion increased over time in both drug and placebo arms, it was positive only in the V2 receptor antagonist-treated group (B, the response to the 250-mg dose is shown). These results confirm that AVP secretion contributes significantly to the water retention seen in CHF. *Asterisk* indicates *P<0.05*. (*Adapted from* Martin *et al.* [25].)

FIGURE 6-30. Renal effects of arginine vasopressin (AVP) in congestive heart failure. AVP prevents diuresis by activating V2 receptors on the basolateral surface of the principal cells in the collecting duct. Activation of these receptors leads to the translocation of aquaporin-2 water channels from cytoplasmic vesicles to the apical surface of the collecting duct. These channels then allow water molecules to traverse the apical membrane in response to the

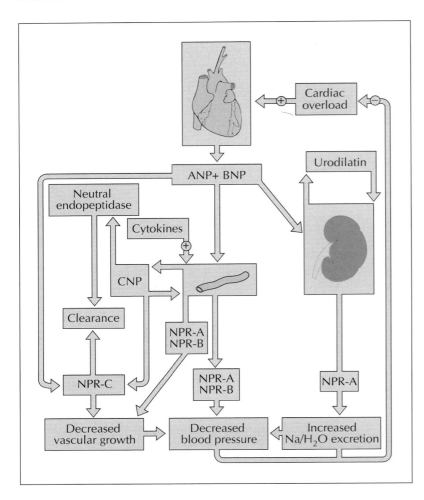

FIGURE 6-31. The natriuretic peptide family. The natriuretic peptides include atrial natriuretic peptide (ANP), brain natriuretic peptide (BNP), C-type natriuretic peptide (CNP), and urodilatin. ANP is derived from a prohormone composed of 126 amino acids, and it is secreted primarily from cardiac atria. The prohormone is cleaved to an *N*-terminal fragment (ANP1-98) and a C-terminal fragment (ANP99-126). BNP, identified initially in brain, is secreted from both atria and ventricles, particularly the latter. CNP has been identified primarily in brain but is also present in vascular endothelial cells. Urodilatin, or ANP95-126, is found in urine. Stretch receptors in the atria and ventricles detect changes in cardiac chamber volume related to increased cardiac filling pressures, resulting in release of both ANP and BNP but not CNP. The natriuretic peptides are inactivated by neutral endopeptidases. The actions of the natriuretic peptides are mediated by natriuretic peptide receptors (NPRs), designated NPR-A, NPR-B, and NPR-C. Both NPR-A and NPR-B are particulate guanylate cyclases, activation of which increases levels of cGMP. Natriuretic peptide receptors have been localized in vascular smooth muscle, endothelium, platelets, the adrenal glomerulosa, and the kidney. ANP and BNP increase urine volume and sodium excretion, decrease vascular resistance, and inhibit release of renin and secretion of aldosterone and vasopressin. CNP reduces vascular resistance but despite its name, does not have natriuretic properties. (*Adapted from* Wilkins *et al.* [24].)

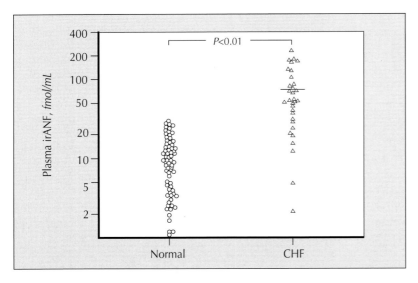

FIGURE 6-32. Cody *et al.* [25] measured plasma immunoreactive atrial natriuretic factor (irANF) in 70 normal subjects and 31 patients with congestive heart failure (CHF). Plasma irANF was 11 ± 0.9 fmol/mL in normal subjects and 71 ± 9.9 fmol/mL in patients with CHF ($P<0.01$). These results demonstrate a significant elevation of circulating atrial natriuretic factor in patients with CHF. Despite high circulating levels of ANF, patients with CHF demonstrate marked sodium retention, possibly reflecting downregulation of ANF receptors or a persistent imbalance between ANF and opposing mechanisms. (*Adapted from* Cody *et al.* [25].)

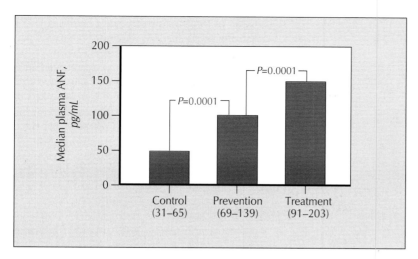

FIGURE 6-33. In the Studies of Left Ventricular Dysfunction (SOLVD), atrial natriuretic factor (ANF) levels were measured in patients with asymptomatic left ventricular (LV) dysfunction and mild congestive heart failure. Plasma ANF was measured in 54 control subjects, 147 patients with LV dysfunction but no evidence of congestive heart failure (prevention group), and 80 patients with mild congestive heart failure (treatment group). The median ANF level was 48 pg/mL in the control group, 103 pg/mL in the prevention group, and 146 pg/mL in the treatment group (interquartile ranges are shown in parentheses). Mean values for plasma ANF were significantly higher in patients with LV dysfunction compared with normal control subjects and were higher in the treatment arm compared with the prevention. Thus, increased release of ANF may be an early response to LV dysfunction. (*Adapted from* Francis *et al.* [1].)

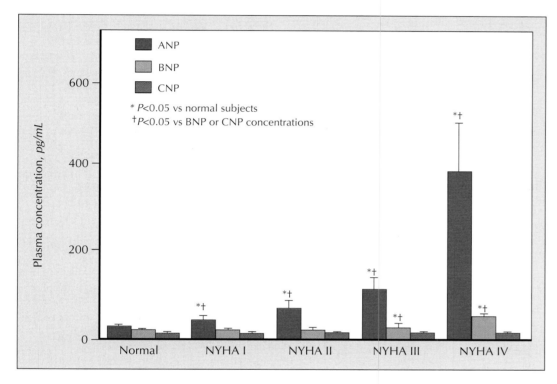

FIGURE 6-34. Plasma concentrations of atrial natriuretic peptide (ANP), brain natriuretic peptide (BNP), and C-type natriuretic peptide (CNP) in patients with congestive heart failure and in normal persons. Whereas plasma ANP concentration was elevated in groups of patients with heart failure whose symptoms ranged from mild to severe, plasma BNP concentration was significantly increased only in patients with severe heart failure. Plasma CNP concentrations were not elevated in any group of patients with heart failure compared with normal subjects. NYHA—New York Heart Association. (*Adapted from* Wei *et al.* [26].)

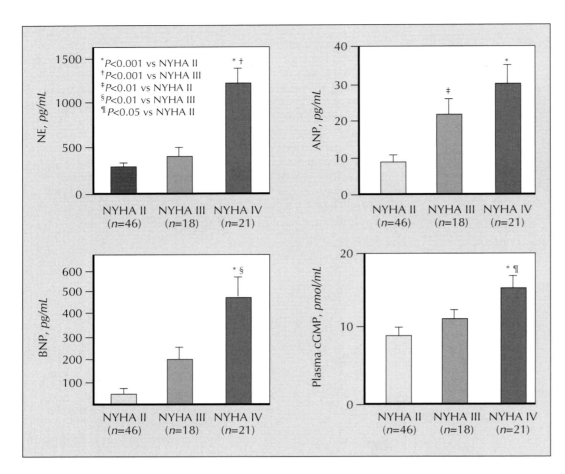

FIGURE 6-35. Measurement of natriuretic peptides in patients with heart failure. The prognostic information derived from measurement of natriuretic peptides in patients with heart failure was assessed by Tsutamoto *et al.* [27]. Plasma levels of atrial natriuretic peptide (ANP), brain natriuretic peptide (BNP), cGMP, and norepinephrine (NE) were measured in 85 patients with chronic congestive heart failure who were followed for 2 years. The concentrations of ANP, BNP, cGMP and norepinephrine increased proportionally with the functional severity of heart failure. In a Kaplan-Meyer analysis of the cumulative rates of survival in patients with heart failure stratified into two groups on the basis of the median plasma concentration of BNP (73 pg/mL), it was shown that survival was significantly worse in the group with the higher plasma BNP levels (*see* Fig. 8-10*B*). A stepwise multivariate analysis, which included ANP, BNP, norepinephrine, New York Heart Association (NYHA) functional class, selected hemodynamic indices, and demographic features, found that only a high concentration of plasma BNP (*P*<0.0001) and pulmonary capillary wedge pressure (*P*=0.003) were significant independent predictors of mortality. (*Adapted from* Tsutamoto *et al.* [27].)

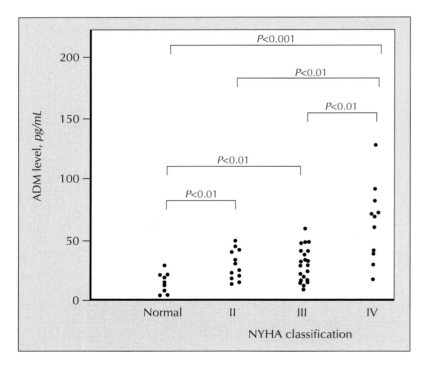

FIGURE 6-36. Adrenomedullin (ADM). A peptide with vasodilating and natriuretic properties, ADM was initially isolated from extracts of human pheochromocytoma. It is present in heart, kidney, vascular smooth muscle, and endothelial cells. Jougasaki *et al.* [28] measured circulating AMD levels in normal subjects and in patients with congestive heart failure, and found that the plasma concentration of ADM increased as the severity of heart failure worsened. Moreover, the study demonstrated evidence of cardiac secretion of ADM based on measurement of plasma samples obtained in the aorta, coronary sinus, and anterior interventricular vein. This study raises the possibility that ADM may participate in the regulation of vascular function and sodium excretion in patients with heart failure. NYHA—New York Heart Association. (*Adapted from* Jougasaki *et al.* [28].)

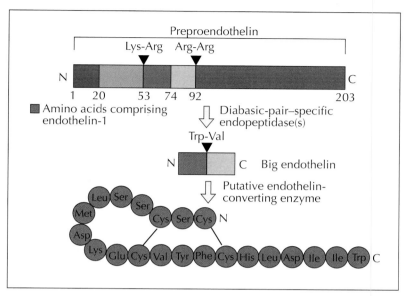

FIGURE 6-37. Endothelin, a 21-amino-acid peptide hormone, is a potent endogenous vasoconstrictor substance produced by endothelial cells. Preproendothelin, a 203-amino-acid peptide, is the endothelin precursor. Initial cleavage by endogenous endopeptidases forms a 39-amino-acid residue called *proendothelin* or *big endothelin*, which is then cleaved to the active endothelin-1 by an endothelin-specific converting enzyme. This enzyme is predominantly bound to the cell membrane but is also present within the cytoplasm. C—carboxyl terminal; N—amino terminal. (*Adapted from* Yanagisawa *et al.* [29].)

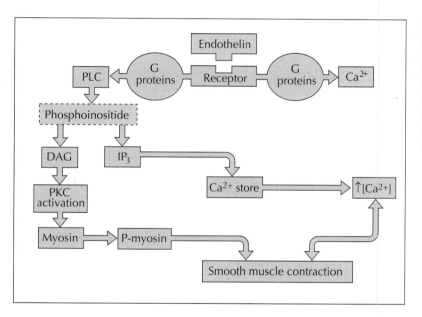

FIGURE 6-38. Endothelin exerts its action via binding with a specific receptor on the cell membrane, which is linked via guanine nucleotide regulatory binding proteins (G proteins) to stimulation of phospholipase C (PLC) and opening of voltage-dependent calcium channels. Activation of PLC degrades phosphoinositide to form inositol trisphosphate (IP_3) and diacylglycerol (DAG), second messengers that release calcium from intracellular stores and promote the activation of protein kinase C (PKC), respectively. (*Adapted from* Masaki *et al.* [30].)

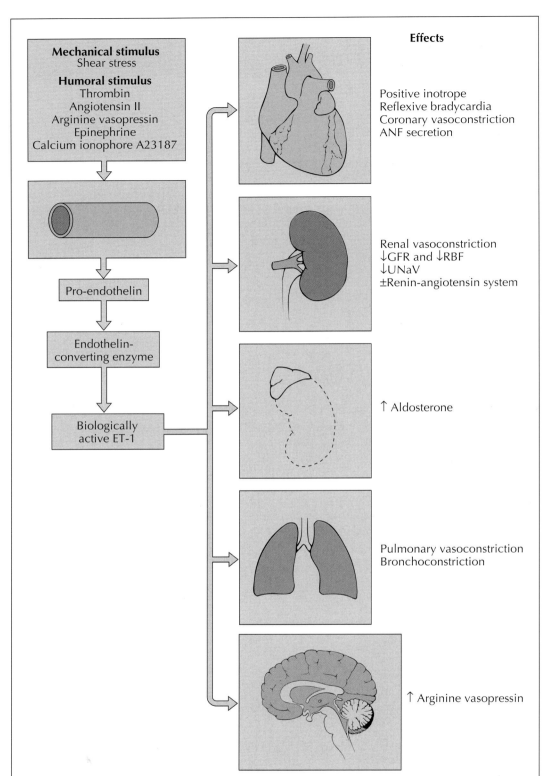

FIGURE 6-39. Summary of the stimuli for endothelin secretion and effects of endothelin in several organs. Mechanical (shear stress) and humoral (thrombin, angiotensin II, vasopressin, epinephrine, calcium ionophore A23187) stimuli may cause the release of endothelin-1 (ET-1). Endothelin increases circulating levels of atrial natriuretic factor (ANF), vasopressin, and aldosterone. It also modulates renin release. Endothelin has a positive inotropic effect and produces coronary and systemic vasoconstriction. These responses produce an increase in blood pressure that is associated with a reflex decrease in heart rate. ET-1 constricts human pulmonary resistance vessels and has a potent bronchoconstrictor effect. Furthermore, ET-1 causes renal vasoconstriction, leading to a reduction in renal blood flow (RBF) and glomerular filtration rate (GFR) and a decrease in urinary sodium excretion (UNaV). (*Adapted from* Underwood *et al.* [31].)

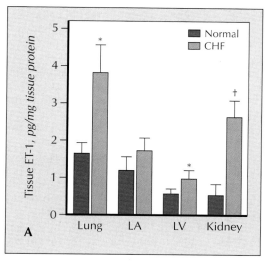

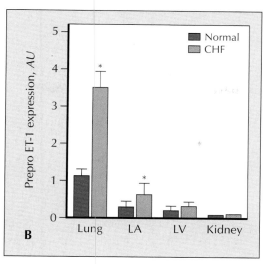

FIGURE 6-40. Tissue-specific distribution of endothelin-1 in congestive heart failure. Endothelin-1 (ET-1) is believed to exert its effects predominantly as an autocrine and

paracrine hormone rather than a circulating hormone. In an canine model of pacing-induced heart failure, ET-1 tissue concentrations and preproendothelin (prepro ET-1) gene expression in the lung, heart, and kidney in heart failure were compared with the levels in normal controls. ET-1 tissue concentrations (**A**) were significantly increased in the lung, left ventricle, and kidney while prepro-ET1 mRNA expression (**B**) was significantly increased only in the lung and left atrium. This suggests that ET-1 exerts its effects in the lung in an autocrine fashion, in the left ventricle as a paracrine hormone, and in the kidney as a circulating hormone. *Asterisk* indicates $P<$ 0.05. *Daggers* indicate $P<$ 0.01. (*Adapted from* Luchner *et al.* [32].)

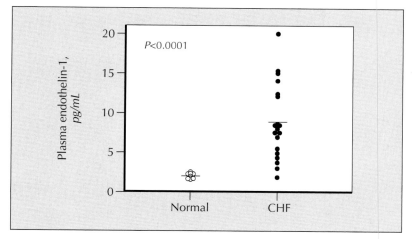

FIGURE 6-41. Cody *et al.* [33] measured immunoreactive circulating endothelin-1 in 12 normal control subjects and in 20 patients with congestive heart failure (CHF). Plasma endothelin-1 was 3.7±0.6 pg/mL in the control group and 9.1±4.1 pg/mL in the CHF group. Increased endothelin synthesis by angiotensin I and vasopressin stimulation and decreased endothelin clearance may contribute to the increased plasma endothelin levels in CHF. Of note, there was a strong positive correlation between endothelin levels and the severity of pulmonary hypertension. (*Adapted from* Cody *et al.* [33].)

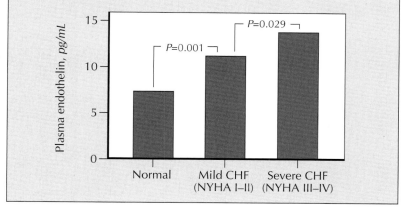

FIGURE 6-42. Rodeheffer *et al.* [34] measured plasma endothelin in 71 normal subjects, 24 patients with mild congestive heart failure (CHF), and 32 patients with severe congestive heart failure (New York Heart Association [NYHA] functional classes are shown in parentheses). The mean plasma concentration of endothelin was 7.1±0.1 pg/mL in the control group, 11.1±0.7 pg/mL in the mild heart failure group, and 13.8±0.9 pg/mL in the severe heart failure group. These data demonstrate that plasma endothelin is significantly increased in patients with CHF and that the level is correlated with the severity of the disease. (*Adapted from* Rodeheffer *et al.* [34].)

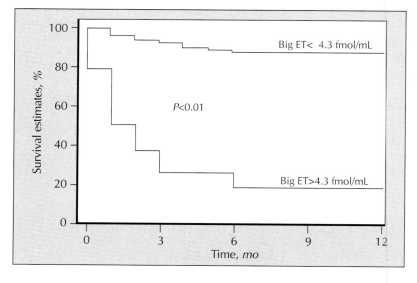

FIGURE 6-43. The prognostic implications of endothelin-1 for patients with congestive heart failure. Pacher *et al.* [35] measured plasma big endothelin-1 (Big ET) concentrations and 16 clinical, hemodynamic, and neurohumoral variables in 113 patients with left ventricular ejection fraction (LVEF) less than 20%, and related these to 1-year mortality. Of the 113 patients, there were 58 1-year survivors, 29 nonsurvivors, and 26 heart transplant recipients. Plasma Big ET concentrations were lower in 1-year survivors than in nonsurvivors (2.6±0.1 vs 5.9±0.4 fmol/mL; P=0.0001). Cumulative rates of survival over 1 year in 87 patients with severe chronic heart failure (excluding 26 transplant recipients) were stratified into two groups according to Big ET concentration. Survival rates were significantly lower in the patients whose plasma endothelin-1 levels were greater than 4.3 fmol/mL. By multivariate analysis, taking into consideration plasma endothelin 1 concentration, functional class, furosemide dose, LVEF, hemodynamic variables, and plasma atrial natriuretic peptide, renin activity, and aldosterone levels, only plasma Big ET and functional class predicted 1-year mortality (P<0.0001). (*Adapted from* Pacher *et al.* [35].)

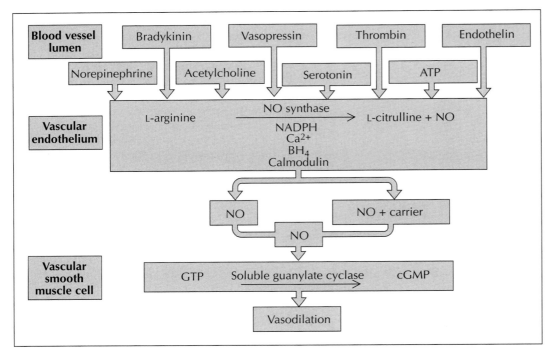

FIGURE 6-44. Vascular endothelial cells synthesize both vasodilators (nitric oxide [NO] and prostacyclin) and vasoconstrictors (*eg*, endothelin and vasoconstrictor prostanoids). NO is released in response to a wide variety of stimuli (acetylcholine, norepinephrine, vasopressin, thrombin, endothelin, ATP, serotonin, bradykinin, calcium ionophore A23187). NO is derived from the metabolism of the amino acid L-arginine, a reaction that is catalyzed by the enzyme NO synthase and requires the presence of calcium, NADPH (nicotinamide adenine dinucleotide phosphate), tetrahydrobiopterin (BH_4), and calmodulin as cofactors. NO synthase is competitively inhibited by L-arginine analogues. NO is released from the endothelium either as a free radical or combined with a carrier molecule. NO activates the vascular smooth muscle–soluble enzyme guanylate cyclase, increases cGMP, and thereby causes vasodilation.

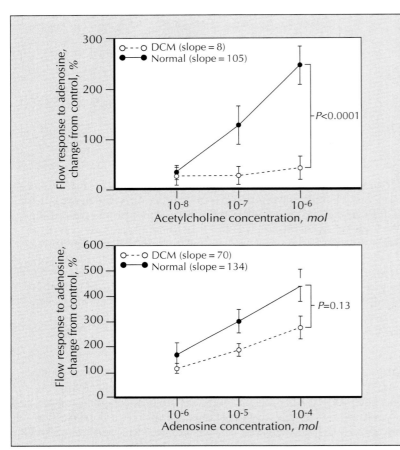

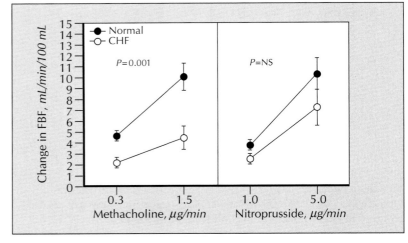

FIGURE 6-46. Abnormal endothelium-dependent relaxation of forearm resistance vessels in patients with congestive heart failure (CHF). Kubo *et al*. [37] measured the forearm blood flow (FBF) response to methacholine, an endothelium-dependent vasodilator, and nitroprusside, an endothelium-independent vasodilator, in eight normal subjects and in 10 patients with CHF. There was a significant decrease in the response to methacholine in heart failure patients compared with normal subjects. There was no significant difference in the response to nitroprusside. These data suggest that endothelium-dependent relaxation is impaired in patients with CHF. (*Adapted from* Kubo *et al*. [37].)

FIGURE 6-45. Endothelium-dependent relaxation of the coronary arteries in congestive heart failure. Treasure *et al*. [36] studied the coronary blood flow responses to serial infusions of acetylcholine and adenosine in seven normal subjects and eight patients with dilated cardiomyopathy (DCM). Infusion of acetylcholine produced a dose-dependent increase in coronary blood flow in normal subjects but not in patients with congestive heart failure. Infusion of adenosine produced a dose-dependent increase in coronary blood flow in both groups. Thus, endothelium-dependent vasodilatation was significantly diminished in heart failure patients, but the maximal vasodilator response to adenosine was similar in both groups. (*Adapted from* Treasure *et al*. [36].)

POTENTIAL MECHANISMS FOR IMPAIRED ENDOTHELIUM-MEDIATED VASODILATION IN HEART FAILURE

Impaired endothelial cell receptor function or postreceptor signaling
Deficiency of L-arginine substrate
Abnormal nitric oxide synthase expression or function
Deficient or abnormal nitric oxide synthase cofactors
Impaired release or diffusion of EDRF
Increased degradation of EDRF
Concomitant release of EDCFs
Abnormal cGMP or cGMP-dependent protein phosphorylation
Nonspecifically impaired smooth muscle vasodilator response

FIGURE 6-47. Potential mechanisms for impaired endothelium-mediated vasodilatation in heart failure. The postulated mechanisms for impaired endothelium-mediated vasodilation include impaired endothelial cell receptor function or postreceptor signaling; deficiency of L-arginine substrate; abnormal nitric oxide (NO) synthase expression or function; deficient or abnormal nitric oxide synthase cofactor, such as calcium, calmodulin, or NADPH; impaired release or diffusion of nitric oxide; increased degradation of NO, concomitant release of endothelium-derived contracting factors (EDCFs), such as thromboxane A_2 and prostaglandin H_2; abnormal cGMP or cGMP-dependent protein phosphorylation; or a nonspecifically impaired smooth–muscle vasodilator response. (*Adapted from* Kubo and Bank [38].)

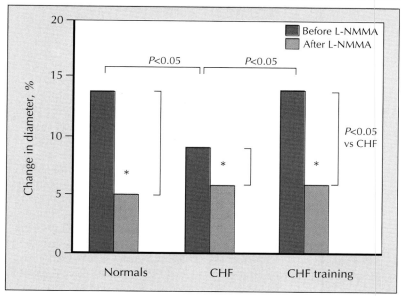

FIGURE 6-48. Increase in shear stress, as occurs when flow is accelerated, stimulates the release of endothelium-derived nitric oxide

from blood vessels. Flow-mediated, endothelium-dependent vasodilation, as assessed by vascular ultrasonography, is reduced in limb arteries of patients with congestive heart failure (CHF). Hornig *et al.* [39] studied the effect of physical training on flow-mediated endothelium-dependent vasodilation in patients with heart failure and age-matched healthy subjects. Flow-mediated vasodilation, induced by reactive hyperemia, was assessed in each group of subjects before and after administration of the nitric oxide synthase antagonist, N^G-monomethyl-L-arginine (L-NMMA). Measurements were made at baseline, after 4 weeks of handgrip training, and 6 weeks after the training program was discontinued. Prior to training, flow-mediated vasodilation was reduced in patients with heart failure compared with healthy subjects ($8.6\% \pm 0.9\%$ versus $13.5\% \pm 0.7\%$; $P<0.05$). After 4 weeks of handgrip training, flow-mediated vasodilation in the patients with heart failure increased to $13.6\% \pm 0.9\%$. After training, the portion of flow-mediated vasodilation inhibited by L-NMMA was significantly increased compared with baseline and was similar to that observed in healthy subjects. These findings indicate that physical training improves flow-mediated vasodilation in patients with CHF, most likely by enhancing endothelial release of nitric oxide. *Asterisks* indicate $P<0.05$ versus corresponding value before L-NMMA. (*Adapted from* Hornig *et al.* [39].)

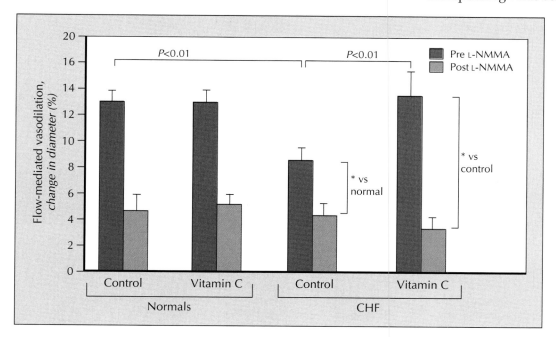

FIGURE 6-49. Oxidative stress contributes to endothelial dysfunction in congestive heart failure (CHF). Oxidative stress is increased in CHF. The NADPH–NADH oxidase system in endothelial cells, smooth muscle cells, and phagocytes has been suggested as a source of increased oxygen free radicals in CHF. These free radicals can contribute to endothelial dysfunction by reducing nitric oxide (NO) synthase activity and by inactivating NO to form

peroxynitrite. Hornig *et al.* [39] demonstrated the contribution of oxidative stress to endothelial dysfunction by administering the antioxidant, vitamin C, intravenously in 10 patients with CHF and 5 healthy controls. They evaluated flow-mediated endothelium-dependent vasodilatation (FMD) induced by reactive hyperemia at baseline and in the presence of N-monomethyl-L-arginine (L-NMMA), an NO synthase antagonist. These measurements were repeated in both groups after intra-arterial infusion of vitamin C. FMD was impaired at baseline in the CHF group compared to normal controls (8.42% vs 12.9%). L-NMMA decreased flow-mediated vasodilatation to a lesser extent in the CHF group than in controls (4.2% vs 8.4%), indicating reduced bioavailability of NO in CHF. After the administration of vitamin C, FMD was restored to normal levels in the CHF group and was then suppressed by the addition of L-NMMA. These results suggest that vitamin C, by restoring NO, improves endothelial function in CHF via its antioxidant effects. *Asterisk* indicates $P<0.01$. (*Adapted from* Hornig *et al.* [39].)

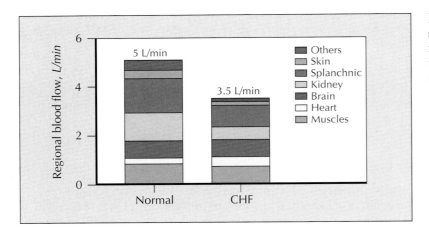

FIGURE 6-50. Distribution of regional blood flow at rest in normal subjects and in patients with congestive heart failure (CHF). The net effect of the various vasoconstricting and vasodilating systems that are activated in CHF is to redistribute the cardiac output. (*Adapted from* Zelis *et al.* [41].)

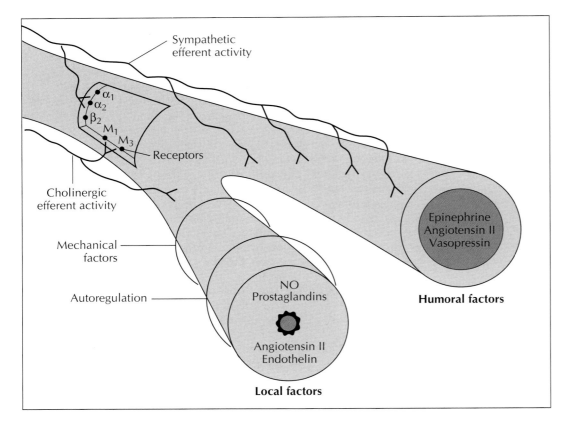

FIGURE 6-51. Peripheral blood flow is determined by the interaction of multiple factors. These factors include sympathetic efferent activity (modulated by baroreceptors, chemoreceptors, and somatic receptors), cholinergic efferent activity, humoral factors (such as nitric oxide [NO]), local factors (such as endothelium-derived relaxing factor [EDRF], endothelin, angiotensin II, prostaglandins, and kinins), mechanical factors (such as muscle activity and cutaneous thermoregulation), and autoregulatory mechanisms (including myogenic reflexes and metabolism-induced responses). Increased sympathetic efferent activity modulated by blunted baroreceptors, systemic increases in angiotensin II and vasopressin, local increases in endothelin and prostaglandins, local reduction of NO, and mechanical factors, such as increased arterial wall sodium and extravascular tissue edema, all contribute to the decreased peripheral blood flow associated with congestive heart failure [42].

REFERENCES

1. Francis GS, Benedict C, Johnstone DE, *et al.*: Comparison of neuroendocrine activation in patients with left ventricular dysfunction with and without congestive heart failure. *Circulation* 1990, 82:1724–1729.

2. Vanhoutte PM, Luscher TF: Peripheral mechanisms in cardiovascular regulation: transmitters, receptors and the endothelium. In *Handbook of Hypertension*, vol 8. Edited by Tarazi RC, Zanchetti A. Amsterdam: Elsevier Science Publishers; 1986:96–123.

3. Davis D, Baily R, Zelis R: Abnormalities in systemic norepinephrine kinetics in human congestive heart failure. *Am J Physiol* 1988, 254 (suppl E):760–766.

4. Leimbach WN Jr, Wallin BG, Victor RG, *et al.*: Direct evidence from intraneural recordings for increased central sympathetic outflow in patients with heart failure. *Circulation* 1986, 73:913–919.

5. Paganelli WC, Creager MA, Dzau VJ: Cardiac regulation of renal function. In *The International Textbook of Cardiology*. Edited by Cheng TO. New York: Pergammon Press; 1986:1010–1020.

6. Dibner-Dunlap ME, Thames MD: Baroreflex control of renal sympathetic nerve activity is preserved in heart failure despite reduced arterial baroreceptor sensitivity. *Circ Res* 1989, 65:1526–1535.

7. Sopher SM, Smith ML, Eckberg DL, *et al.*: Autonomic pathophysiology in heart failure: carotid baroreceptor-cardiac reflexes. *Am J Physiol* 1990, 259:H689–H696.

8. Creager MA: Baroreceptor reflex function in congestive heart failure. *Am J Cardiol* 1992, 69:10G–16G.

9. Ferguson DW, Abboud FM, Mark AL: Selective impairment of baroreflex mediated vasoconstrictor responses in patients with ventricular dysfunction. *Circulation* 1984, 69:451–460.

10. Kaye DM, Jennings GL, Dart AM, Esler MD: Differential effect of acute baroreceptor unloading on cardiac and systemic sympathetic tone in congestive heart failure. *J Am Coll Cardiol* 1998, 31:583–587.

11. Floras JS: Clinical aspects of sympathetic activation and parasympathetic withdrawal in heart failure. *J Am Coll Cardiol* 1993, 22:72A–84A.

12. Cohn JN, Levine B, Olivari MT, *et al.*: Plasma norepinephrine as a guide to prognosis in patients with chronic congestive heart failure. *N Engl J Med* 1984, 311:819–823.

13. Benedict CR, Shelton B, Johnstone DE, *et al.* for the SOLVD Investigators: Prognostic significance of plasma norepinephrine in patients with asymptomatic left ventricular dysfunction. *Circulation* 1996, 94:690–697.

14. Cody RJ, Laragh JH: The role of the renin-angiotensin-aldosterone system in the pathophysiology of chronic heart failure. In *Drug Treatment of Chronic Heart Failure*. Edited by Cohn J. New York: Advanced Therapeutics Communications; Yorke Medical Publications; 1983:35–51.

15. Hirsch AT, Pinto YM, Schunkert D, *et al.*: Potential role of the tissue renin-angiotensin system in the pathophysiology of congestive heart failure. *Am J Cardiol* 1990, 66:22D–32D.

16. Hirsch AT, Creager MA: The peripheral circulation in heart failure. In *Congestive Heart Failure*. Edited by Hosenpud JD, Greenberg BH. Heidelberg: Springer-Verlag; 1994:145–160.

17. Tsutamoto T, Wada A, and Maeda K, *et al.*: Effect of spironolactone on plasma natriuretic peptide and left ventricular remodeling in patients with congestive heart failure. *J Am Coll Cardiol* 2001,37:1228–1233

18. Dzau VJ: Short- and long-term determinants of cardiovascular function and therapy: contributions of circulating and tissue renin-angiotensin systems. *J Cardiovasc Pharmacol* 1989, 14(suppl 4):T1–T5.

19. Creager MA, Halperin AL, Bernard DB, *et al.*: Acute regional circulatory and renal hemodynamic effects of converting enzyme inhibition in patients with congestive heart failure. *Circulation* 1981, 64:483–489.

20. Packer M: Interaction of prostaglandins and angiotensin II in the modulation of renal function in congestive heart failure. *Circulation* 1988, 77:I64–I73.

21. Francis GS, Goldsmith SR, Levine BT, *et al.*: The neurohumoral axis in congestive heart failure. *Ann Intern Med* 1984, 101:370–377.

22. Creager MA, Faxon DP, Cutler SS, *et al.*: Contribution of vasopressin to vasoconstriction in patients with congestive heart failure: comparison with the renin angiotensin system and the sympathetic nervous system. *J Am Coll Cardiol* 1986, 7:758–765.

23. Martin PY, Abraham WT, Lieming X, *et al.*: Selective V2-receptor antagonism decreases urinary aquaporin-2 excretion in patients with chronic heart failure. *J Am Soc Nephrol* 1999,10:2165–2170.

24. Wilkins MR, Redondo J, Brown LA: The natriuretic-peptide family. *Lancet* 1997, 349:1307–1310.

25. Cody RJ, Atlas SA, Laragh JH, *et al.*: Atrial natriuretic factor in normal subjects and heart failure patients. *J Clin Invest* 1986, 78:1362–1374.

26. Wei C-M, Lerman A, Rodeheffer RJ, *et al.*: Endothelin in human congestive heart failure. *Circulation* 1994, 89:1580–1586.

27. Tsutamoto T, Wada A, Maeda K, *et al.*: Attenuation of compensation of endogenous cardiac natriuretic peptide system in chronic heart failure. *Circulation* 1997, 96:509–516.

28. Jougasaki M, Rodeheffer RJ, Redfield MM, *et al.*: Cardiac secretion of adrenomedullin in human heart failure. *J Clin Invest* 1996, 97:2370–2376.

29. Yanagisawa M, Kurihara S, Kimura S, *et al.*: A novel potent vasoconstrictor peptide produced by vascular endothelial cells. *Nature* 1988, 332:411–415.

30. Masaki T, Yanagisawa M, Goto K, *et al.*: Cardiovascular significance of endothelin. In *Cardiovascular Significance of Endothelium-Derived Vasoactive Factors*. Edited by Rubanyi GM. Mt. Kisco, NY: Futura Publishing; 1991:65–81.

31. Underwood RD, Chan DP, Burnett JC: Endothelin: an endothelium derived vasoconstrictor peptide and its role in congestive heart failure. *Heart Failure* 1991, 7:50–58.

32. Luchner A, Jougasaki M, Friedrich E, *et al.*: Activation of cardiorenal and pulmonary tissue endothelin-1 in experimental heart failure. *Am J Physiol Regulatory Integrative Comp Physiol* 2000, 279:R974–R979.

33. Cody RJ, Haas GJ, Binkley PF, *et al.*: Plasma endothelin correlates with the extent of the pulmonary hypertension in patients with chronic congestive heart failure. *Circulation* 1992, 85:504–509.

34. Rodeheffer RJ, Lerman A, Heublein DM, *et al.*: Increased plasma concentrations of endothelin in congestive heart failure in humans. *Mayo Clin Proc* 1992, 67:719–724.

35. Pacher R, Stanek B, Hülsmann M, *et al.*: Prognostic impact of big endothelin-1 plasma concentrations compared with invasive hemodynamic evaluation in severe heart failure. *J Am Coll Cardiol* 1996, 27:633–641.

36. Treasure CB, Vita JA, Cox DA, *et al.*: Endothelium dependent dilation of the coronary microvasculature is impaired in dilated cardiomyopathy. *Circulation* 1990, 81:772–779.

37. Kubo SH, Rector TS, Bank AJ, *et al.*: Endothelium dependent vasodilation is attenuated in patients with heart failure. *Circulation* 1991, 84:1589–1596.

38. Kubo SH, Bank AJ: Endothelium dependent vasodilation in heart failure. *Heart Failure* 1992, 8:142–153.

39. Hornig B, Maier V, Drexler H: Physical training improves endothelial function in patients with chronic heart failure. *Circulation* 1996, 93:210–214.

40. Hornig B, Arakawa N, Kohler C, *et al.*: Vitamin C improves endothelial function of conduit arteries in patients with chronic heart failure. *Circulation* 1998,97:363–368.

41. Zelis R, Nellis S, Longhurst J, *et al.*: Abnormalities in the regional circulations accompanying congestive heart failure. *Prog Cardiovasc Dis* 1975, 18:181–199.

42. Hirsch AT, Dzau VJ, Creager MA: Baroreceptor function in congestive heart failure: effect on neurohumoral activation and regional vascular resistance. *Circulation* 1987, 75 (suppl IV):36–48.

ASSESSMENT OF HEART FAILURE

James B. Young

The clinical syndrome of heart failure may result from cardiac disease of many different etiologies. It reflects both the primary hemodynamic abnormalities caused by cardiac dysfunction and the consequences of multiple secondary compensatory systems (*eg*, vasoconstriction, neurohormonal activation, metabolic imbalance). Not surprisingly, the clinical manifestations of heart failure show a striking heterogeneity and, as a consequence, the clinical assessment of patients with heart failure is among the most challenging in medicine [1–3].

Traditionally, physicians have looked for symptoms and signs that reflect abnormal fluid retention or organ congestion [4,5]. Although many patients present with these "congestive" findings, it has become apparent that many more patients with heart failure can be diagnosed earlier in the course of the illness, with symptoms secondary to reduced exercise capacity, fatigue, or arrhythmia [6–10]. Particularly challenging is the treatment of elderly patients [3] and those with occult or minimally symptomatic left ventricular systolic dysfunction [7,10].

The signs and symptoms of heart failure may present acutely, as with the fulminant onset of myocarditis, or they may develop gradually, such as several years after an uncomplicated myocardial infarction. Pulmonary or systemic congestion may appear suddenly in a patient with previously undetected or compensated heart failure (*eg*, due to a change in salt intake or the initiation of a nonsteroidal anti-inflammatory drug). The presentation of signs and symptoms of heart failure may also reflect the nature of the underlying cardiac dysfunction (*eg*, right versus left heart failure), and there is increasing awareness that many patients with heart failure have predominantly diastolic (versus systolic) ventricular dysfunction [11]. Such patients may present with marked clinical symptoms and signs, despite a normal or nearly normal left ventricular ejection fraction. The prevalence of symptomatic heart failure is increasing because of the growing population of elderly individuals predisposed to this condition by the long-term effects of coronary heart disease, valvular disease, or systemic conditions such as hypertension and diabetes mellitus [12–14]. In these patients, heart failure is often due predominantly to diastolic dysfunction and is frequently undetected because the symptoms are attributed to the normal consequences of aging or other coexistent illnesses.

The assessment of patients with heart failure should include efforts to characterize the etiology, determine the severity, and identify factors that may have precipitated clinical decompensation. Several questions should be posed during the evaluation of a patient for heart failure: Are the symptoms and signs caused by heart failure or by any of several noncardiac conditions that can cause similar findings? What is the etiology of cardiac dysfunction? What is the severity of the cardiac dysfunction? What is the level of functional impairment? What is the prognosis? What is the optimal therapeutic approach? Arriving at the correct answers to these questions begins with taking a complete history and conducting a full physical examination, supplemented by appropriate hematologic and blood chemistry determinations, an electrocardiogram, and chest radiograph. In the large majority of patients in whom there is a suspicion of heart failure, an echocardiogram is important to clarify cardiac anatomy and function. An assessment of exercise capacity is also frequently helpful to quantify the level of functional impairment, detect inducible myocardial ischemia, exclude noncardiac (*eg*, pulmonary) causes of dyspnea, and determine prognosis. Additional tests, including radionuclide studies, cardiac catheterization, and myocardial biopsy, may be needed to complete the evaluation in selected patients.

Perhaps the most important and significant development with respect to diagnosing and staging the severity of the congestive heart failure syndrome is the recent introduction of a point-of-care serum brain natriuretic peptide assay. Brain natriuretic peptide, (BNP) is a 32-amino-acid peptide secreted primarily from the ventricles of the heart. This hormone is released in response to stretch and increased volume in the ventricles. BNP levels correlate with left ventricular and diastolic pressure and volume and New York Heart Association classification of congestive heart failure. A rapid, point-of-care assay for BNP (Triage BNP Test, Biosite Incorporated, San Diego, CA) is now available to facilitate diagnosis of congestive heart failure and can be used as a prognostic marker [15–17].

It is now recognized that asymptomatic cardiac dysfunction can be present for long periods prior to the development of clinically evident signs and symptoms of decompensation [7–14]. Because there is evidence (*see* Chapter 5) that treatment of asymptomatic individuals can delay or even prevent the progression to symptomatic disease and improve prognosis, early diagnosis of asymptomatic or minimally symptomatic ventricular dysfunction is of paramount importance.

OVERVIEW

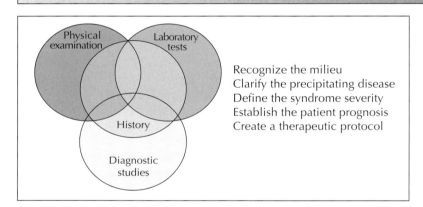

FIGURE 7-1. Specific goals of patient evaluation when heart failure is suspected. First, one must appropriately recognize the heart failure syndrome and differentiate heart and circulatory failure from problems that cause similar complaints and findings. Second, by staging the severity of heart failure, the clinician can establish prognosis with reasonable accuracy. This is important in the design of therapeutic protocols to treat certain aspects of the syndrome. Finally, identifying the primary etiology of myocardial dysfunction and determining the precipitating causes of decompensation are extremely important. The interplay of patient history, physical examination, laboratory tests, and specific diagnostic studies helps the clinician achieve these goals.

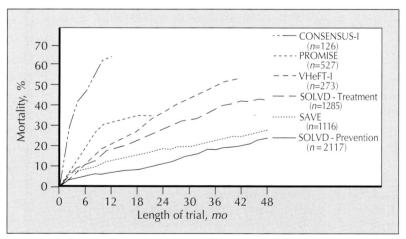

FIGURE 7-2. Clinical heart failure trials: placebo mortality curves. The data from several large, now classic placebo-controlled clinical trials emphasize that patients with heart failure or asymptomatic ventricular dysfunction represent a wide spectrum of morbidity and mortality risks. The CONSENSUS-I (Cooperative North Scandinavian Enalapril Survival Study) trial evaluated patients with New York Heart Association (NYHA) class IV congestive heart

failure treated with diuretics and digitalis [18]. The placebo cohort demonstrated a mortality at 12 months in excess of 60%. Patients in this trial had ejection fractions of 35% or less.

These patients should be compared with the placebo cohorts of the SOLVD (Studies of Left Ventricular Dysfunction)-Prevention trial [19] and SAVE (Survival and Ventricular Enlargement) Trial [20]. These studies were also performed in patients with ventricular dysfunction (ejection fraction of ≤35% in SOLVD and <40% in SAVE). Patients were asymptomatic after myocardial infarction in SAVE, and either asymptomatic or minimally symptomatic (NYHA class I and II) in SOLVD-Prevention. Twelve-month placebo mortality rates in these groups, in contrast to the CONSENSUS-I cohort, were around 10%. At the 48-month follow-up point, mortality was substantial (about 20%), but was still dramatically less than that typically noted in patients with symptomatic congestive heart failure.

The first Veterans Administration Heart Failure Trial (VHeFT-I) [21], SOLVD Treatment Trial [22], and PROMISE (Prospective Randomized Milrinone Survival Evaluation) Trials [23] included patients with mild to moderate congestive heart failure (usually NYHA class II or III). In these trials, a gradation in placebo group mortality can be noted, with the curves falling between the less ill SAVE or SOLVD-Prevention trial cohorts and the more ill CONSENSUS-I patients.

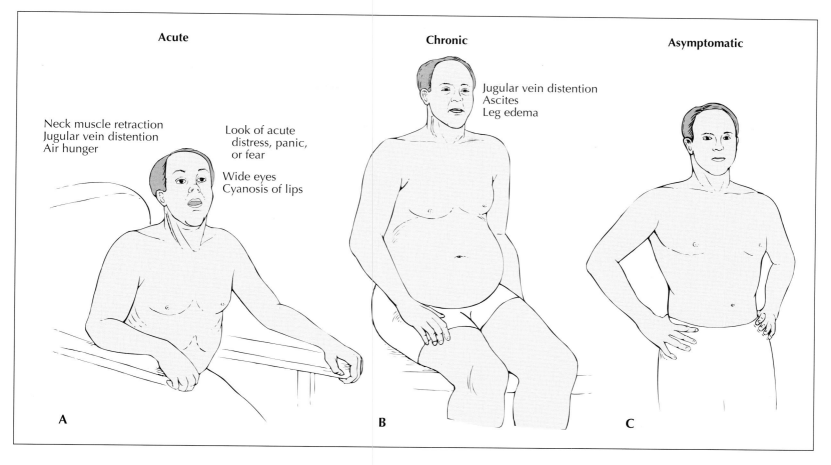

Acute   Chronic   Asymptomatic

Neck muscle retraction
Jugular vein distention
Air hunger

Look of acute
distress, panic,
or fear

Wide eyes
Cyanosis of lips

Jugular vein distention
Ascites
Leg edema

A   B   C

FIGURE 7-3. The varied faces of heart failure. When heart failure is discussed, patients with pulmonary edema, such as the patient with acute, distressing air hunger (**A**), or those with chronic congestive heart failure, such as the patient with edema (**B**), often come to mind. This is not unreasonable, because heart failure traditionally was diagnosed when congestion developed [14].

We now know that the patient who appears fit and has few complaints (**C**) may also have heart failure. In fact, the majority of patients with left ventricular dysfunction do not manifest congestive symptomatology or findings. The detection of heart failure in such patients is challenging.

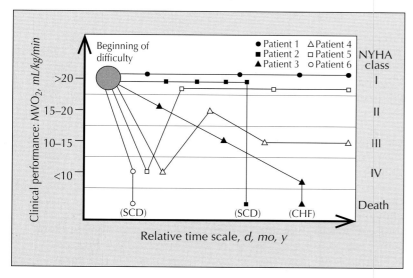

FIGURE 7-4. Variability of natural history of congestive heart failure (CHF). Patients can present at a variety of points during their illness. Initial patient contact may be triggered by an episode of acute pulmonary edema caused by severe diastolic dysfunction (perhaps precipitated by hypertension or ventricular ischemia), or symptoms may have been developing insidiously over several

months as the heart dilates slowly in response to chronic alcohol toxicity. A variety of theoretic courses are plotted in this figure; a patient might present at any of the marked points. Patient 1, for example, is one in whom myocardial infarction has caused asymptomatic left ventricular (LV) dysfunction. In this patient, clinical compensation is present, ongoing ischemia is absent, and exercise performance is adequate. The patient is discovered to have systolic LV dysfunction during echocardiography performed before hospital discharge, and remains asymptomatic throughout long-term follow-up. Patient 2 has ischemic heart disease, myocardial infarction, mild to moderate LV dysfunction, and adequate exercise performance. This patient, without preceding congestive decompensation, suffers sudden cardiac death (SCD). Patient 3 is one in whom myocardial injury is steadily progressive over time, causing gradual clinical deterioration until death from CHF ensues. Patients 4 and 5 develop substantive and debilitating CHF but improve with treatment. However, whereas patient 4, despite aggressive therapy, continues to experience moderately severe CHF (New York Heart Association [NYHA] class III), patient 5 does not exhibit recurrence of congestive symptomatology and achieves adequate exercise performance during long-term follow-up. Patient 6 deteriorates dramatically, with SCD occurring soon after the diagnosis of CHF has been made. MVO2—myocardial oxygen consumption.

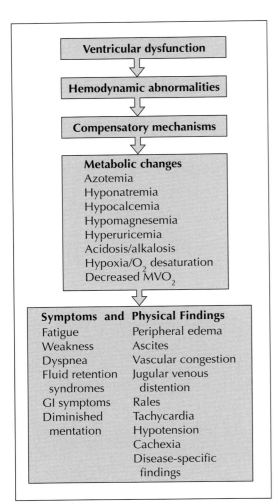

FIGURE 7-5. Clinical presentation of heart failure. The primary myocardial injury (multiple different diseases) produces ventricular dysfunction, resulting in subsequent hemodynamic abnormalities that eventually cause clinical manifestations of heart failure. A period of clinical compensation is often observed, during which patients are asymptomatic. A variety of symptoms, physical findings, and metabolic abnormalities may occur in heart failure. Symptoms can be exacerbated or attenuated, depending on fluctuations in hemodynamic abnormalities, adequacy of physiologic compensatory mechanisms, and the success of therapeutic intervention. Death in patients with heart failure can result from systemic organ failure (caused by hypoperfusion or congestion) or from sudden cardiac death (caused by the lethal arrhythmias that commonly accompany heart failure). Pulmonary embolism, stroke, or concurrent diseases that precipitate heart failure can also cause death. GI—gastrointestinal; MVO_2—myocardial oxygen consumption.

ASSESSING THE PATIENT

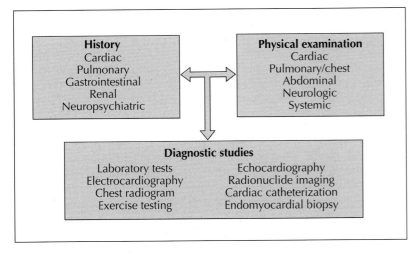

FIGURE 7-6. Approach to the problem of assessing heart failure. To adequately assess patients with heart failure, historical information, data from the physical examination, and diagnostic study information should be obtained and integrated. It should be emphasized that although information from all three categories may be used in the evaluation, not every test needs to be, or should be, performed. In most patients, an electrocardiogram, a chest radiograph, and an echocardiogram are performed. Additional diagnostic studies should be tailored to the patient. Echocardiography could include M-mode, two-dimensional, and Doppler studies. Radionuclide examination might consist of perfusion, performance, or positron emission tomographic studies. Cardiac catheterization could include angiography, hemodynamics, or endomyocardial biopsy in certain circumstances. Computed tomography and magnetic resonance imaging are sometimes useful, as is determination of maximal exercise oxygen consumption. Information obtained from the history and physical examination should dictate the need for and type of ancillary testing.

THE CLINICAL HISTORY IN ASSESSING HEART FAILURE

CARDIOVASCULAR	SYSTEMIC	PULMONARY	RENAL	GASTROENTEROLOGIC	NEUROLOGIC AND NEUROPSYCHIATRIC
Angina pectoris	Edema	Dyspnea on exertion	Nocturia	Abdominal pain	
Nonspecific chest pain	Petechiae or ecchymosis	Orthopnea	Oliguria	Abdominal bloating	Anxiety or panic attacks
Fatigue	Diet	Paroxysmal nocturnal dyspnea	Anuria	Constipation	Depression
Weakness	Medication use	Pleurisy		Anorexia	Syncope
Orthostatic faintness		Cough		Nausea	Confusion
Palpitations		Hemoptysis		Vomiting	Decreased mental activity
		Wheezing		Diarrhea	

FIGURE 7-7. Use of clinical history in assessing heart failure. Gathering historical information that documents and clarifies the clinical presentation is the first important task when heart failure is suspected. Although dyspnea is a hallmark of heart failure, it can also be characteristic of other conditions [24]. During history taking, a cardinal issue is the attempt to quantify the exertion level required to produce symptoms [25]. By eliciting the factors that cause symptoms, insight into the syndrome's severity can be gained. The assessment of heart failure focuses on objectively measured parameters that quantify cardiac dysfunction and subsequent physical limitations. Weakness, fatigue, dyspnea, and edema are considered the most common symptoms of heart failure. Obtaining an ancillary history that elucidates concomitant cardiovascular and noncardiovascular illnesses is also critical, as is assessment of medication use [26]. Many drugs can exacerbate heart failure (eg, antiarrhythmic drugs, β-adrenergic blockers, calcium channel blockers, and nonsteroidal anti-inflammatory agents), depending on the clinical situation, and thus their use should be characterized.

PHYSICAL FINDINGS TO PURSUE WHEN EXAMINING PATIENTS WITH HEART FAILURE

VITAL SIGNS	PULMONARY SIGNS
Positional blood pressure	Rales
Pulse rate, rhythm, and quality	Rhonchi
Respiratory rate and pattern	Friction rub
Temperature	Wheezes
Blood pressure response to Valsalva's maneuver	Dullness to percussion
Determination of proportional pulse pressure	Diaphragmatic impairment

CARDIOVASCULAR SIGNS / **ABDOMINAL SIGNS**

CARDIOVASCULAR SIGNS	ABDOMINAL SIGNS
Neck-vein distention	Ascites
Abdominal-jugular neck-vein reflex	Hepatosplenomegaly
Cardiomegaly on palpation or percussion	Decreased bowel sounds
Chest wall pulsatile activity	Ileus
Gallop rhythm on auscultation	
Heart murmurs	**NEUROLOGIC SIGNS**
Diminished S_1 or S_2	Mental status abnormalities
Prominent P_2	**SYSTEMIC SIGNS**
Friction rub	Edema
	Cachexia
	Petechiae or ecchymosis
	Rash
	Arthritis

FIGURE 7-8. Physical findings to pursue when examining patients with heart failure. The physical examination of heart failure patients provides critical information that supplements data from the patient's history. Vital signs should be carefully measured. Positional blood pressure is important in patients receiving vasodilator drugs, as are pulse rate and rhythm. The presence of atrial fibrillation or frequent premature ventricular contractions has significant prognostic and therapeutic implications and can be suspected from analysis of the cardiac rhythm. The respiratory rate and pattern are important because tachypnea may reflect the severity of pulmonary congestion or compromise, and certain periodic respiratory patterns can be seen in the later stages of severe circulatory failure (eg, Cheyne-Stokes respirations).

Assessment of the blood pressure response to Valsalva's maneuver [27–29], calculation of proportional pulse pressure (pulse pressure divided by systolic pressure) [24], determination of augmented jugular vein distention after abdominal compression (hepatojugular reflux) [2–5,30,31], and thoracic percussion to identify cardiomegaly [34] are simple procedures that should be performed in every patient suspected of having heart failure or ventricular dysfunction. Distension of normally filled jugular veins or further distention of already filled jugular veins after gentle abdominal pressure suggests central venous congestion with volume overload. A proportional pulse pressure less than 0.25 has an 88% accuracy in predicting cardiac index less than 2.21/min/m². Cardiomegaly is suggested by a laterally displaced heart border detected by percussion [34]. The usual abnormalities searched for during cardiac examination, such as murmurs, rubs, and gallop sounds, must be sought.

Many findings that are routinely sought are well known and described, such as pulmonary rales, wheezes ("cardiac asthma"), ascites, and peripheral edema. Other findings, however, may be equally important and can provide insight into both the chronicity and the severity of disease. Cachexia, for example, points to long-standing heart failure that is often end-stage. Petechiae or ecchymoses suggest coagulopathy secondary to hepatic congestion. Examination of the integument can point toward the presence of systemic disease (eg, scleroderma, myxedema).

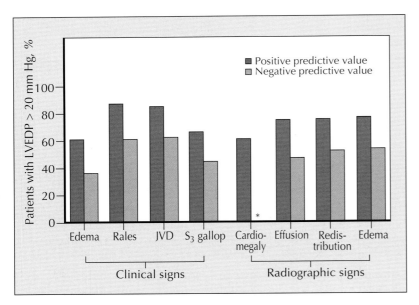

FIGURE 7-9. Predictive values of clinical findings in congestive heart failure (CHF) patients. Many studies have reviewed the clinical and radiographic findings often used to diagnose CHF [2–5,26,35–40]. These reports have consistently emphasized that, although in certain circumstances clinical findings might be quite accurate in the diagnosis of CHF, their reliability in predicting hemodynamics is limited. Absence of radiographic or physical signs of congestion does not necessarily ensure a normal pulmonary capillary wedge pressure, for example, and may lead to either an inaccurate diagnosis of heart failure or inadequate therapy [33].

This figure demonstrates that in one study of 52 consecutive patients with chronic CHF [33], detection of peripheral edema, pulmonary rales, jugular venous distension (JVD), and an S_3 gallop had positive predictive values ranging from 61% to 87%. Chest radiographic findings, such as cardiomegaly, pleural effusion, vascular redistribution suggesting congestion, and frank pulmonary edema, had similar positive and negative predictive values. The negative predictive value of cardiomegaly on chest radiography was not calculated (*asterisk*) because all but three patients had this finding. Thus, no single finding alone can be used to make the diagnosis [34–38]. LVEDP—left ventricular end-diastolic pressure.

LABORATORY TESTS TO CONSIDER DURING ASSESSMENT OF PATIENTS WITH HEART FAILURE

Complete blood count (including white blood cell differential and platelet count)
Serum electrolyte level
Blood urea nitrogen
Serum creatinine (and clearance) level
Liver function tests
Prothrombin time
Erythrocyte sedimentation rate
Arterial blood gases (possibly with exercise) levels
Urinalysis
Biochemistry screen (*ie*, magnesium, uric acid, calcium, and phosphorus levels)
Thyroid function studies
Serum drug levels (*ie*, digoxin and anti-arrhythmic drugs)
BNP level

FIGURE 7-10. Laboratory tests for assessment of patients with heart failure. A variety of laboratory studies should be considered during assessment of the patient with heart failure. In general, these studies help in estimating the severity of heart failure and provide information regarding problems that can be anticipated with therapeutic interventions. Some of these studies should be obtained (*eg*, thyroid function studies) in an attempt to diagnose causes of left ventricular dysfunction. Others are ordered to give insight into therapeutic or toxic effects of drugs commonly administered to patients with heart failure. Not all tests listed are necessary in every patient with heart failure. Ordinarily, sophisticated measures of plasma neurohumors, such as epinephrine, norepinephrine, vasopressin, renin, and so on, are not necessary or helpful in the diagnosis and management of individual patients with heart failure (although their importance with respect to the pathophysiology of the syndrome is unquestioned). Cowie *et al.* [10] demonstrated that in patients with symptoms suspected by a primary care physician to be due to heart failure, brain natriuretic peptide seemed a useful predictor of which patients are likely to have heart failure and require further clinical evaluation.

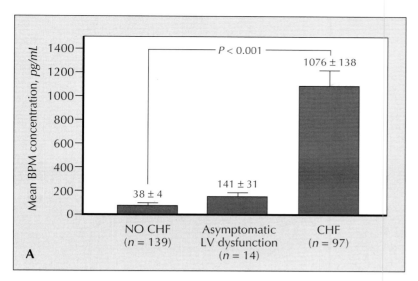

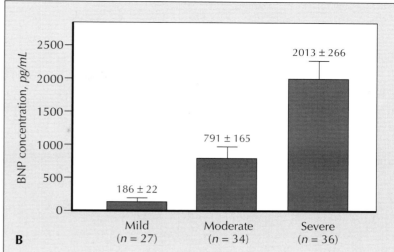

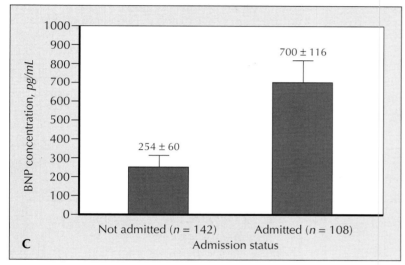

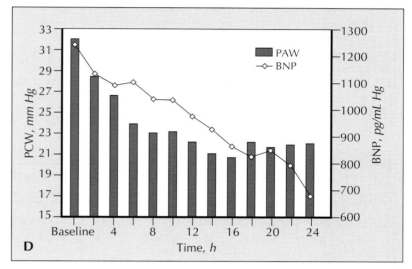

FIGURE 7-11. Brain natriuretic peptide (BNP) as a diagnostic tool in heart failure (*see also* Fig. 7-12). Point-of-care BNP levels have been studied by Maisel *et al.* [15], Kazanegra *et al.* [16], and Cheng *et al.* [17] extensively. **A,** BNP levels were stratified quite dramatically according to whether patients presenting to an emergency department with symptoms possibly related to heart failure were evaluated. The mean BNP concentration in patients with no congestive heart failure, in the end, was $38 \geq 4$ pg/mL compared to those patients with manifest congestive heart failure (BNP level of $1076 \geq 138$ pg/mL). Patients with left ventricular systolic dysfunction but no significant symptoms or findings of congestion have elevated BNP levels, but not

nearly to the point noted in individuals with manifest congestive heart failure (**A**).

B, BNP concentrations in comparison to the severity of congestive heart failure with those most limited and congested having the highest serum BNP level. **C,** Higher BNP levels in patients admitted to the hospital from the emergency department for therapy of decompensated congestive heart failure. **D,** The correlation between BNP level and pulmonary capillary wedge pressure during treatment with diuretics and vasodilators in the hospital. Interestingly, there is a close correlation between BNP and pulmonary artery wedge pressure that can be tracked as close as every 15 minutes.

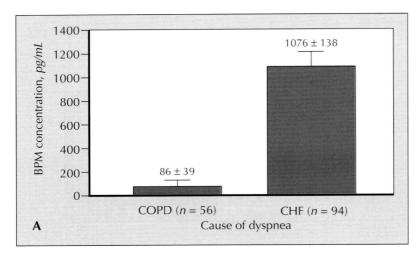

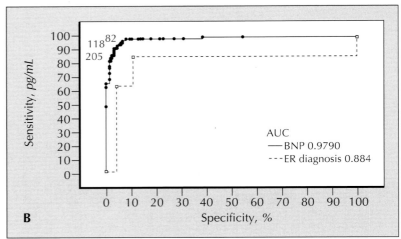

FIGURE 7-12. Brain natriuretic peptide (BNP) as a diagnostic tool in heart failure (*see also* Fig. 7-11). **A,** The utility of point-of-care BNP levels used in an emergency department setting to clarify confusing presentations. Patients with dyspnea secondary to chronic obstructive pulmonary disease had low BNP levels versus those individuals having a significant component of congestive heart failure, as demonstrated by Maisel *et al.* [15], Kazanegra *et al.* [16], and Cheng *et al.* [17]. **B,** Receiver-operator curve (ROC) data for BNP levels and the emergency department diagnosis of

congestive heart failure suggesting that a BNP level greater than 80 pg/mL could, with a diagnostic accuracy of 95%, differentiate congestive heart failure from other problems presenting in a similar vein. **C,** Patients under- and over-diagnosed in the Maisel *et al.* study [15]. Studies to date of point-of-care BNP assays suggest that a level greater than 80 pg/mL is an important discriminator between congestive heart failure and other clinical problems. As discussed in chapter 8, BNP levels also can provide prognostic information.

DIAGNOSTIC PROCEDURES TO CONSIDER DURING ASSESSMENT OF PATIENTS WITH HEART FAILURE

Aerobic exercise capacity testing	Chest radiography	Electrocardiogram
Oxygen utilization at maximal exertion	Cardiac fluoroscopy	Ambulatory electrocardiogram
Time to anaerobic threshold	CT	Electrophysiologic study
Cardiac catheterization		Magnetic resonance imaging
Aortography	Echocardiogram	Positron-emission tomography
Coronary angiography	M-mode	Pulmonary function testing
Hemodynamic assessment	Pulsed Doppler	Radionuclide angiogram
Ventriculography	Two-dimensional	Scintigraphic perfusion studies

FIGURE 7-13. Diagnostic procedures for assessment of patients with heart failure. There are many ancillary diagnostic tests to be considered during evaluation of the heart failure patient. These range from rather simple procedures, such as chest radiography and electrocardiography, to sophisticated studies, such as magnetic resonance imaging and positron-emission tomography.

Whereas some are noninvasive, others, such as cardiac catheterization, require central vascular access. In planning assessment of the patient with heart failure, the risks, costs, and the type of information they can provide should dictate the selection of diagnostic tests.

DIAGNOSTIC TESTS AND THE INFORMATION THEY PROVIDE DURING ASSESSMENT OF HEART FAILURE

CHEST RADIOGRAPHY AND
CARDIAC FLUOROSCOPY

Cardiothoracic ratio
Selective chamber size and shape
Cardiac or great vessel calcification
Pulmonary vascularity and congestion
Pleural effusions
Mass lesions or infiltrates
Mediastinal configuration
Great vessel abnormality

ELECTROCARDIOGRAPHY

Rhythm
  Atrial fibrillation
  Ventricular arrhythmias
  Atrioventricular conduction
Heart rate
Evidence of hypertrophy
Q waves
"P" mitrale or pulmonale
Conduction disturbances
Metabolic and drug effects (ST, T changes)

ECHOCARDIOGRAPHY
(TWO-DIMENSIONAL AND M-MODE)

Chamber size and shape
Valve integrity and motion
Fractional shortening of ventricles
Mean circumferential fiber shortening
Mitral E-point to septal separation
Systolic wall thickening
Wall motion analysis
Estimation of wall stress
Endomyocardial biopsy guidance
Exercise and pharmacologic stress (wall
  motion)
Tissue characterization
Pericardial effusion
Pericardial restriction

DOPPLER ECHOCARDIOGRAPHY
(PULSED AND CONTINUOUS WAVE)

Quantification of valve stenosis and
  regurgitation
  Estimation of pulmonary artery pressure
  Estimation of stroke volume and cardiac
  output
Determination of diastolic filling
  characteristics
Detection of shunts

FIGURE 7-14. Common ancillary diagnostic tests. The most commonly requested diagnostic tests in patients with heart failure are chest radiography, electrocardiography, and echocardiography (including M-mode, two-dimensional, and Doppler studies).

The chest radiogram can provide insight into cardiac size, pleural effusions, pulmonary congestion, and mediastinal configuration. Electrocardiography may suggest ischemic heart disease.

Echocardiography (M-mode, two-dimensional, or Doppler) provides an evaluation of the valves, chambers, pericardium, myocardium, and global function. More information is probably gained by echocardiographic examination of heart failure patients than by any other tests available.

A. NONINVASIVE IMAGING TECHNIQUES FOR ASSESSMENT OF PATIENTS WITH HEART FAILURE

OBSERVATION	FIRST-PASS RNVG	EQUILIBRIUM RNVG	MRI	CT
Anatomic relationships	0/+	+	++++	+++
Tissue characterization	0	0	+++	+++
Wall motion	++	++++	+++	+++
Hypertrophy	0	0/+	++++	+++
Wall thickening	0	0	++++	++
Valvular regurgitation and stenosis	0	0	++	+
Hemodynamics	0	0	0	0
Diastolic function	++	++	+	0
Stress exercise	++++	++++	0	0
Pharmacologic stress	++++	++++	+	+
Lower cost and easy availability	+++	+++	+	+

B. NONINVASIVE IMAGING TECHNIQUES FOR ASSESSMENT OF PATIENTS WITH HEART FAILURE

OBSERVATION	M-MODE ECHOCARDIOGRAPHY	TWO-DIMENSIONAL ECHOCARDIOGRAPHY	DOPPLER
Anatomic relationships	+	+++	0/+
Tissue characterization	++	++	0
Wall motion	+	++++	0
Hypertrophy	+++	++++	0
Wall thickening	+++	+++	0
Valvular regurgitation and stenosis	++	++	++++
Hemodynamics	+	+	++++
Diastolic function	++	+++	++++
Stress exercise	++++	++++	++++
Pharmacologic stress	+	++++	++
Lower cost and easy availability	++++	++++	+++

FIGURE 7-15. Noninvasive imaging techniques for assessment of patients with heart failure. A variety of noninvasive techniques can be used to provide greater insight into ventricular performance and to aid in the assessment of heart failure.

A, In addition to radionuclide techniques and echocardiography, magnetic resonance imaging (MRI) and computed tomographic (CT) studies can be valuable. MRI defines cardiac anatomy, clarifies anatomic relationships, characterizes tissue patterns, and may be the best method to quantify cardiac mass and chamber dimensions. It is, however, expensive. The major limitation of CT scans of the heart are the long exposure times required for the motion artifacts to be great. The major advantage of this form of cardiac imaging is that cross-sectional views with spatial and density orientation can be produced and appear to be better than echocardiographic or radionuclide studies. CT scans also provide precise images of great-vessel orientation. Performance of stress testing, either physiologic or pharmacologic, can be difficult in the MRI or CT facility.

B, In general, echocardiography is readily available and costs less than radionuclide, MRI, or CT procedures. Echocardiography may be valuable and cost-effective when simple questions such as normal versus abnormal ventricular function or presence of pericardial effusion are asked. *Zero* represents no value; *plus signs* represent the relative value, *one plus sign* meaning minimal value and *four plus signs* meaning very valuable. RNGV—radionuclide ventriculography. (*Adapted from* Young and Farmer [1].)

NYHA CLASS (SYMPTOM SEVERITY)	METS (mL O_2/kg/min)	WEBER-JANICKI STAGE (min)	SPEED, mph	ELEVATION, %	BRUCE STAGE (min)	SPEED, mph	ELEVATION, %	NAUGHTON STAGE (min)	SPEED, mph	ELEVATION, %
IV — Severe	1.0(3.5)									
III — Moderate to severe	1.5(5.3)									
II — Mild to moderate	2.0(7.0)									
I — Minimal or asymptomatic	2.5(8.8)	1(2)	1.0	0				1(3)	1.0	0
	3.0(10.5)							2(3)	1.5	0
	3.5(12.3)	2(2)	1.5	0				3(3)	2.0	0
	4.0(14.0)							4(3)	2.0	3.5
	4.5(15.8)	3(2)	2.0	3.5				5(3)	2.0	7.0
	5.0(17.5)									
	5.5(19.3)	4(2)	2.0	7.0	1(3)	1.7	10.0	6(3)	3.0	5.0
	6.0(21.0)									
	6.5(22.8)	5(2)	2.0	10.5				7(3)	3.0	7.5
	7.0(24.5)									
	7.5(26.3)	6(2)	3.0	7.5				8(3)	3.0	10.0
	8.0(28.0)									
	8.5(29.8)	7(2)	3.0	10.0	2(3)	2.5	12.0	9(3)	3.0	12.5
	9.0(31.5)									
	9.5(33.3)	8(2)	3.0	12.5	3(3)	3.4	14.0	10(3)	3.0	15.0
	10.0(35.0)									
	10.5(36.8)	9(2)	3.0	15.0						
	11.0(38.5)	10(2)	3.4	14.0						
	11.5(40.3)									
	12.0(42.0)									
	12.5(43.8)									
	13.0(45.5)				4(3)	4.2	16.0			

FIGURE 7-16. Exercise testing in patients with heart failure. Maximal myocardial oxygen consumption (MVO$_2$) is defined as the greatest amount of oxygen a patient can utilize while performing dynamic aerobic exercise that utilizes large muscle masses. It reflects oxygen transport and cellular metabolism. MVO$_2$ is usually expressed as milliliters of oxygen consumed per kilogram of body weight per minute. Exercise performance can be described in "metabolic equivalents" (METS). One MET is defined as 3.5 mL O$_2$/kg/min and reflects the quantity of oxygen utilized when an individual is sitting or resting quietly. World-class endurance athletes can achieve 18 METS during maximal exercise (reflecting 60 mL O$_2$/kg/min MVO$_2$). Patients with coronary heart disease capable of achieving 10 METS (or 35 mL O$_2$/kg/min MVO$_2$) have excellent prognoses. On the other hand, patients able to obtain peak exercise of 5 METS or less have poor prognoses [39–41]. Exercise testing in heart failure is performed to quantify functional capacity. Shown are six commonly used exercise protocols. In general, the best estimate of MVO$_2$ in a heart failure patient can be accomplished with protocols that increase physical stress loads gradually, such as the Weber-Janicki and Naughton protocols (A), and the Balke and Branching protocols (B). (continued)

NYHA CLASS (SYMPTOM SEVERITY)	METS (mL O₂/kg/min)	ELLESTAD STAGE (min)	ELLESTAD SPEED, mph	ELLESTAD ELEVATION, %	BALKE STAGE (min)	BALKE SPEED, mph	BALKE ELEVATION, %	BRANCHING STAGE (min)	BRANCHING SPEED, mph	BRANCHING ELEVATION, %
IV Severe / III Moderate to severe / II Mild to moderate / I Minimal or asymptomatic	1.0(3.5)									
	1.5(5.3)									
	2.0(7.0)							BRANCH I		
	2.5(8.8)				1(2)	3.0	0	1(2)	1.9	0
	3.0(10.5)									
	3.5(12.3)							2(2)	2.6	0
	4.0(14.0)				2(2)	3.0	2.5	3(2)	2.6	3.0
	4.5(15.8)							4(2)	2.6	6.0
	5.0(17.5)	1(3)	1.7	10.0	3(2)	3.0	5.0	5(2)	2.6	9.0
	5.5(19.3)							6(2)	2.6	12.0
	6.0(21.0)				4(2)	3.0	7.5	7(2)	2.6	15.0
	6.5(22.8)							8(2)	2.6	17.5
	7.0(24.5)	2(2)	3.0	10.0	5(2)	3.0	10.0	9(2)	2.6	20.0
	7.5(26.3)							10(2)	2.6	22.0
	8.0(28.0)				6(2)	3.0	12.0			
	8.5(29.8)	3(2)	4.0	10.0				BRANCH II		
	9.0(31.5)				7(2)	3.0	15.0	3.4–4.4 METs		
	9.5(33.3)							BRANCH III		
	10.0(35.0)				8(2)	3.0	17.5	3.9–4.9 METs		
	10.5(36.8)							BRANCH IV		
	11.0(38.5)				9(2)	3.0	20.0	4.5–5.3 METs		
	11.5(40.3)									
	12.0(42.0)				10(2)	3.0	22.5			
	12.5(43.8)									
	13.0(45.5)	4(3)	5.0	10.0						

FIGURE 7-16. (*continued*) Protocols that rapidly increase stress levels, such as the Bruce (**A**) and Ellstead (**B**) protocols, are more suitable for the screening of patients for the presence of ischemic heart disease than for quantifying functional limitations resulting from ventricular dysfunction. Although values for peak oxygen uptake can be estimated from exercise workload, online measured values of oxygen consumption may more accurately reflect cardiac impairment and allow differentiation between cardiac and pulmonary pathophysiology. Several additional parameters are important to take into consideration during exercise. These include ability to augment systolic blood pressure, the onset of the anaerobic threshold (when gas exchange is measured online), and electrocardiographic changes such as ST-segment abnormalities (possibly reflecting ischemia) or development of cardiac arrhythmias. NYHA—New York Heart Association. (*Adapted from* Young and Farmer [1].)

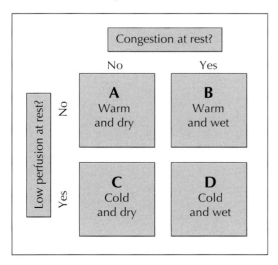

	Congestion at rest?	
	No	Yes
No (Low perfusion at rest?)	**A** Warm and dry	**B** Warm and wet
Yes	**C** Cold and dry	**D** Cold and wet

FIGURE 7-17. Rapid classification of hemodynamic states. Stevenson [42] popularized the concept of tailoring therapies to hemodynamic status of patients. This approach can be coupled to a noninvasive diagnostic evaluation of patients admitted to the hospital with congestive heart failure with therapeutic approaches, perhaps, directed by varying combinations of fluid retention states and peripheral organ perfusion. The two basic components outlined in this figure are, indeed, congestion (B and C) and low perfusion (C and D). Perhaps the most complex patient is the individual who is substantially volume overloaded with low flow states (D). These patients as well as those with simply low perfusion states are generally in cardiogenic shock. Signs and symptoms of congestion to review include orthopnea, paroxysmal nocturnal dyspnea, jugular venous distention, hepatomegaly, particularly with hepatojugular reflux, peripheral edema, presence of rales (remembering that they can be rare in chronic heart failure), and the Valsalva square wave blood pressure sign. Signs of low perfusion include a narrow pulse pressure, a sleepy or obtunded patient, periodic respirations, cool extremities, hypotension after angiotensin-converting enzyme inhibitor introduction, and renal dysfunction or a low serum sodium [42].

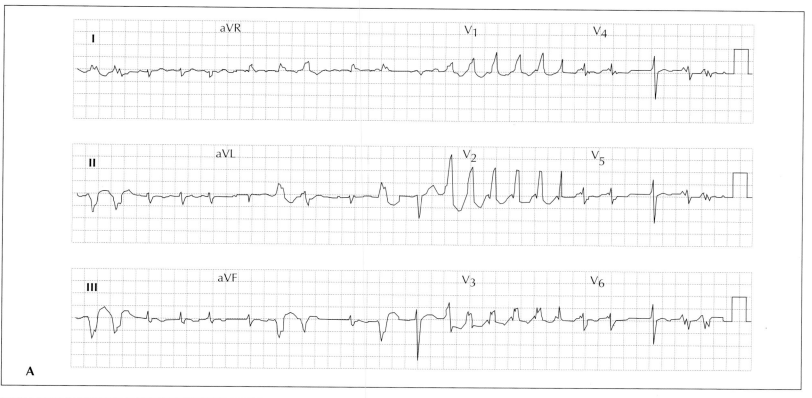

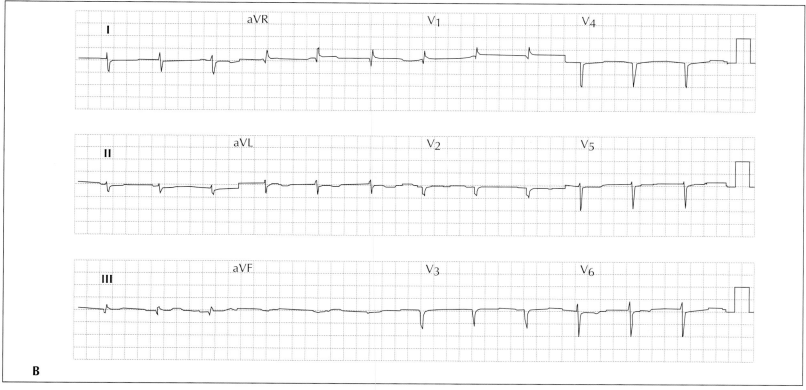

FIGURE 7-18. Electrocardiography in heart failure patients. An electrocardiogram (ECG) can provide valuable information in the assessment of patients with heart failure. These examples represent commonly observed findings in severe heart failure. **A,** Low voltage and arrhythmia. This ECG demonstrates a right bundle branch block pattern and low voltage throughout the limb leads and precordium. Premature ventricular contractions, couplets, and nonsustained ventricular tachycardia are also seen. This patient has severe coronary heart disease with multiple myocardial infarctions and an ejection fraction of 15%. **B,** Cardiomyopathy. Patients with dilated cardiomyopathy may have Q waves (*see* precordial leads), which can lead to the mistaken diagnosis of myocardial infarction. This patient did not have coronary heart disease. The tracing also shows low voltage throughout, an interventricular conduction defect pattern, and nonspecific ST-T wave changes.

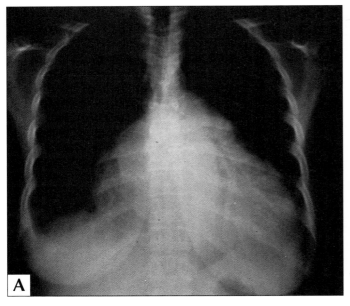

A

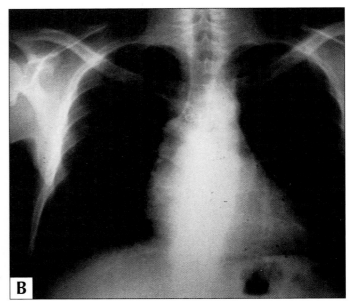

B

FIGURE 7-19. Chest radiographs of patients with heart failure. **A,** Congestive heart failure with cardiomegaly. This radiograph demonstrates cardiomegaly (cardiothoracic ratio, 0.77), pulmonary congestion, and bilateral pleural effusions (note blunted costophrenic angles). The cardiac silhouette may indicate the existence of a pericardial effusion. Also note the thin chest wall and osteopenia suggesting cachexia.

B, Congestive heart failure with left ventricular hypertrophy. This radiograph demonstrates mild pulmonary congestion with a high-normal cardiothoracic ratio of 0.53. These radiographic findings are typical of patients with hypertensive heart disease or hypertrophic cardiomyopathy resulting in diastolic dysfunction in the presence of a normal ejection fraction.

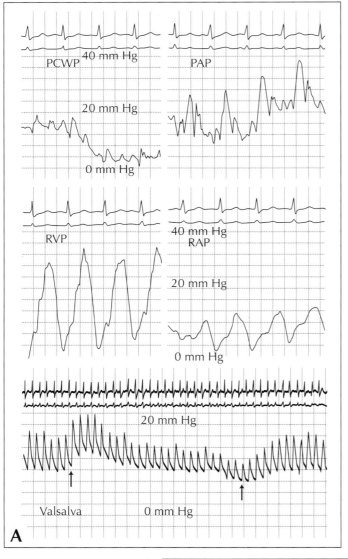

A

FIGURE 7-20. Hemodynamics in heart failure patients. **A,** Hemodynamic findings obtained during routine surveillance by right heart catheterization and endomyocardial biopsy in a patient 5 years after heart transplantation. The patient complained of mild dyspnea on exertion, but was well compensated and could perform ordinary daily activities. During maximal exercise, he achieved a myocardial oxygen consumption (MVO_2) of 18 mL O_2/kg/min. Although the patient was moderately hypertensive (blood pressure, 170/100 mm Hg), intracardiac and pulmonary pressures were at the upper limits of normal. Right atrial pressure (RAP) was slightly elevated with a paradoxic increase during inspiration, a characteristic finding with orthotopic allografts. The patient's cardiac output was 4.7 L/min. Valsalva's maneuver in this patient is not entirely normal, since it does not exhibit the "overshoot" phenomenon seen in patients with normal ventricular function. This patient's ejection fraction was 47%. *(continued)*

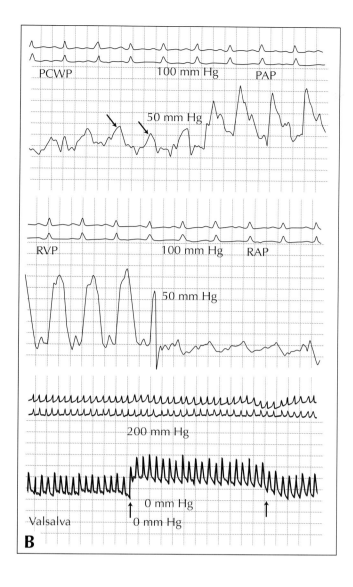

B

FIGURE 7-20. *(continued)* **B,** Hemodynamic findings from a patient with cardiomyopathy and severe systolic and diastolic dysfunction: a 45-year-old man with end-stage cardiomyopathy believed to be caused by excessive alcohol consumption. The patient's ejection fraction is 15%. Cardiac output is 2.9 L/min, and the systemic blood pressure is 103/82 mm Hg. The patient has severe pulmonary hypertension (pulmonary artery pressure [PAP] of 87/35 mm Hg with pulmonary capillary wedge pressure [PCWP] of 35 mm Hg). Valsalva's maneuver in this patient is markedly abnormal, demonstrating the "square wave" pattern characteristic of severe left ventricular dysfunction. RVP—right ventricular pressure.

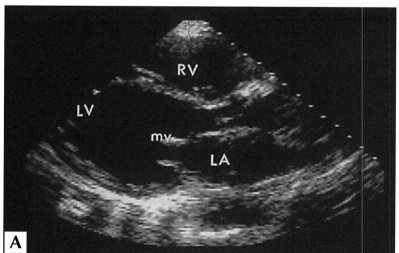

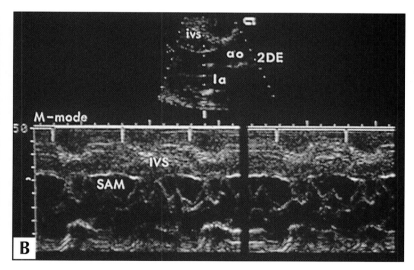

FIGURE 7-21. Echocardiographic patterns in heart failure. Information obtained with an echocardiogram can help clarify a patient's complaints and certain physical findings. **A,** Dilated cardiomyopathy. This long-axis parasternal view from a two-dimensional echocardiogram demonstrates the multichamber enlargement characteristic of dilated cardiomyopathy. No evidence of pericardial effusion is present, even though the patient had a paradoxical drop in systolic blood pressure of 10 mm Hg with inspiration (systolic pressure starting at 90 mm Hg). The left ventricular (LV) wall is symmetrically thin, and in real time, no focal wall motion abnormalities are seen. Rather, the entire LV is hypokinetic, and the ejection fraction is calculated to be only 15%.

B, Hypertrophic cardiomyopathy. M-mode and two-dimensional (2DE) echocardiographic findings of severe LV hypertrophy with evidence of outflow tract obstruction (systolic anterior motion [SAM] of the mitral valve). In systole, the LV cavity becomes virtually obliterated, and the ejection fraction is calculated to be greater than 75%. The interventricular septum (IVS) is dramatically thickened. The patient complained of chest pain and severe dyspnea on exertion, and he also had syncope. *(continued)*

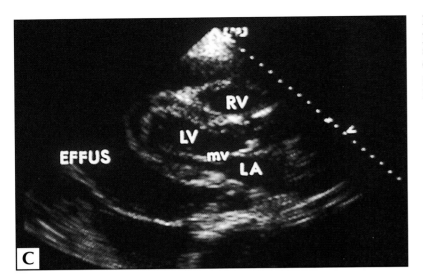

FIGURE 7-21. *(continued)* **C,** Pericardial effusion (EFFUS). This patient has normal right and left ventricular chamber size and systolic function, but a large pericardial effusion is present. Clinically, the patient was hypotensive and complained of shortness of breath. ao—aorta; LA—left atrium; mv—mitral valve; RV—right ventricle.

DESIGNING A THERAPEUTIC PLAN

QUESTIONS AFTER ASSESSMENT TO DETERMINE THERAPEUTIC STRATEGY

Is heart failure present?

Is the problem primarily systolic or diastolic dysfunction?

What caused the problem?

What precipitated deterioration?

How severe is the heart failure?

What is the prognosis?

What is the best acute therapeutic strategy?

What is the best chronic therapeutic strategy?

Can the initiating/precipitating problem be cured or eliminated, and can the state of heart failure be ameliorated or attenuated?

FIGURE 7-22. Integration of diagnostic evaluation in the assessment of patients with heart failure. Data obtained during the assessment of patients with heart failure can be used to answer several key questions. It is critical to determine if heart failure is present, what caused the difficulty or precipitated deterioration, and how severe the syndrome is. When these questions are answered, insight into the patient's long-term prognosis can be gained and therapeutic strategies can be designed to address both acute and chronic problems as well as the initiating or precipitating causes.

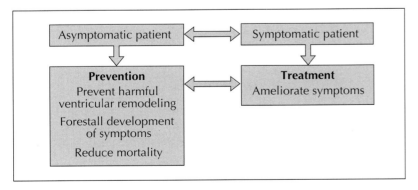

FIGURE 7-23. Coupling heart failure assessment with therapeutic philosophy. Therapy of heart failure should be designed to prevent ventricular remodeling, forestall development of clinical symptoms, ameliorate symptoms, and reduce mortality. Treatment strategies are based on data obtained during clinical assessment, particularly during risk stratification of both symptomatic and asymptomatic patients. Patients sometimes alternate between compensation and decompensation or asymptomatic and symptomatic states, and treatment protocols should reflect an ongoing assessment of a patient's clinical status.

REFERENCES

1. Young JB, Farmer JA: The diagnostic evaluation of patients with heart failure. In *Congestive Heart Failure: Pathophysiology, Diagnosis, and Comprehensive Approach to Management*. Edited by Hosenpud JD, Greenberg BH. New York: Springer-Verlag; 1994:597–621.

2. Badgett RG, Lucey CR, Mujrow CD: Can the clinical examination diagnose left sided heart failure in adults? *JAMA* 1997, 277:1712–1719.

3. Tresch DD: The clinical diagnosis of heart failure in older patients. *J Am Geriatr Soc* 1997, 45:1128–1133.

4. Cohn JN: Jugular venous pressure monitoring: a lost art? *J Cardiac Failure* 1997, 3:71–73.

5. McGee SR: Physical examination of venous pressure: a critical review. *Am Heart J* 1998, 136:10–18.

6. Armstrong PW, Moe GW: Medical advances in the treatment of congestive heart failure. *Circulation* 1994, 88:2941–2952.

7. Cohn JN: The prevention of heart failure: a new agenda [editorial]. *N Engl J Med* 1992, 327:725–726.

8. Feldman AM: Can we alter survival in patients with congestive heart failure? *JAMA* 1992, 267:1956–1961.

9. Parrish DL, Grayburn PA: Use of echocardiography in patients with congestive heart failure. *Cardiol Rev* 1998, 6:203–212.

10. Cowie MR, Struthers AD, Wood DA, *et al.*: Volume of natriuretic peptides in assessment of patients with possible new heart failure in primary care. *Lancet* 1997, 350:1349–1353.

11. Gaasch WH: Diagnosis and treatment of heart failure based on left ventricular systolic or diastolic dysfunction. *JAMA* 1994, 271:1276–1280.

12. Ghali JK, Cooper R, Ford E: Trends in hospitalization rates for heart failure in the United States, 1973–1986. *Arch Intern Med* 1992, 152:649–655.

13. Kannel WB, Belanger AJ: Epidemiology of heart failure. *Am Heart J* 1991, 121:951–957.

14. McKee PA, Castelli WP, McNamara PM, *et al.*: The natural history of congestive heart failure: the Framingham Study. *N Engl J Med* 1971, 285:1441–1446.

15. Maisel A: B-type natriuretic peptide levels: a potential novel "white count" for congestive heart failure. *J Card Fail* 2001, 7:183–193.

16. Kazanegra R, Cheng V, Garcia A, *et al.*: A rapid test for B-type natriuretic peptide correlates with falling wedge pressures in patients treated for decompensated heart failure: a pilot study. *J Card Fail* 2001, 7:21–29.

17. Cheng V, Kazanegra R, Garcia A, *et al.*: A rapid bedside test for B-type peptide predicts treatment outcomes in patients admitted for decompensated heart failure. *J Am Coll Cardiol* 2001, 37:386–391.

18. The CONSENSUS Trial Study Group: Effects of enalapril on mortality in severe congestive heart failure. *N Engl J Med* 1987, 316:1429–1435.

19. The SOLVD Investigators: Effect of enalapril on mortality and the development of heart failure in asymptomatic patients with reduced left ventricular ejection fractions. *N Engl J Med* 1992, 327:685–691.

20. Pfeffer MA, Braunwald E, Moyé LA, *et al.*: Effect of captopril on mortality and morbidity in patients with left ventricular dysfunction after myocardial infarction: results of the Survival and Ventricular Enlargement Trial. *N Engl J Med* 1992, 327:668–677.

21. Cohn JN, Archibald DG, Ziesche S, *et al.*: Effect of vasodilator therapy on mortality in chronic congestive heart failure: results of a Veterans Administration Cooperative Study. *N Engl J Med* 1986, 314:1547–1552.

22. The SOLVD Investigators: Effect of enalapril on survival in patients with reduced left ventricular ejection fractions and congestive heart failure. *N Engl J Med* 1991, 325:293–302.

23. Packer M, Carver JR, Rodeheffer RJ, *et al.*: Effect of oral milrinone on mortality in severe chronic heart failure. *N Engl J Med* 1991, 325:1468–1475.

24. Stevenson LW, Perloff JK: The limited reliability of physical signs for estimating hemodynamics in chronic heart failure. *JAMA* 1989, 261:884–888.

25. Szlachcic J, Massie BM, Kramer BL, *et al.*: Correlates and prognostic implication of exercise capacity in chronic congestive heart failure. *Am J Cardiol* 1985, 55:1037–1042.

26. Young JB, Weiner DH, Pratt CM, *et al.*: Relationship of ejection fraction and symptomatic status to medication use in patients with heart failure: a report from Studies of Left Ventricular Dysfunction (SOLVD) Registry. *South Med J* 1994, 88:414–423.

27. Zema MJ, Caccovano M, Kligfield P: Detection of left ventricular dysfunction in ambulatory subjects with the bedside Valsalva maneuver. *Am J Med* 1983, 75:241–248.

28. Zema MJ, Restivo Bernard, Sos T, *et al.*: Left ventricular dysfunction: bedside Valsalva manoeuvre. *Br Heart J* 1980, 44:560–590.

29. Zema MJ, Masters AP, Margouleff D: Dyspnea: the heart or the lungs? Differentiation at bedside by use of the simple Valsalva maneuver. *Chest* 1984, 85:59–64.

30. Ewy GA: The abdominojugular test: technique and hemodynamic correlates. *Ann Intern Med* 1988, 109:456–460.

31. Butman SM, Ewy GA, Standen JR, *et al.*: Bedside cardiovascular examination in patients with severe chronic heart failure: importance of rest or inducible jugular venous distension. *J Am Coll Cardiol* 1993, 22:968–974.

32. Heckerling PS, Wiener SL, Wolfkiel CJ, *et al.*: Accuracy and reproducibility of precordial percussion and palpation for detecting increased left ventricular end-diastolic volume and mass: a comparison of physical findings and ultrafast computed tomography of the heart. *JAMA* 1993, 270:1943–1948.

33. Chakko S, Woska D, Martinez H, *et al.*: Clinical, radiographic, and hemodynamic correlations in chronic congestive heart failure: conflicting results may lead to inappropriate care. *Am J Med* 1991, 90:353–359.

34. Gahli JK, Kadakia S, Cooper RS, Liao Y: Bedside diagnosis of preserved versus impaired left ventricular systolic function in heart failure. *Am J Cardiol* 1991, 67:1002–1006.

35. Goldman L, Hashimoto B, Cook EF, Loscalzo A: Comparative reproducibility and validity of systems for assessing cardiovascular functional class: advantages of a new specific activity scale. *Circulation* 1981, 64:1227–1234.

36. Remes J, Miettinen H, Reunanen A, *et al.*: Validity of clinical diagnosis of heart failure in primary health care. *Eur Heart J* 1991, 12:315–321.

37. Packer M: Clinical trials in congestive heart failure: why do studies report conflicting results [editorial]? *Ann Intern Med* 1988, 109:3–5.

38. Marantz PR, Alderman MH, Tobin JN: Diagnostic heterogeneity in clinical trials for congestive heart failure. *Ann Intern Med* 1988, 109:55–61.

39. Morris CK, Ueshima K, Kawaguchi T, *et al.*: The prognostic value of exercise capacity: a review of the literature. *Am Heart J* 1991, 122:1423–1431.

40. Mancini DM, Eisen H, Kussmaul W, *et al.*: Value of peak exercise oxygen consumption for optimal timing of cardiac transplantation in ambulatory patients with heart failure. *Circulation* 1991, 83:778–786.

41. Mills RM Jr, Haught WH: Evaluation of heart failure patients: objective parameters to assess functional capacity. *Clin Cardiol* 1996, 19:455–460.

42. Stevenson LW: Tailored therapy to hemodynamic goals for advanced heart failure. *Eur J Heart Failure* 1999, 1:251–257.

PROGNOSTIC INDICATORS AND ASSESSMENT OF THERAPEUTIC RESPONSES

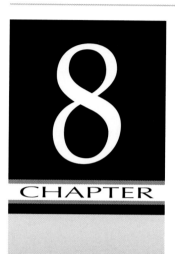

8

CHAPTER

Henry Ooi and Jay N. Cohn

The diagnosis of heart failure carries a risk of mortality comparable to that of the major malignancies. In the past 20 years, advances in understanding the pathophysiology of heart failure and new developments in treatment have added substantially to the physician's ability to alleviate the symptoms of this disease, slow the natural progression of the underlying myocardial process, and improve survival. However, the prognosis remains generally poor, and the expanding range of therapeutic options has greatly increased the complexity of treating these patients. It has become increasingly important to identify factors that may predict clinical outcome or response to therapy, thus allowing rational selection of therapy for individual patients.

Heart failure deaths increase exponentially with age, and deaths occur suddenly and unexpectedly without any evidence of recent hemodynamic or functional deterioration in about 30% to 50% of patients with chronic heart disease. The proportion of deaths that are sudden tend to be higher during earlier stages of the disease, *ie*, in patients with mild to moderate symptoms of chronic heart failure. However, the reliable identification of patients at increased risk of sudden death remains a problem.

Numerous hemodynamic, structural, biochemical, and functional variables have been identified as prognostic markers that can be used to place patients in different risk strata. Predictions regarding life expectancy are best made by considering several prognostic variables, but useful statistical models are not available. Therefore, in evaluating the cost-effective use of medications and surgical interventions, the physician must make qualitative assessments of the patient's risk and likelihood of benefiting from therapy.

Assessment of therapeutic response entails the examination of multiple endpoints. Two of the most important potential benefits of medical therapy—the prevention of premature mortality and hospital admissions for heart failure—are impossible for the physician to assess in patient management. Surrogate endpoints for these important benefits would be helpful, and monitoring changes in plasma brain natriuretic peptide (BNP) levels with treatment has shown promise. Nevertheless, patients should be treated with interventions that have been shown to reduce the incidence of death and hospitalization when the potential for benefit outweighs the adverse effects and costs. The effects of heart failure and its treatment on a patient's quality of life can and should be evaluated by systematic inquiry. A self-administered questionnaire has been developed and validated as a measure of therapeutic response. Use of a peak exercise test to evaluate the response to therapy may provide data supporting an effect, but may not necessarily reflect a symptomatic or clinically important benefit of therapy.

Looking to the future, genetic polymorphisms, for example of the β_2-adrenergic receptor, have been identified that may significantly impact on the pathophysiology of heart failure or predict an individual's response to drug therapy. Further study is required to validate these results before they can be widely applied to predict outcome or response to treatment.

MORTALITY IN PATIENTS WITH HEART FAILURE

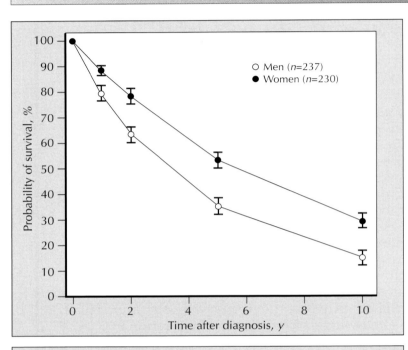

FIGURE 8-1. Survival after the clinical diagnosis of congestive heart failure from 1948 to 1988 in the Framingham Heart Study [1]. Even though individuals who died within 90 days of the diagnosis were excluded, median survival after recognition of heart failure in men was only 3.2 years. Women also had a poor, but better, survival rate, with a median survival time of 5.4 years. Although the difference in survival compared with a control group without heart failure (similar in age and concurrent diseases) was not established, development of clinical heart failure clearly is associated with a poor prognosis. There were no differences in survival between the cohorts who developed heart failure from 1948 to 1974 and those who developed heart failure from 1975 to 1988. Standard error bars are shown.

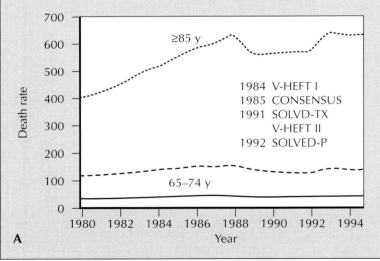

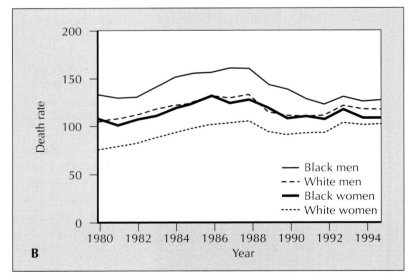

FIGURE 8-2. Changes in death rate for heart failure in the United States between 1980 and 1995. **A,** Age-specific death rate for persons aged 65 years or older, by age group and year [2]. The death rates from heart failure reflect the known age-related increases in the incidence and prevalence of heart failure. The death rate for persons aged 85 years or older increased during 1980 to 1988, but declined from 1989 to 1992 with similar small declines for the other age groups. **B,** Age-adjusted death rates for persons aged 65 years or older, by race, sex, and year, with publication dates of results from some of the major heart failure trials during this period. Death rates increased during 1980 to 1988 and declined after 1988 in all gender and racial groups with the greatest decrease being among black men. The decline in death rates may represent not only advances in the prevention and treatment of heart failure, but also improvements in control of hypertension and access to medical care among older black adults. CONSENSUS—Cooperative North Scandinavian Survival Study; SOLVD-P—Studies of Left Ventricular Dysfunction Prevention; SOLVD-TX—Studies of Left Ventricular Dysfunction Treatment; V-HeFT I—Vasodilator Heart Failure Trial I; V-HeFT II—Vasodilator Heart Failure Trial II. (*Adapted from* the *Morbidity and Mortality Weekly Report* [2].)

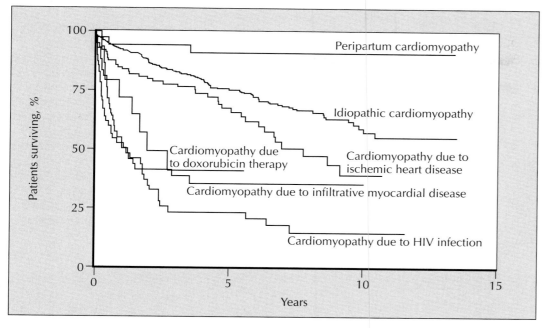

FIGURE 8-3. Survival according to the underlying cause of heart failure. A total of 1230 patients referred to John Hopkins Hospital for assessment of unexplained

cardiomyopathy underwent a comprehensive diagnostic evaluation including endomyocardial biopsy, enabling identification of an underlying etiology in 50% of cases [3]. Patients with peripartum cardiomyopathy had the best prognosis, whereas patients with an ischemic etiology did worse than those with idiopathic cardiomyopathy, consistent with the results of previous studies [4]. This study is limited by the referral nature of the study population, resulting in underrepresentation of patients with common causes of heart failure. Further, the poor outcome seen among patients with doxorubicin cardiotoxicity, infiltrative myocardial disease, and HIV infection may relate more to the underlying disease process than to cardiac involvement. Nevertheless, this study provides important information on survival, and demonstrates the prognostic value of identifying the underlying cause of cardiomyopathy.

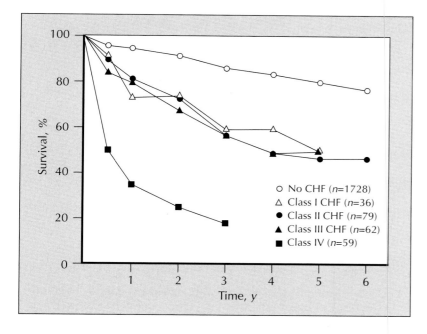

FIGURE 8-4. Survival among patients with different degrees of heart failure symptoms compared with similar patients without congestive heart failure (CHF) [5]. Classification of heart failure was based on the worst clinical condition 6 weeks prior to cardiac catheterization at Duke University Medical Center (1969 to 1981). All patients had coronary artery disease that was managed medically. These data demonstrate the effect, per se, of heart failure on mortality. The difference in survival between groups with a recent history of CHF and patients without overt heart failure was 27% after 3 years of follow-up. Patients who were symptomatic with any physical activity (class IV) had a very poor prognosis. (*Adapted from* Califf *et al.* [5].)

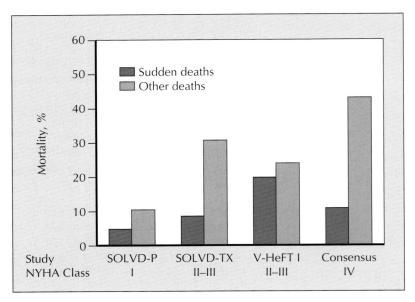

FIGURE 8-5. Proportion of deaths that occurred suddenly in the placebo arms of several large clinical trials that enrolled patients with heart failure [6–9]. *Sudden deaths* were defined generally as those that occurred a short time after the onset of symptoms in the absence of signs or symptoms of worsening heart failure. However, it is likely that there are inconsistencies in the classification of deaths by different investigators. Sudden deaths were common, comprising 20% to 45% of the total deaths. A prognostic variable that is specific for sudden deaths has not been established because the incidences of deaths from both pump failure and sudden deaths, which are presumably caused by abnormal rhythms, tend to increase with the severity of cardiac dysfunction. CONSENSUS—Cooperative North Scandinavian Enalapril Survival Study; SOLVD P—Studies of Left Ventricular Dysfunction Prevention; SOLVD-Tx—Studies of Left Ventricular Dysfunction Treatment; V-HeFT I—Vasodilator Heart Failure Trial I.

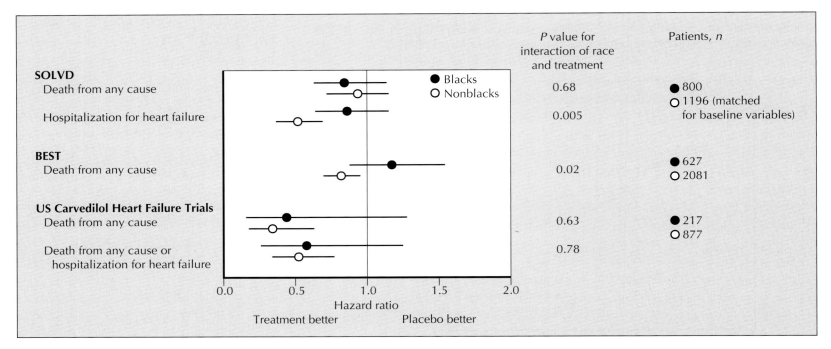

FIGURE 8-6. Effects of race on response to treatment for heart failure. In an analysis of pooled data from the Studies of Left Ventricular Dysfunction (SOLVD) and an analysis of the Beta-Blocker Evaluation of Survival Trial (BEST), benefits of treatment with enalapril and with bucindolol, respectively, were mainly seen in nonblack patients [10,11]. In contrast, carvedilol produced equal benefit across racial groups in the US Carvedilol Heart Failure Trials [12]. Several caveats apply to these data: there were relatively few black patients in the US Carvedilol Heart Failure Trials, and the event rate was low among these patients. Further, only the BEST subgroup analysis was prospectively planned, and it is possible the differences seen were caused by chance alone. It is important to recognize that racial groups and genetic pools are highly mixed and skin color alone cannot serve as an adequate discriminator. Nevertheless, it is important to consider the possibility of racial differences in therapeutic response to drugs commonly used to treat heart failure, and perhaps the need to tailor therapy according to racial background.

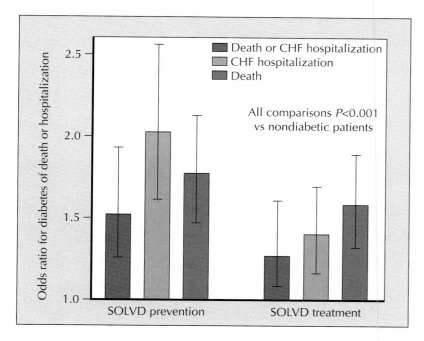

FIGURE 8-7. Survival among patients with heart failure stratified by presence of diabetes. The incidence of complications after myocardial infarction is known to be increased in diabetics. After adjustment for baseline characteristics including etiology of heart failure, diabetes remained a significant predictor of death and hospitalizations in the 6797 patients recruited into the Studies of Left Ventricular Dysfunction (SOLVD) [13]. The risk of death was higher in both asymptomatic and symptomatic patients, and increased with the duration of diabetes; however, diabetic and nondiabetic patients derived equivalent benefit from treatment with enalapril.

USE OF PROGNOSTIC VARIABLES

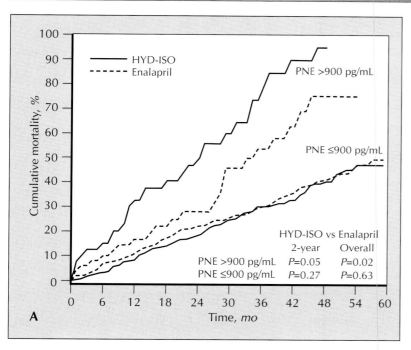

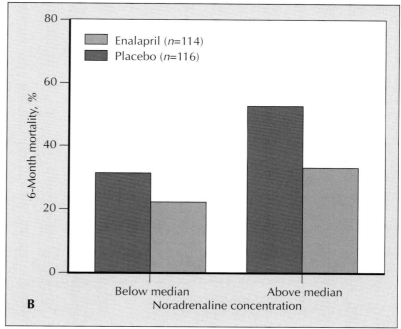

FIGURE 8-8. Effect of enalapril on survival within strata of plasma norepinephrine concentration (PNE). **A,** The Vasodilator Heart Failure Trial (V-HeFT II), in which improved survival with enalapril compared with hydralazine plus isosorbide dinitrate (HYD-ISO) was found in patients with PNE greater than 900 pg/mL [14].

B, In the CONSENSUS (Cooperative North Scandinavian Enalapril Survival Study) trial, which compared enalapril with placebo [9], the median PNE was 772 pg/mL. Once again, the survival benefit was larger in the group with the highest PNEs. These data suggest that the PNE may be useful in identifying patients who are most likely to gain a survival benefit from enalapril. Further studies are needed to determine whether this observation is related to a specific pharmacologic effect that is most likely seen in patients with a high PNE. (Part A *adapted from* Francis *et al.* [14]; part B *adapted from* Swedberg *et al.* [15].)

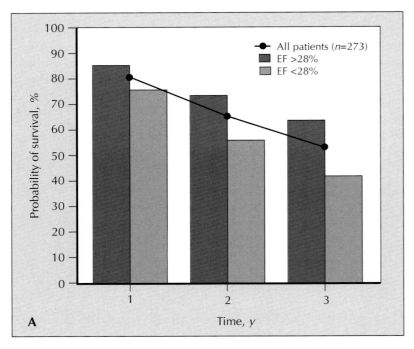

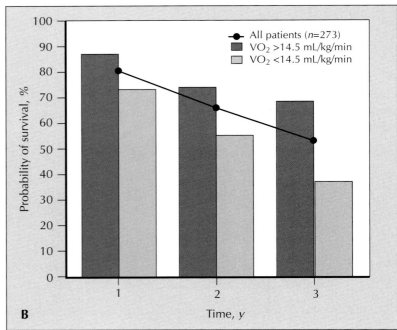

FIGURE 8-9. Examples of the prognostic information available from measurement of the left ventricular ejection fraction (EF; **A**) and peak oxygen consumption (VO$_2$; **B**) in the Vasodilator Heart Failure Trial (V-HeFT I). These data from the placebo group (patients treated with digoxin and diuretic) [16] indicate that the probability of survival over 3 years in different risk strata can differ by 20% to 30%. Strata were defined arbitrarily by the median values in this sample and may not represent the most discriminating cutpoints for these prognostic variables.

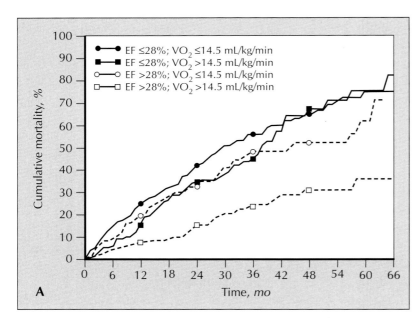

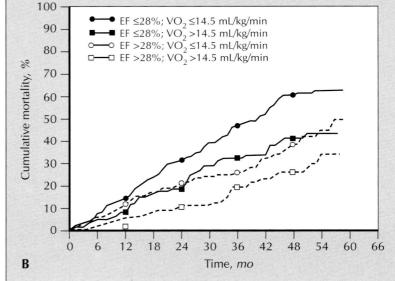

FIGURE 8-10. Prognostic stratification using ejection fraction (EF) and peak oxygen consumption (VO$_2$), which were found to be significant prognostic variables during multivariate analysis. Data are from all patients in the Vasodilator Heart Failure Trials (V-HeFT I in **A** and II in B) [16]. Patients who had relatively good EF and VO$_2$ clearly had a better prognosis than those who fell into the higher risk strata of both variables. For example, the difference in the probability of survival between these two strata after 3 years of follow-up was approximately 30%.

Patients in the higher risk strata of only one of these prognostic variables had an intermediate survival. These trends were evident in both studies even though the overall prognosis tended to be better in V-HeFT II. This was in part because all patients in V-HeFT II received medications that prolong survival (hydralazine plus isosorbide dinitrate or enalapril), whereas the majority of patients in V-HeFT I received placebo or prazosin, which did not improve survival. (*Adapted from* Cohn *et al.* [16].)

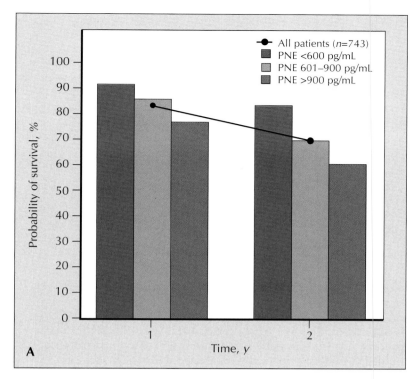

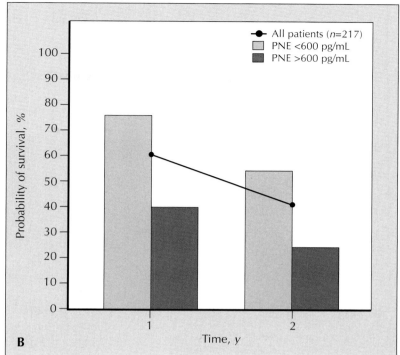

FIGURE 8-11. **A** and **B**, Probability of survival in two studies stratified by measurement of supine resting plasma norepinephrine concentration (PNE) [14,17]. These are among several studies associating PNE with the likelihood of survival in patients with heart failure. The overall prognosis of the group in **B** [17] was worse than that in **A** [14], as was the prognosis within similar strata of PNE. These data highlight the difficulty in making a quantitative prognosis. Several prognostic variables need to be taken into consideration because of the complex pathophysiology and multiple modes of death in patients with heart failure. Multivariate predictive models have not been developed and validated.

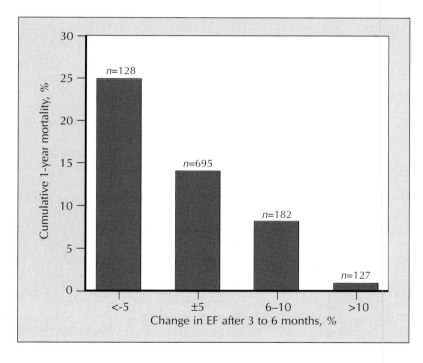

FIGURE 8-12. Survival among patients stratified by changes in ejection fraction (EF) 3 to 6 months after baseline in the Vasodilator Heart Failure Trials (V-HeFT) I and II [18]. EF did not differ by more than 5% in the majority of patients (61%), and mortality 1 year after the second assessment in this subgroup was 14%. The small subgroup whose EF improved by more than 10% had a very low mortality of 1% after 1 year. In contrast, a fall in the EF of more than 5% was associated with a 25% mortality after 1 year. The changes in EF were not strongly associated with several other prognostic variables, including baseline EF and treatment. Further, the second measurement tended to be more informative than the baseline assessment and change from baseline. Data that establish change in any prognostic variable as a surrogate for a beneficial effect of a treatment on survival have not been reported.

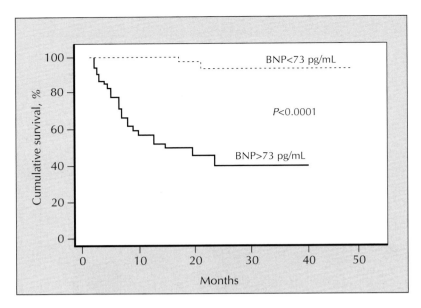

FIGURE 8-13. Survival in patients with congestive heart failure (CHF) stratified by levels of BNP (B-type or brain natriuretic peptide). BNP is secreted mainly from the ventricular myocytes in proportion to the degree of left ventricular dysfunction. Patients who have relatively high BNP levels clearly have worse prognosis. This suggests that downregulation of natriuretic peptide receptors coupled with attenuation of the compensatory activity of the cardiac natriuretic peptide system may increase the mortality of CHF patients with high levels of plasma cardiac natriuretic peptides [19].

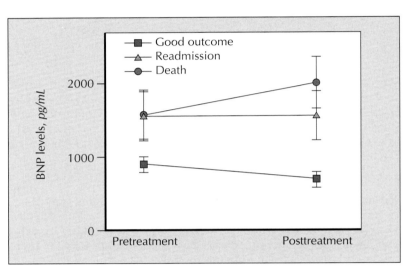

FIGURE 8-14. Changes in brain natriuretic peptide (BNP) levels predict outcomes in patients admitted with decompensated heart failure [20]. BNP levels were measured daily in 72 patients following admission; a decrease in BNP levels following treatment for decompensated heart failure predicts a good outcome. Conversely, BNP levels increased or did not change in patients who died or were readmitted early, and univariate analysis showed the last measured BNP strongly predicted outcome. These results suggest that changes in BNP levels may offer a convenient biochemical marker to assess control of heart failure, and could be used to guide treatment of patients admitted with decompensated heart failure. (*Adapted from* Cheng *et al.* [20].)

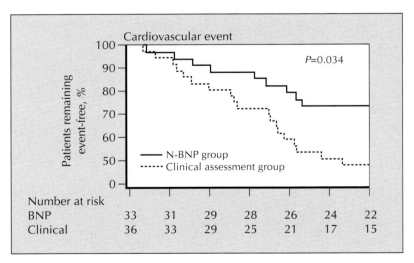

FIGURE 8-15. Use of brain natriuretic peptide (BNP) levels to titrate treatment for heart failure [21]. Sixty-nine patients with left ventricular ejection fraction of 40% or lower and symptomatic heart failure were randomly assigned to receive treatment guided by either plasma N-terminal BNP levels (N-BNP group) or clinical assessment alone. Patients with plasma N-BNP levels higher than 200 pmol/L received intensified treatment according to a predetermined protocol until the target level was met. N-BNP levels fell 79 pmol/L below baseline in the N-BNP group and significantly fewer cardiovascular events (cardiovascular death, hospital admission, or worsening heart failure) were seen compared with the clinical assessment group (*P*<0.05) in whom N-BNP levels fell by only 3 pmol/L. This study suggests that patients with raised N-BNP levels are at higher risk of cardiovascular events, and therapy directed at reducing the N-BNP level is more effective than clinical assessment alone in preventing cardiovascular events. (*Adapted from* Troughton *et al.* [21].)

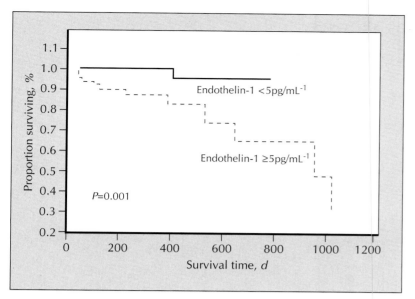

FIGURE 8-16. Survival stratified by assessment of plasma endothelin system. Pousset *et al.* [22] studied the association of plasma endothelin-1 as a predictor of cardiac death in 120 congestive heart failure patients with ischemic or nonischemic cardiomyopathy by using an assay with very low cross-reactivity to big endothelin. This is among several studies associating high plasma levels of both endothelin-1 and the propeptide big endothelin-1 (Big ET) with strong predictors of mortality in severe heart failure. Several studies have now demonstrated improved hemodynamics in patients with heart failure receiving endothelin receptor antagonists, suggesting a role for endothelin in the pathophysiology of heart failure. (*Adapted from* Pousset *et al.* [22].)

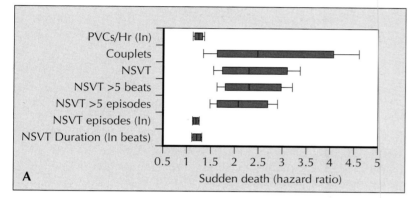

FIGURE 8-17. Sudden death in patients with chronic heart failure (HF). Ventricular arrhythmias are common in chronic heart failure (HF) patients, but their importance in predicting sudden death in these patients remains uncertain. **A,** In the Prospective Randomized Milrinone Survival Evaluation (PROMISE) trial, nonsustained ventricular tachycardia (NSVT) on baseline ambulatory ECGs from 1080 patients with HF (54% ischemic cardiomyopathy) and New York Heart Association (NYHA) class III/IV symptoms predicted sudden death [23]. **B,** Univariate

logistic analysis showed false-positive rates of greater than 80% at all sensitivity levels of 50% or greater for NSVT episodes, the best of the ECG variables, in predicting sudden death [23]. This demonstrates that NSVT on ambulatory ECGs has poor sensitivity and specificity for discriminating between sudden death and all-cause mortality. Ventricular arrhythmias are likely a marker for more severe HF and thus increased mortality. *NSVT episodes* indicates number of NSVT episodes (ln transformed); *NSVT duration* indicates longest number of continuous beats of NSVT (ln transformed).

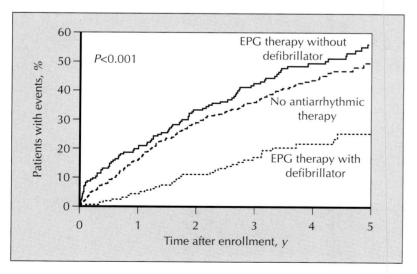

FIGURE 8-18. Effects of electrophysiologically guided antiarrhythmic therapy on mortality in patients with ischemic left ventricular dysfunction and asymptomatic, unsustained ventricular tachycardia (VT). A total of 704 patients (New York Heart Association functional class I–III) in whom sustained VT could be induced at electrophysiologic (EPG) testing were assigned to receive antiarrhythmic therapy including drugs (predominantly class I agents) and implantable defibrillators, or no antiarrhythmic therapy [24]. Eighteen percent of patients randomly assigned to receive no antiarrhythmic therapy had a cardiac arrest or death from arrhythmia during a median follow-up period of 39 months. Rates of cardiac arrest, death from arrhythmia, and overall mortality were reduced only by treatment with a defibrillator. The results of this study suggest that it is reasonable to perform electrophysiologic testing in patients with ischemic left ventricular dysfunction and asymptomatic VT, with implantation of a defibrillator if sustained VT can be induced.

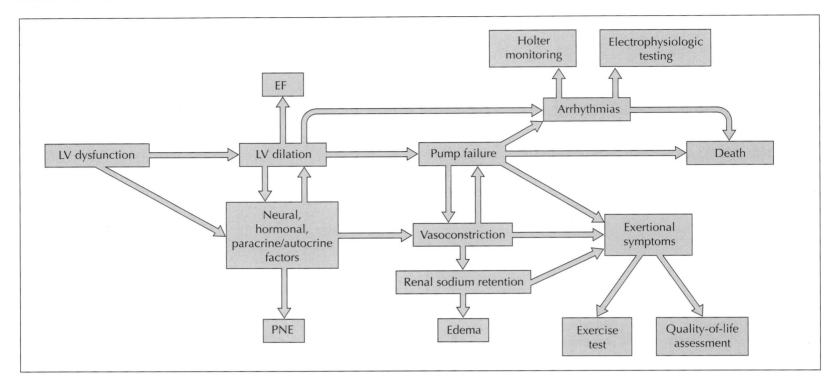

FIGURE 8-19. Physiologic mechanisms leading to markers for the severity of heart failure. Left ventricular (LV) dysfunction progresses through ventricular remodeling to chamber enlargement that can be detected by echocardiographic, radionuclide, or angiographic measurement of reduced LV ejection fraction (EF) or an increased chamber volume. LV dysfunction and chamber dilation result in activation of neural, hormonal, and local tissue paracrine and autocrine processes, which contribute to vasoconstriction, renal sodium retention, and aggravation of LV dysfunction. The neurohormonal abnormality can be detected by elevated circulating levels of norepinephrine, renin activity, atrial natriuretic peptide, or other hormonal markers of the process. The sodium retention is manifested by edema or pulmonary congestion. The LV pump failure combined with the neurohormonal and vasocon-strictor mechanisms contribute to symptoms that can be quantitated by a formal exercise test, often supplemented by measurement of gas exchange.

Quality of life instruments provide a more global assessment of the functional impairment produced by the disease and its treatment. Pump failure may progress to death, but ventricular arrhythmias that are frequent accompaniments of LV dilation and pump failure may contribute independently to sudden death and may be assessed by Holter monitoring and electrophysiologic testing. In the treatment of heart failure, an improvement in any of these clinical markers may be used as a guide to a therapeutic response, but the relationship of any of these markers to clinical benefit, including life prolongation, has not yet been validated empirically. PNE—plasma norepinephrine concentration.

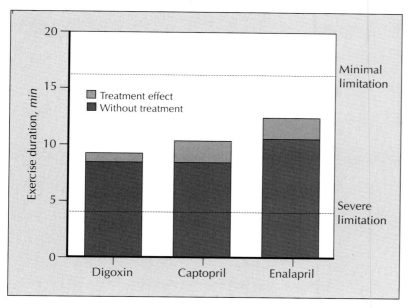

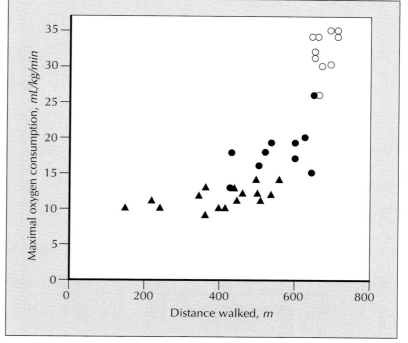

FIGURE 8-20. The magnitude of changes in exercise duration observed after 12 weeks in controlled clinical trials of commonly used medications [25–27]. All of these studies used a modified Naughton treadmill protocol in which the workload was increased every 2 minutes, beginning with a very easy workload of 1 mph (slow walk) on a level grade. Severely limited (able to complete less than two stages) or minimally impaired (able to complete more than eight stages) patients are often excluded from trials in an effort to select those thought to be most amenable to treatment. These particular medications have increased exercise duration by 2 minutes (one stage) or less on average compared with control groups in several studies. However, individual responses have been highly variable. In addition, patients often have substantial intolerance to exercise despite these improvements, and changes in exercise duration have not been established as reliable markers of changes in quality or quantity of life.

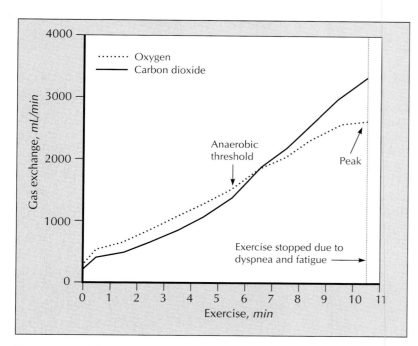

FIGURE 8-21. The most commonly used endpoints to ascertain changes in cardiopulmonary functional status during an exercise tolerance test. Patients exercise on a treadmill or bicycle against a gradually increasing workload until they stop because of dyspnea and fatigue. The most frequently used measure is total exercise time. Peak oxygen consumption is readily determined with equipment to monitor breath-by-breath respiratory gases and air flow. The anaerobic threshold that indicates excess carbon dioxide production from anaerobic metabolism is determined by the examination of several criteria such as a disproportionate increase in carbon dioxide production and ventilatory exchange relative to oxygen uptake, but this threshold is difficult to identify in many patients with heart failure.

Some of the problems with using a peak exercise test to assess the response to treatment include the following: 1) patient's routine daily activities usually do not involve this level of stress; 2) concurrent conditions such as angina, peripheral claudication, and arrhythmias may interfere with an assessment of dyspnea and fatigue; and 3) improvements have often occurred while the patient is taking placebo because of learning effects, training effects, and motivational factors.

FIGURE 8-22. Results of a 6-minute walk test in relation to peak oxygen consumption on a treadmill and New York Heart Association classification [28]. Patients were asked to walk as far as they could in 6 minutes on a level corridor. They could slow down or stop if necessary and were told when 3 and 5 minutes had elapsed. Some encouragement was given (this needs to be standardized to avoid biasing the results of the test). *Closed circles* represent patients whose ordinary physical activity caused symptoms such as dyspnea and fatigue (class II), and *closed triangles* represent patients who became symptomatic during less than ordinary physical activity (class III). *Open circles* represent normal subjects. There were no subjects in this study who were symptomatic with any physical activity or at rest (class IV) or who were not unduly symptomatic during ordinary physical activities (class I). Self-paced walking tests are being evaluated in clinical trials and may serve as a simple measure of the effects of heart failure on daily physical activity (*Adapted from* Lipkin *et al.* [28].)

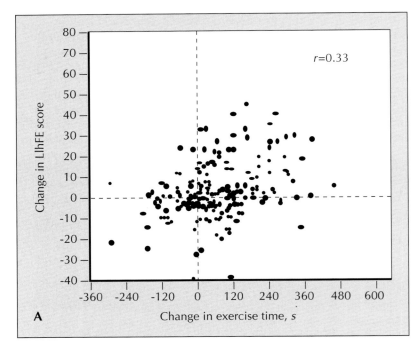

A

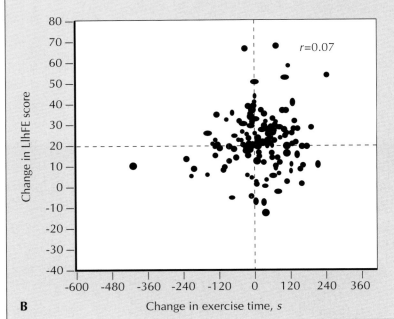

B

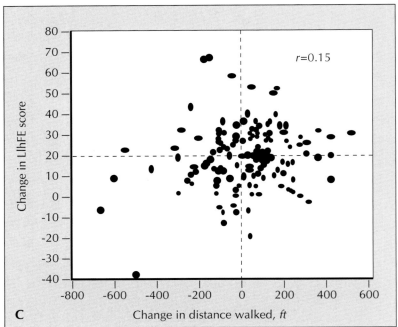

C

FIGURE 8-23. Correlations between changes in exercise variables and changes in quality of life as measured by the Minnesota Living with Heart Failure (LIhFE) questionnaire in the pimobendan (**A**) and digoxin withdrawal (**B** and **C**) studies [25,29]. Changes in exercise time for peak exercise tests done according to a modified Naughton protocol are shown in *A* and *B* . Changes in the distance walked for the 6-minute walk test are shown in *C*. The association between these variables was modest at best even though there were significant changes on average in each variable during these studies. These data and similar observations in other studies indicate that exercise tests and quality of life questionnaires provide distinctly different information about a patient's heart failure. Both types of measures are needed for a comprehensive evaluation.

LIVING WITH HEART FAILURE QUESTIONNAIRE

These questions concern how your heart failure (heart condition) has prevented you from living as you wanted during the last month. The items listed below describe different ways some people are affected. If you are sure an item does not apply to you or is not related to your heart failure then circle 0 (No) and go on to the next item. If an item does apply to you, then circle the number rating how much it prevented you from living as you wanted. Remember to think about ONLY THE LAST MONTH.

DID YOUR HEART FAILURE PREVENT YOU FROM LIVING AS YOU WANTED DURING THE LAST MONTH BY:	NO	VERY LITTLE				VERY MUCH
1. causing swelling in your ankles, legs, etc?	0	1	2	3	4	5
2. making you sit or lie down to rest during the day?	0	1	2	3	4	5
3. making your walking about or climbing stairs difficult?	0	1	2	3	4	5
4. making your working around the house or yard difficult?	0	1	2	3	4	5
5. making your going places away from home difficult?	0	1	2	3	4	5
6. making your sleeping well at night difficult?	0	1	2	3	4	5
7. making your relating to or doing things with your friends or family difficult?	0	1	2	3	4	5
8. making your working to earn a living difficult?	0	1	2	3	4	5
9. making your recreational pastimes, sports or hobbies difficult?	0	1	2	3	4	5
10. making your sexual activities difficult?	0	1	2	3	4	5
11. making you eat less of the foods you like?	0	1	2	3	4	5
12. making you short of breath?	0	1	2	3	4	5
13. making you tired, fatigued, or low on energy?	0	1	2	3	4	5
14. making you stay in a hospital?	0	1	2	3	4	5
15. costing you money for medical care?	0	1	2	3	4	5
16. giving you side effects from medications?	0	1	2	3	4	5
17. making you feel you are a burden to your family or friends?	0	1	2	3	4	5
18. making you feel a loss of self-control in your life?	0	1	2	3	4	5
19. making you worry?	0	1	2	3	4	5
20. making it difficult for you to concentrate or remember things?	0	1	2	3	4	5
21. making you feel depressed?	0	1	2	3	4	5

FIGURE 8-24. The Minnesota Living with Heart Failure questionnaire. Improvement in quality of life is one of two primary goals of therapy (prolonged survival being the other). This measure of quality of life, which has been used in many investigations of treatments for heart failure, defines *quality of life* as living as one wants with minimal limitations secondary to heart failure and its treatment. Physical, social, emotional, and economic limitations are included. Patients self-administer the questions after listening to a standard set of instructions. The score is the sum of the responses for all 21 questions. Eight questions including dyspnea and fatigue are highly interrelated and their sum is called the *physical dimension* [29]. Similarly, five interrelated questions comprise an emotional dimension. (*Adapted from* Rector and Cohn [29].)

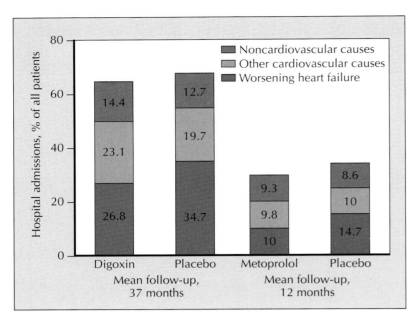

FIGURE 8-25. Hospitalizations during the Digitalis Investigators Group (DIG) trial and the Metoprolol CR/XL Randomized Intervention Trial in Congestive Heart Failure (MERIT-HF) [30,31]. Digoxin significantly reduced hospitalizations for heart failure in the DIG trial during a mean follow up period of 37 months, although this was partially offset by a small increase in hospitalizations for other cardiovascular causes. Total hospitalizations remained significantly reduced. Similarly, metoprolol reduced the number of patients who were hospitalized, mainly due to a fall in the number hospitalized for heart failure during a mean follow-up period of one year. Reducing the frequency of hospital admissions would be expected to translate into lower costs, better quality of life, and perhaps prolonged life.

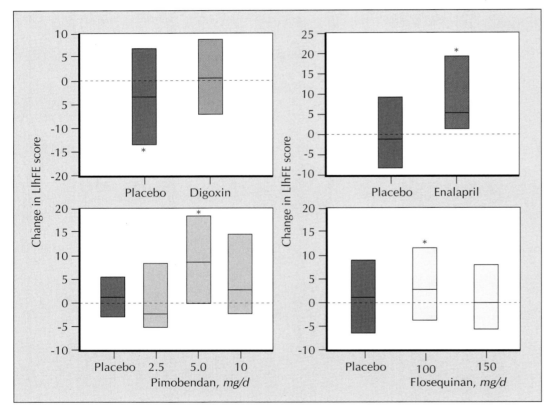

FIGURE 8-26. Responses to different medications as determined by the Minnesota Living with Heart Failure (LIhFE) questionnaire in four randomized, double-blinded clinical trials [25,29,32,33]. The placebo groups did not exhibit significant changes in any of these trials, and there was a significant difference between the treatment and control arms in each study. The top and bottom of each rectangle represent the 75th and 25th percentiles of the changes in the LIhFE score from baseline, respectively. The horizontal line within each rectangle is the median change score. In the *upper left*, placebo was substituted for digoxin. *Asterisks* indicate *P*<0.05.

REFERENCES

1. Ho KK, Anderson KM, Kannel WB, et al.: Survival after the onset of congestive heart failure in Framingham Heart Study subjects. *Circulation* 1993, 88:107–115.

2. Changes in mortality from heart failure: United States, 1980–1995. *MMWR Morbid Mortal Wkly Rep* 1998, 47:633–637.

3. Felker GM, Thompson RE, Hare JM, et al.: Underlying causes and long-term survival in patients with initially unexplained cardiomyopathy. *N Engl J Med* 2000, 342: 1077–1084.

4. Bart BA, Shaw LK, McCants CB, Jr., et al.: Clinical determinants of mortality in patients with angiographically diagnosed ischemic or nonischemic cardiomyopathy. *J Am Coll Cardiol* 1997, 30:1002–1008.

5. Califf RM, Bounous P, Harrell FE, et al.: The prognosis in the presence of coronary artery disease. In *Congestive Heart Failure: Current Research and Clinical Applications*. Edited by Braunwald E, Mock B, Watson JT. New York: Grune & Stratton; 1982:31–40.

6. The SOLVD Investigators: Effect of enalapril on mortality and the development of heart failure in asymptomatic patients with reduced left ventricular ejection fractions. *N Engl J Med* 1992, 327:685–691.

7. The SOLVD Investigators: Effect of enalapril on survival in patients with reduced left ventricular ejection fractions and congestive heart failure. *N Engl J Med* 1991, 325:293–302.

8. Cohn JN, Archibald DG, Ziesche S, et al.: Effect of vasodilator therapy on mortality in chronic congestive heart failure: results of a Veterans Administration Cooperative Study. *N Engl J Med* 1986, 314:1547–1552.

9. The CONSENSUS Trial Study Group: Effects of enalapril on mortality in severe congestive heart failure: results of the Cooperative North Scandinavian Enalapril Survival Study. *N Engl J Med* 1987, 316:1429–1435.

10. Exner DV, Dries DL, Domanski MJ, Cohn JN: Lesser response to angiotensin-converting-enzyme inhibitor therapy in black as compared with white patients with left ventricular dysfunction. *N Engl J Med* 2001, 344:1351–1357.

11. A trial of the beta-blocker bucindolol in patients with advanced chronic heart failure. *N Engl J Med* 2001, 344:1659–1667.

12. Yancy CW, Fowler MB, Colucci WS, et al.: Race and the response to adrenergic blockade with carvedilol in patients with chronic heart failure. *N Engl J Med* 2001, 344:1358–1365.

13. Shindler DM, Kostis JB, Yusuf S, et al.: Diabetes mellitus, a predictor of morbidity and mortality in the Studies of Left Ventricular Dysfunction (SOLVD) Trials and Registry. *Am J Cardiol* 1996, 77:1017–1020.

14. Francis GS, Cohn JN, Johnson G, et al.: Plasma norepinephrine, plasma renin activity, and congestive heart failure: relations to survival and the effects of therapy in V-HeFT II. The V-HeFT VA Cooperative Studies Group. *Circulation* 1993, 87:VI40–VI48.

15. Swedberg K, Eneroth P, Kjekshus J, Wilhelmsen L: Hormones regulating cardiovascular function in patients with severe congestive heart failure and their relation to mortality: CONSENSUS Trial Study Group. *Circulation* 1990, 82:1730–1736.

16. Cohn JN, Johnson GR, Shabetai R, et al.: Ejection fraction, peak exercise oxygen consumption, cardiothoracic ratio, ventricular arrhythmias, and plasma norepinephrine as determinants of prognosis in heart failure: the V-HeFT VA Cooperative Studies Group. *Circulation* 1993, 87:VI5–V16.

17. Rector TS, Olivari MT, Levine TB, et al.: Predicting survival for an individual with congestive heart failure using the plasma norepinephrine concentration. *Am Heart J* 1987, 114:148–152.

18. Cintron G, Johnson G, Francis G, et al.: Prognostic significance of serial changes in left ventricular ejection fraction in patients with congestive heart failure. *Circulation* 1993, 87(suppl VI):17–23.

19. Tsutamoto T, Wada A, Maeda K, et al.: Attenuation of compensation of endogenous cardiac natriuretic peptide system in chronic heart failure: prognostic role of plasma brain natriuretic peptide concentration in patients with chronic symptomatic left ventricular dysfunction. *Circulation* 1997, 96:509–516.

20. Cheng V, Kazanagra R, Garcia A, et al.: A rapid bedside test for B-type peptide predicts treatment outcomes in patients admitted for decompensated heart failure: a pilot study. *J Am Coll Cardiol* 2001, 37:386–391.

21. Troughton RW, Frampton CM, Yandle TG, et al.: Treatment of heart failure guided by plasma aminoterminal brain natriuretic peptide (N-BNP) concentrations. *Lancet* 2000, 355:1126–1130.

22. Pousset F, Isnard R, Lechat P, et al.: Prognostic value of plasma endothelin-1 in patients with chronic heart failure. *Eur Heart J* 1997, 18:254–258.

23. Teerlink JR, Jalaluddin M, Anderson S, et al.: Ambulatory ventricular arrhythmias in patients with heart failure do not specifically predict an increased risk of sudden death. PROMISE (Prospective Randomized Milrinone Survival Evaluation) Investigators. *Circulation* 2000, 101:40–46.

24. Buxton AE, Lee KL, Fisher JD, et al.: A randomized study of the prevention of sudden death in patients with coronary artery disease: Multicenter Unsustained Tachycardia Trial Investigators. *N Engl J Med* 1999, 341:1882–1890.

25. Packer M, Gheorghiade M, Young JB, et al.: Withdrawal of digoxin from patients with chronic heart failure treated with angiotensin-converting-enzyme inhibitors: RADIANCE Study. *N Engl J Med* 1993, 329:1–7.

26. Captopril Multicenter Research Group: A placebo-controlled trial of captopril in refractory chronic congestive heart failure. *J Am Coll Cardiol* 1983, 2:755–763.

27. Enalapril Congestive Heart Failure Investigators: Long-term effects of enalapril in patients with congestive heart failure; a multicenter, placebo-controlled trial. *Heart Failure* 1987, 1:102–107.

28. Lipkin DP, Scriven AJ, Crake T, Poole-Wilson PA: Six minute walking test for assessing exercise capacity in chronic heart failure. *Br Med J (Clin Res Ed)* 1986, 292:653–655.

29. Rector TS, Cohn JN: Assessment of patient outcome with the Minnesota Living with Heart Failure questionnaire: reliability and validity during a randomized, double-blind, placebo-controlled trial of pimobendan. Pimobendan Multicenter Research Group. *Am Heart J* 1992, 124:1017–1025.

30. The Digitalis Investigation Group: The effect of digoxin on mortality and morbidity in patients with heart failure. *N Engl J Med* 1997, 336:525–533.

31. Hjalmarson A, Fagerberg B: MERIT-HF mortality and morbidity data. *Basic Res Cardiol* 2000, 95 (Suppl 1):I98–I103.

32. Rector TS, Kubo SH, Cohn JN: Validity of the Minnesota Living with Heart Failure questionnaire as a measure of therapeutic response to enalapril or placebo. *Am J Cardiol* 1993, 71:1106–1107.

33. Massie BM, Berk MR, Brozena SC, et al.: Can further benefit be achieved by adding flosequinan to patients with congestive heart failure who remain symptomatic on diuretic, digoxin, and an angiotensin converting enzyme inhibitor? Results of the flosequinan-ACE inhibitor trial (FACET). *Circulation* 1993, 88:492–501.

UNSTABLE HEART FAILURE

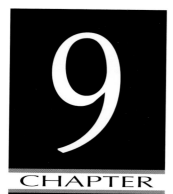

CHAPTER

Carl V. Leier and David A. Orsinelli

Unstable heart failure represents the clinical state of progressively worsening or decompensated heart failure, which, if not improved within a reasonable time (usually minutes to hours), often evolves into markedly symptomatic heart failure, cardiovascular collapse, and shock or death. The clinical settings include, among others, the patient who arrives in the emergency room in acute pulmonary edema, the patient with postinfarction cardiogenic shock, the patient who cannot be weaned from cardiopulmonary bypass after cardiac surgery, or the chronic heart failure patient who is experiencing a rather abrupt worsening of symptoms. Most patients with unstable heart failure must be approached with a certain sense of urgency.

The management approach to unstable heart failure is directed specifically at improving the tenuous clinical condition and suffering that many of these patients are experiencing, and promptly correcting or reversing the underlying cause of the unstable, decompensated cardiac condition. The 1-year mortality rate for patients who present with acute pulmonary edema and whose underlying lesion or condition is not determined, corrected, or properly treated exceeds 50% and is worse for those who go on to develop cardiogenic shock [1–5]. For many patients, unstable or decompensated cardiac failure cannot be improved without definitive correction of the underlying lesion (*eg*, acute valvular regurgitation, high-grade obstructive disease of a major coronary artery).

Atherosclerotic coronary artery disease is the most common etiology for acute and chronic heart failure in Western societies. The short- and long-term clinical courses of patients with atherosclerotic heart disease are strongly dependent on the relative amounts of well-perfused viable myocardium, reversibly ischemic myocardium, and infarcted (irreversibly necrotic or fibrotic) myocardium. Methods are now available to save jeopardized, ischemic myocardium from infarction and to bring it back to a viable, functional state; these methods include thrombolysis, interventional coronary catheterization (*eg*, angioplasty with stent placement), and bypass surgery. For the patient who presents with unstable heart failure secondary to acute myocardial infarction, the concept of "time is muscle" is extremely important. Detection of myocardial infarction, followed by definitive diagnostic and therapeutic interventions (medical or surgical), must take place as soon as possible after patient presentation. A delay in or inefficient delivery of definitive cardiovascular services in this setting unequivocally jeopardizes the immediate and long-term outcome of the patient who presents with symptomatic heart failure caused by occlusive coronary artery disease.

From the standpoint of clinical relevance and application and for the sake of clarity, unstable heart failure is presented here as acute heart failure and decompensated chronic heart failure. The views presented in this chapter are consistent with the most current heart failure guidelines [6,7].

ACUTE HEART FAILURE

COMPARISONS OF UNSTABLE VS CHRONIC HEART FAILURE

FEATURE	ACUTE HEART FAILURE	DECOMPENSATED CHRONIC HEART FAILURE	CHRONIC HEART FAILURE
Symptom severity	Marked	Marked	Mild to moderate
Pulmonary edema	Frequent	Frequent	Rare
Peripheral edema	Rare	Frequent	Occasional
Weight gain	None to mild	Frequent	Frequent
Whole-body fluid volume load	No change or mild increase	Markedly increased	Increased
Cardiomegaly	Uncommon	Usual*	Common*
Ventricular systolic function	Hypo-, normo-, or hypercontractile	Reduced*	Reduced*
LV wall stress	Elevated	Markedly elevated	Elevated
Activation of sympathetic nervous system	Marked	Marked	Mild to marked
Activation of renin-angiotensin-aldosterone axis	Often increased	Marked	Mild to marked
Reparable, remedial causative lesion(s)	Common	Occasional	Occasional

*Patients with diastolic dysfunction heart failure may have little to no cardiomegaly and normal systolic function.

FIGURE 9-1. Comparisons of unstable versus chronic heart failure. Clinical and pathophysiologic characteristics of the two major categories of unstable heart failure (acute heart failure and decompensated chronic heart failure) are compared with those of chronic heart failure. Chronic heart failure (compensated and decompensated) is accompanied by total volume overload, weight gain, and edema. In contrast, acute heart failure is less characterized by total volume overload but is often accompanied by a shift of intravascular volume centrally to cardiac chambers and pulmonary vasculature. Therefore, diuretics, angiotensin-converting enzyme inhibitors, β-blockers, and digitalis represent rational pharmacotherapy for chronic heart failure. Acute preload and afterload reduction (sublingual and intravenous nitroglycerin, nitroprusside, or nesiritide), supplemented by intravenous diuretic administration and occasionally by positive inotropic or vasopressor support (*eg*, dobutamine, milrinone, dopamine), represent the proper pharmacotherapeutic approach to most patients with acute heart failure. A combination of these strategies is often necessary to stabilize and improve decompensated chronic heart failure. An important feature that distinguishes the management approach to acute heart failure from that of chronic heart failure is the high incidence of reparable lesions (*eg*, acute occlusion of a major coronary artery, ruptured chordae tendineae) causing acute heart failure, although an occasional patient with chronic heart failure may also require definitive intervention.

MAJOR CAUSES OF ACUTE HEART FAILURE

Myocardial ischemia-infarction

    Ventricular systolic or diastolic dysfunction

    Mitral valve regurgitation

    Ventricular rupture (septum, free wall)

Disruption of valvular apparatus (aortic, mitral)

Myocarditis or cardiomyopathy

Uncontrolled, severe systemic hypertension

Others, *eg,* cardiac dysrhythmias, pulmonary emboli, pulmonary hypertension, pericardial tamponade

FIGURE 9-2. Major causes of acute heart failure. Acute heart failure is often caused by one or more of these common conditions. It is apparent that many of these disorders and lesions can be definitively treated. Therefore, in addition to clinical and hemodynamic stabilization, the approach to acute heart failure includes an active search and specific intervention for reparable lesions with the dual intent of improving the patient's short- and long-term course and averting a recurrence of acute heart failure and evolution into chronic heart failure.

STEPS IN CLINICAL AND HEMODYNAMIC STABILIZATION OF ACUTE HEART FAILURE

1. Administer oxygen ($\uparrow F_iO_2$)

2. When accompanied by fluid volume overload or a "congestive" component

    Sublingual nitroglycerin

    Intravenous furosemide

    Consider morphine sulfate

    Consider additional preload-afterload reduction

3. Evaluate early for

    Readily reversible causes of acute heart failure (*eg,* cardiac dysrhythmias, pericardial tamponade); if present, initiate appropriate intervention

    Myocardial ischemia-infarction; if present, promptly initiate appropriate interventions (*eg,* thrombolytic therapy, urgent angioplasty)

4. If patient is refractory to above therapies, hypotensive, or in cardiogenic shock

    Intravenous fluid administration if no evidence is found for fluid volume overload

    Consider intravenous inotropic or vasopressor agents

    Consider catheter placement (pulmonary and systemic arterial)

    Obtain echocardiogram to assist in diagnosis, evaluation, and determining reparability of the culprit lesion or condition

    Consider need for mechanical circulatory assistance (intra-aortic balloon counterpulsation)

5. Proceed to definitive diagnostic and interventional procedures

6. Be prepared to administer advanced cardiovascular life support (ACLS) at any point as needed

FIGURE 9-3. General management of acute heart failure. Because of the high likelihood of an underlying reparable lesion or condition, the general management approach to acute heart failure emphasizes definitive diagnostic studies. The patient's hemodynamic and clinical status are improved and stabilized to allow safe passage through definitive diagnostic testing (*eg,* echocardiography, cardiac catheterization) and intervention (*eg,* surgery, coronary angioplasty). Major steps in the initial management of acute heart failure [2,5–34] are arranged in the general order of application and according to the general types of acute heart failure encountered:

1) When possible, it is informative to obtain pulse oximetry or arterial blood for gas analysis before oxygen administration.

2) Sublingual nitroglycerin can be administered at a dose of one tablet (one or two sprays) every 5 minutes three or four times until intravenous nitroglycerin, nitroprusside, or nesiritide can take effect. Furosemide is usually administered in a dose range of 20 to 80 mg intravenously. Preload-afterload reduction beyond sublingual nitroglycerin is best achieved by intravenous administration of nitroglycerin, nitroprusside or nesiritide.

3) The medical history and electrocardiogram are obtained early in the evaluation of the patient with acute heart failure to determine whether myocardial ischemia-infarction is the underlying cause for the acute event and whether the patient is a candidate for acute intervention (*eg,* thrombolytic therapy, coronary angioplasty with stent).

4) Dobutamine, milrinone, dopamine, and norepinephrine represent the principal inotropic or vasopressor agents used in this acute care setting.

5) Once the patient's condition is stabilized, diagnostic and interventional procedures can be performed.

CONSIDERATIONS IN ADMINISTERING MORPHINE SULFATE FOR ACUTE HEART FAILURE

DOSE

2–6 mg intravenously

OPTIONAL THERAPY

Consider in the patient with pulmonary edema who is still dyspneic after admin- istration of sublingual nitroglycerin (× 3–4)

PRECAUTIONS IN PATIENTS WITH HEART FAILURE

Acidosis or marginally compensated acidosis

Chronic lung disease

Inadequate availability of prompt ventilatory support, if needed

FIGURE 9-4. Considerations in administering morphine sulfate for acute heart failure. With the appropriate use of sublingual and intravenous nitroglycerin, morphine sulfate should no longer be viewed as a routine step in the management of acute heart failure, particularly in the presence of the precautions noted.

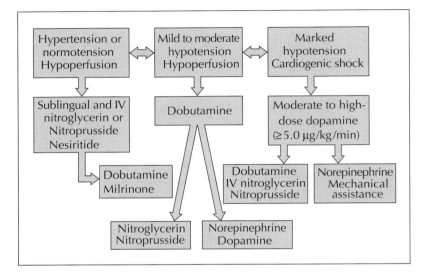

FIGURE 9-5. A practical working diagram of the cardiovascular support drugs commonly employed in the initial short-term management of acute or severe heart failure. It is assumed that patients who require these support drugs have adequate to high left ventricular diastolic filling pressures (≥ 18 mm Hg) or clinical evidence of fluid volume overload. Systemic hypoperfusion and hypotension in a patient without evidence of volume overload or with filling pressures of less than 18 mm Hg should be approached with a fluid volume challenge as the first step. On the basis of the clinical presentation and the state of systemic perfusion and blood pressure, the initial drug of choice is selected and its dosage is increased until clinical or hemodynamic endpoints are achieved or adverse effects appear. At this point, inadequate improvement of clinical status and systemic perfusion usually requires either the addition of a second agent as combination therapy or mechanical assistance. IV—intravenous.

PRINCIPAL PRELOAD- AND AFTERLOAD-REDUCING DRUGS FOR ACUTE OR SEVERE HEART FAILURE

DRUG	DOSING	POTENTIAL ADVANTAGE	POTENTIAL DISADVANTAGES
Nitroglycerin	Sublingual: 1 tablet (or 1–2 sprays) × 3–4 at 5-min intervals Intravenous: 0.4 µg/kg/min initially; increase as needed	Favorable effect on coronary vasculature and in myocardial ischemia-infarction	Tolerance during prolonged infusion Fluid retention Inadequate afterload reduction in catastrophic cardio- vascular disorders (eg, acute valvular insufficiency, ventricular rupture)
Nitroprusside	Intravenous: 0.1 µg/kg/min initially; increase as needed	Relatively powerful afterload reduction	Less favorable effect on coronary vasculature and myocardial ischemia; administration must be closely monitored to avoid marked hypotension; thiocyanate or cyanide toxicity during high-dose or prolonged infusions, particularly in patients with renal failure
Nesiritide	0.01 µg/kg/min initially (± bolus at onset of infusion); increase as needed	Favorable renal profile	Bradycardia (infrequent), hypotension

FIGURE 9-6. Principal preload- and afterload-reducing drugs for acute or severe heart failure. Nitroglycerin and nitroprusside are the primary vasodilators employed to reduce excessive preload and afterload in acute or severe heart failure [8,9]. Nitroglycerin is used most often, particularly in conditions caused by occlusive athero- sclerotic coronary artery disease. Nitroprusside is the drug of choice when more aggressive afterload and preload reduction are needed; examples include catastrophic cardiovascular events (eg, acute,

severe mitral, or aortic regurgitation), hypertensive emergencies (eg, aortic dissection, pulmonary edema), and inadequate response to nitroglycerin. Nesiritide (BNP) was recently approved by the US Food and Drug Administration for acute management of severe congestive heart failure [10,11]. Widespread clinical experience with this agent is still somewhat limited. These agents have obviated volume phlebotomy as an intervention for the vast majority of patients who present with acute pulmonary edema.

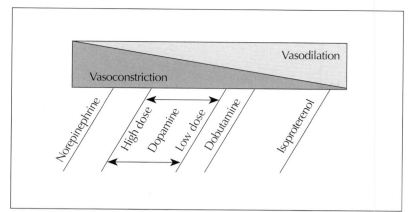

FIGURE 9-7. Comparative systemic vascular responses to the major sympathomimetic amines most commonly employed in acute or severe heart failure. Low-dose (<5.0 µg/kg/min) dopamine has significant visceral and renal vasodilatory properties but behaves as a vasoconstrictor at higher doses (>6.0 µg/kg/min) [12–17]. Norepinephrine is used primarily for its vasoconstrictor properties and dobutamine for its positive inotropic and favorable vascular effects (decreasing vascular resistance). Because vasodilatation is more predictably and safely achieved with nitroglycerin and nitroprusside, isoproterenol is at present rarely used in the management of acute heart failure.

A. PHARMACOLOGIC PROPERTIES AND THERAPEUTIC CONSIDERATIONS IN USING INOTROPIC AGENTS

PHARMACOLOGIC FEATURE	DOBUTAMINE	DOPAMINE LOW DOSE	DOPAMINE HIGH DOSE	NOREPINEPHRINE
General description	Positive inotrope with balanced peripheral vascular effects	Dopaminergic vasodilator, "renal" dopaminergic dose	Vasopressor with some positive inotropic effects	Vasopressor
Dose, µg/kg/min				
Initial	2.0	1.0	5.0	0.03
Usual range	2–20	1–5	5–20	0.02–0.20
Most common adverse effects	Tachycardia	Dysrhythmias	Tachycardia	Intense vasoconstriction
	Dysrhythmias		Dysrhythmias	Dysrhythmias
	Angina		Intense vasoconstriction	Angina
			Angina	

B. PHARMACOLOGIC PROPERTIES AND THERAPEUTIC CONSIDERATIONS IN USING INOTROPIC AGENTS

PHARMACOLOGIC FEATURE	DOBUTAMINE	MILRINONE	DOPAMINE LOW DOSE	DOPAMINE HIGH DOSE	NOREPINEPHRINE
Receptor agonism					
α	+	0	+	+++	++++
β_1	++++	0	+	++	+
β_2	++	0	0	0	0
Dopaminergic	0	0	+++	++	0
Systemic vascular resistance	↓↓	↓↓↓	↓	↑↑	↑↑↑↑
Stroke volume and cardiac output	↑↑↑↑	↑↑↑↑	↑	↑↑	↑
Ability to increase systemic blood pressure	→ to ↑	→ to ↓	→	↑↑↑	↑↑↑↑
Ventricular filling pressure	↓↓	↓↓↓	↓ to →	→ to ↑↑	→ to ↑↑
Chronotropic	→ to ↑↑	→ to ↑↑	→	→ to ↑↑↑	→ to ↑
Myocardial oxygen demand/supply	→ to ↑	→ to ↓	→	↑↑	↑↑

FIGURE 9-8. A and **B,** Principal pharmacologic properties and therapeutic considerations in the use of the major inotropic and vasopressor agents in acute heart failure. [12–18]. Milrinone delivers most of its hemodynamic properties through phosphodiesterase inhibition.

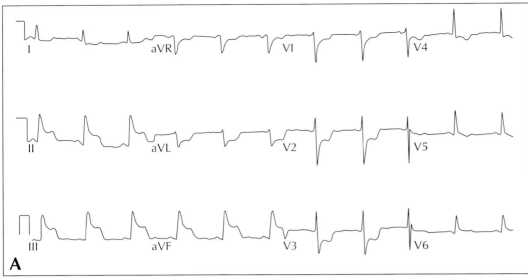

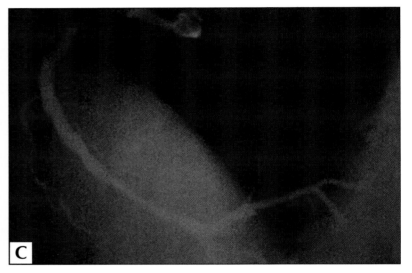

FIGURE 9-9. Electrocardiographic diagnosis of acute myocardial ischemia-infarction as a cause of acute or decompensated heart failure. **A,** Electrocardiographic tracing obtained in the emergency room showing inferoposterior injury in a 61-year-old woman who presented with a 45-minute history of marked dyspnea, chest discomfort, and nausea.

B and **C,** Angioplasty of the acutely thrombosed, high-grade right coronary artery obstruction (*arrow* in **B** depicts point of obstruction) reestablished patency and flow (**C**), and symptoms resolved within 1 hour of presentation.

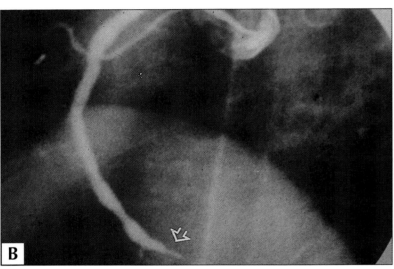

MANAGEMENT OF ACUTE MYOCARDIAL INJURY–ISCHEMIA–INFARCTION IN THE PRESENTATION OF ACUTE HEART FAILURE

Early detection with successful treatment is crucial for favorable short- and long-term clinical course and prognosis; "time is muscle"

Thrombolytic therapy

    Presentation within 12 h of the onset of angina or angina-equivalent symptoms with ECG changes of injury-ischemia

    Angina or angina-equivalent symptoms and ECG changes of injury-ischemia ± infarction that recur or persist beyond 6 h since the onset of symptoms

Emergent cardiac catheterization + intervention

    If readily accessible, can be the initial approach to acute myocardial injury-ischemia (catheterization laboratory modalities: angioplasty + stent placement, assessment for urgent bypass surgery)

    Ischemic symptoms or signs (ECG) that persist or recur beyond initial management and thrombolytic therapy

    Cardiogenic shock or near-shock

    Refractory or recurrent acute heart failure

    Evaluation of clinical events that have a high likelihood of evolving into heart failure (*eg*, new systolic murmur)

FIGURE 9-10. Major issues in the management of myocardial injury-ischemia-infarction in the setting of acute heart failure [2–5,19–34]. The important principles of general management include prompt detection and management of myocardial injury-ischemia-infarction; prompt detection and treatment of the lesions underlying the development of acute heart failure; and vigilance for the complications of ischemia or infarction (*eg*, ruptured myocardium), which can potentially evolve into cardiovascular decompensation and failure. ECG—electrocardiogram.

A. INDWELLING PULMONARY ARTERY CATHETERS (SWAN-GANZ CATHETER)

APPLICATIONS IN ACUTE HEART FAILURE

Acute heart failure not responsive to standard, initial measures

Cardiogenic shock and near-shock not responsive to initial management

Uncertain status of intravascular volume and ventricular filling pressures

Monitor and guide the administration of fluid volume and cardioactive drugs (eg, nitroprusside, dobutamine, dopamine, milrinone)

Assessment of dyspnea and other potential symptoms of heart failure in patients with other conditions (eg, chronic lung disease, marked obesity)

Assist in the determination of whether pulmonary edema is of cardiogenic or noncardiogenic origin

Evaluation of a new systolic murmur when echocardiography is not available or diagnostic

GENERAL REQUIREMENTS

Experienced, proficient operator

Trained personnel to assist in catheter insertion, use, and maintenance

Compatible, accurate amplification-recording equipment

Catheterization laboratory, emergency department, or intensive care unit setting

B. INDWELLING SYSTEMIC ARTERIAL CATHETERS

APPLICATIONS IN ACUTE HEART FAILURE

Continuous monitoring and recording of systemic blood pressure

Conduit for frequent, repeated blood gas determinations

FIGURE 9-11. General indications and other issues of practical application for the pulmonary artery (Swan-Ganz) catheter (**A**) and systemic arterial catheter (**B**). Indwelling vascular catheters may be necessary for the optimal management of acute or severe heart failure. The pulmonary artery catheter can provide useful data to assist in the diagnosis of certain threatening lesions and conditions (*eg*, right ventricular infarction, ruptured ventricular septum) in addition to its use in monitoring fluid and drug therapy.

ECHOCARDIOGRAPHY

GENERAL APPLICATIONS FOR ECHOCARDIOGRAPHY IN ACUTE HEART FAILURE

Part of the overall diagnostic evaluation of acute heart failure

Emergently in

Cardiogenic shock and near-shock

Refractory pulmonary edema

When the underlying etiology is not clear or requires confirmation or the differential diagnoses include major, often masked, reparable lesions

In the assessment of the extent of myocardial involvement in acute ischemia and infarction

As part of the cardiac evaluation of unexplained dyspnea and other symptoms of respiratory failure

In the evaluation of a new systolic murmur and its role in the clinical presentation

FIGURE 9-12. Common clinical reasons for the use of echocardiography in acute heart failure. Examples of major, often masked, reparable lesions include clinically silent aortic stenosis, mitral stenosis or regurgitation, pericardial tamponade, and intracardiac tumor. Assessing the extent of myocardial involvement by echocardiography in acute ischemia and infarction is particularly informative in patients with nondiagnostic electrocardiograms (*eg*, left bundle branch block).

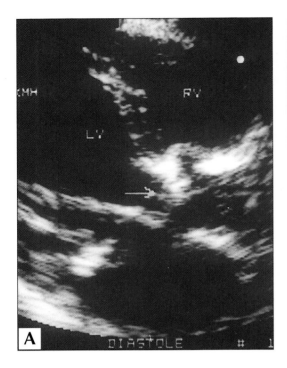

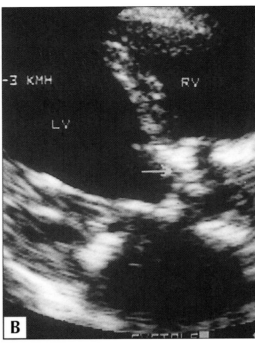

FIGURE 9-13. Echocardiography in the determination of the severity and etiology of ventricular dysfunction and failure. Echocardiograms of a 71-year-old man who presented with acute pulmonary edema after a 4- to 5-month history of dyspnea on exertion. Signs of congestive heart failure were apparent on physical examination. Diastolic (**A**) and systolic (**B**) echocardiograms demonstrated a heavily calcified, poorly mobile, stenotic aortic valve (*arrow*) and consequent ventricular hypertrophy, enlargement, and failure (ejection fraction, 0.24). A systolic murmur was barely audible. This patient represents an example of acute (and chronic) congestive heart failure secondary to silent aortic stenosis. A severely reduced aortic valve area (<0.4 cm^2) was calculated via echo and catheterization. Aortic valve replacement dramatically improved the patient's hemodynamic and clinical condition. LV—left ventricle; RV—right ventricle. (*Courtesy of* Dr. Anthony C. Pearson, Columbus, OH.)

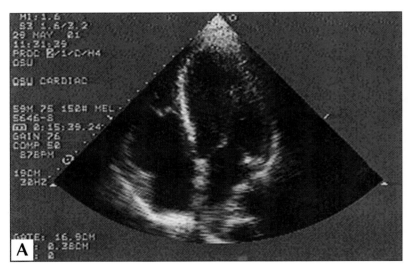

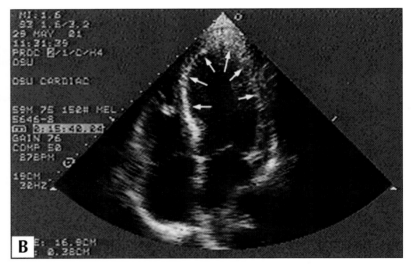

FIGURE 9-14. Echocardiography in the diagnosis of apical contraction abnormality. A 50-year-old man with diabetes mellitus and chronic renal failure underwent three-vessel coronary artery bypass surgery. Several months later, he presented with the clinical picture of acute myocardial infarction and congestive heart failure. The initial echocardiogram demonstrated severe segmental left ventricular dysfunction. Diastolic (**A**) and systolic (**B**) frames from an apical four-chamber view demonstrate a large midseptal and apical contraction abnormality, which in other views also involved the midanterior and inferior segments. Repeat coronary arteriography showed severe occlusive disease of his native coronary arteries and patent grafts; however, the distal run-off of the left anterior descending artery was poor. He was treated rather aggressively with nitrates, angiotensin-converting enzyme inhibitor, β-adrenergic blockade, and other appropriate agents (*eg*, statin, aspirin). Repeat echocardiography 1 month later showed marked improvement in left ventricular systolic function, suggesting that there was a large amount of stunned myocardium present in the initial echocardiogram.

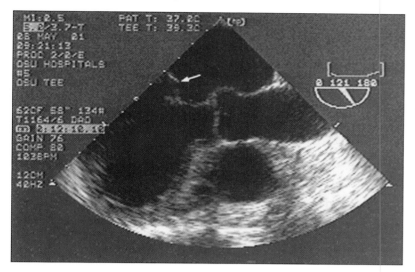

FIGURE 9-15. Echocardiographic imaging of severe mitral valve dysfunction. A 63-year-old woman with a past history of systemic hypertension presented with a 2-week history of increasing dyspnea and fatigue. Her jugular veins were not distended; lungs were clear to auscultation; and a new grade IV/VI holosystolic murmur was readily appreciated over the precordium. A standard transthoracic echocardiogram showed normal left and right ventricular volumes and systolic function, mitral valve prolapse, and substantial mitral regurgitation. Transesophageal echocardiography demonstrated 3 to 4+ (severe) mitral regurgitation, mitral valve prolapse, and flail segments of the posterior leaflet of the mitral valve (*arrow*). She was placed on diuretics, angiotensin-converting enzyme inhibitor, a nitrate preparation, and low-dose β-blockade with clinical improvement. Shortly thereafter, she underwent mitral valve replacement (the valve was not suitable for repair) and clinically she has done well since the operation.

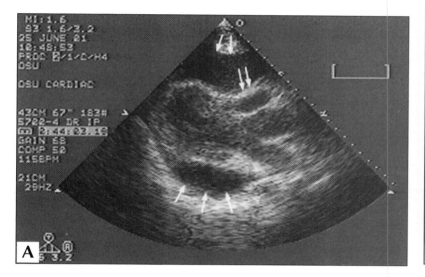

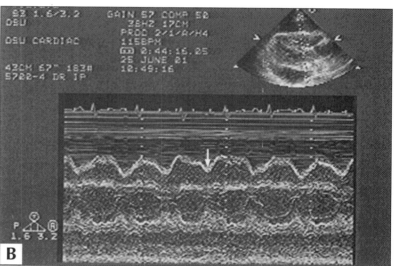

FIGURE 9-16. Echocardiographic imaging of heart failure in systemic lupus erythematosus (SLE). A 43-year-old man with SLE presented to the emergency department with several days of increasing dyspnea, orthopnea, lightheadedness, and chest "pressure." An echocardiogram demonstrated a large pericardial effusion with signs of tamponade. A long parasternal view (**A**) shows a large pericardial effusion anterior and posterior to the heart (*arrows*) with compression of the right ventricle free wall (*double arrow*). The M-mode tracing (**B**) demonstrates diastolic collapse of the right ventricle. The patient underwent pericardiocentesis with symptomatic relief.

INTRA-AORTIC BALLOON COUNTERPULSATION

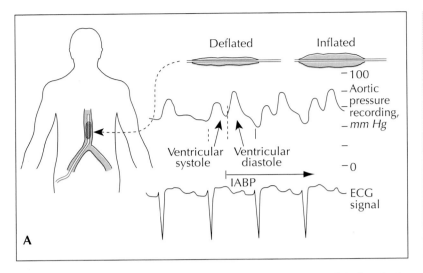

FIGURE 9-17. Intra-aortic balloon counterpulsation. **A,** Mechanical support in acute heart failure via intra-aortic balloon counterpulsation (IABP). By inflating a balloon within the blood-filled aorta during diastole, intra-aortic counterpulsation improves hemodynamics by augmenting coronary or myocardial and peripheral tissue perfusion. Myocardial oxygen consumption and ventricular afterload are reduced as well [19–23]. **B,** General applications in acute heart failure. ECG—electrocardiogram.

B. GENERAL APPLICATIONS FOR INTRA-AORTIC BALLOON COUNTERPULSATION

Cardiogenic shock

Cardiogenic near-shock not responsive to standard therapy

Acute pulmonary edema and other forms of acute cardiac failure not responsive to standard initial therapy

Acute heart failure accompanied by refractory angina or an obstructive lesion of the left main coronary artery

For clinical and hemodynamic stabilization through definitive diagnostic and therapeutic procedures

Relative contraindications

Significant aortic insufficiency

Aortic dissection, aneurysm

DEFINING AND TREATING CAUSATIVE LESIONS

THE MAJOR, DEFINITIVE DIAGNOSTIC, AND INTERVENTIONAL PROCEDURES MOST COMMONLY USED IN THE MANAGEMENT OF ACUTE HEART FAILURE

DIAGNOSTIC	INTERVENTIONAL
Electrocardiography	Thrombolysis
Chest radiography	Coronary angioplasty + stent placement
Echocardiography (transthoracic, transesophageal)	Coronary artery bypass surgery
Cardiac catheterization	Valvular repair or replacement
Coronary arteriography	Repair of ventricular rupture (septal, papillary, free wall)
Contrast ventriculography	Others (*eg*, pericardiocentesis for tamponade, aortic surgery of acute dissection)

FIGURE 9-18. Procedures most commonly used in the management of acute heart failure. Echocardiography and catheterization are the major diagnostic modalities used to define the presence and reversibility of causative lesions in acute heart failure. Other methods, such as nuclear magnetic resonance imaging, may also be useful in certain clinical conditions. Based on the findings of these diagnostic studies, a variety of interventions may be used to reverse and treat the culprit lesions. A crucial component in management of acute heart failure is clinical and hemodynamic stabilization of the patient to allow performance of definitive diagnostic studies and interventional procedures. The short- and long-term outcomes of patients with acute heart failure are directly related to the proficient management of acute heart failure, clinical and hemodynamic stabilization, and definitive diagnosis and intervention.

CAVEATS AND PITFALLS IN THE MANAGEMENT OF ACUTE HEART FAILURE

Misdiagnosis

Delay in the diagnosis and treatment of myocardial ischemia-infarction

Overtreatment

Unattended or unmonitored "gap" in management

FIGURE 9-19. The most common major caveats and pitfalls in the overall management of acute heart failure. A number of other conditions, many readily treatable, can present with symptoms and signs very similar to those of acute heart failure. These include pulmonary embolization, acute asthma, pneumonia, and septicemia, among others. A good medical history and physical examination, selection of key diagnostic studies, and clinical judgment are the best tools available to obviate misdiagnosis.

As noted in Figure 9-10, an immediate effort must be made to exclude or detect the presence of myocardial ischemia or infarction as the underlying cause of acute heart failure. Any delay in this process allows ischemic myocardium to convert to infarction, and thus threatens the short- and long-term clinical course and prognosis. Overtreatment of acute heart failure, particularly acute pulmonary edema, is not uncommon in critical care medicine. The apparent urgency of the clinical presentation creates a sense that the patient has to be treated "fast and hard." Sublingual and intravenous nitroglycerin, high or repeated doses of diuretics, and morphine sulfate usually provide symptomatic relief but occasionally lead to overdiuresis, hypotension, and impaired peripheral perfusion. Good judgment in clinical therapeutics is the best means of prevention. It is not uncommon for the treated acute heart failure patient to pass through an unattended and unmonitored management "gap." This usually occurs after the initial management and before the patient's continued care is assumed by the inpatient medical team. This period represents a vulnerable time in a patient's early course, and is often further complicated by unfavorable logistic situations, such as an interhospital transfer or the transport or transfer from the emergency department to the intensive or coronary care unit. The consequences of misdiagnosis or overtreatment often appear at this particular time.

DECOMPENSATED CHRONIC HEART FAILURE

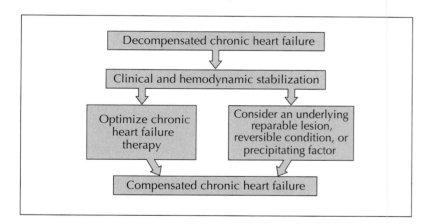

FIGURE 9-20. Management of decompensated chronic heart failure. The majority of patients with chronic heart failure who experience a period of decompensation respond clinically to temporary hemodynamic stabilization or optimization of chronic heart failure therapy (*see* Fig. 9-25). An occasional patient decompensates because of a superimposed lesion or condition, which may be reparable or reversible (*eg*, new-onset atrial fibrillation or flutter, myocardial ischemia, pulmonary embolization, infection).

MAJOR PRECIPITATING FACTORS FOR DECOMPENSATION OF CHRONIC HEART FAILURE

Inadequate therapy or noncompliance

Drug resistance or tolerance

Adverse drug effects
  Negative inotropic properties
  Salt and water retention
  Drug cancellation of a therapeutic effect

Deterioration of underlying cardiac disease

Excessive salt intake

Complicating conditions
  Myocardial ischemia-infarction
  Uncontrolled systemic hypertension
  Dysrhythmias
  Development or exacerbation of valvular dysfunction
  Pulmonary embolization
Renal dysfunction
Infections
Excessive stress
  Others

FIGURE 9-21. Major precipitating factors for decompensation of chronic heart failure. Several reparable lesions, reversible conditions, and precipitating factors should be considered when a patient with heart failure presents with decompensation. Complicating conditions include atrial flutter or fibrillation with or without rapid ventricular response, mitral regurgitation, or renal dysfunction. Among adverse drug effects, certain calcium channel blockers (*eg*, verapamil) and most antiarrhythmic drugs (*eg*, disopyramide) have negative inotropic properties, and nonsteroidal anti-inflammatory drugs can cause salt and water retention. While the patient's decompensated heart failure is being improved and stabilized, the physician should evaluate via medical history and physical examination whether any of these conditions may have led to the decompensation and, when appropriate, obtain specifically directed laboratory tests (*eg*, echocardiography-Doppler studies to assess severity of valvular regurgitation).

CLINICAL FEATURES

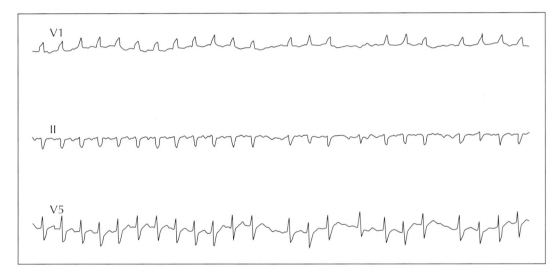

FIGURE 9-22. Electrocardiograpy in assessing decompensated chronic heart failure. A 70-year-old man with chronic, stable systolic and diastolic heart failure presented with increasing dyspnea, fatigue, malaise, and weakness. The rhythm strip of his electrocardiogram on admission showed a rapidly conducting atrial flutter. The dysrhythmia was of recent onset. Slowing the ventricular rate with digitalis and subsequent conversion to sinus rhythm resulted in a return to his usual state of well-compensated heart failure.

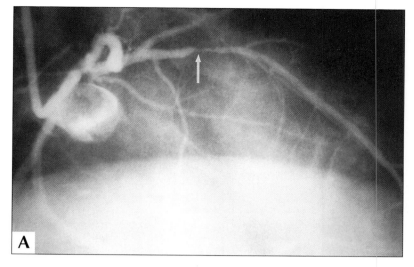

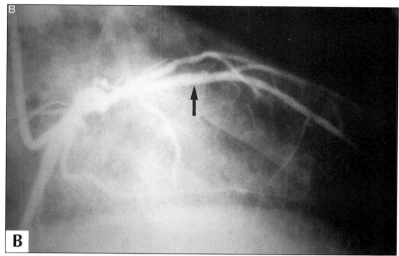

FIGURE 9-23. Recent coronary arteriography in a 70-year-old retired policeman with a 9-year history of left ventricular systolic dysfunction (ejection fraction, 30%) and functional class II heart failure. Coronary arteriography in 1995 showed trivial plaque formation along the left anterior descending coronary artery (LAD).

These angiograms (**A** and **B**) were obtained about 1 month after the patient noticed a progressive increase in dyspnea, first on exertion and eventually at rest (functional class IV congestive heart failure), orthopnea, and paroxysmal nocturnal dyspnea; these symptoms could not be adequately controlled with aggressive medical management. **A,** Injection of the left coronary artery (RAO projection) demonstrated a high-grade proximal stenosis (*white arrow*) of the LAD. He never experienced angina or chest pain. **B,** The LAD lesion shown in **A** was successfully dilated along with stent placement (*black arrow*). The aforementioned symptoms improved rather dramatically over the ensuing 7 to 10 days. The patient currently has a heart failure symptom level of FC II–III.

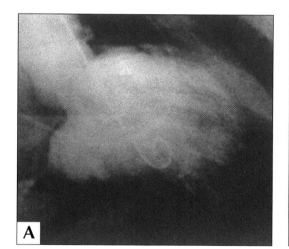

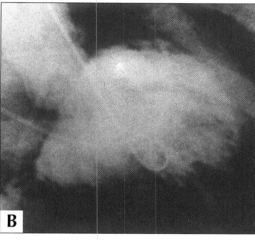

FIGURE 9-24. The systolic (**A**) and diastolic (**B**) frames of a contrast ventriculogram performed on a 47-year-old woman with long-standing systemic hypertension and a 3-year history of chronic heart failure. Discontinuation of her antihypertensive therapy and dietary indiscretion (excessive salt intake during the first week of her new job as a waitress) led to severe decompensated heart failure. After the initial management of decompensated heart failure, reestablishment of her antihypertensive therapy, optimization of her chronic heart failure medication, and dietary measures returned her to a state of stable compensation.

A. THERAPEUTICS FOR CHRONIC HEART FAILURE

STANDARD MAINTENANCE THERAPY

Angiotensin-converting enzyme inhibitors

β-adrenergic blockers

Diuretics, spironolactone

Digoxin

SUPPLEMENTAL AGENTS

Hydralazine-nitrate combination*

Nitrates*

Anticoagulation, antithrombotic agents

Antidysrhythmic intervention

B. THERAPEUTICS FOR CHRONIC HEART FAILURE

SUPPORT DRUGS AVAILABLE FOR USE DURING PERIODS OF DECOMPENSATION IN CHRONIC HEART FAILURE

Diuretics (intravenously administered or ↑ dose)

Positive inotropic agents (± vasodilating properties)

   Dobutamine (*see* Fig. 9-29)

   Dopamine (low to moderate dose)

   Phosphodiesterase inhibitors (*eg*, milrinone)

Vasodilators

   IV nitroglycerin

   Nitroprusside

   Nesiritide

   β-Natriuretic peptide

Vasopressors

   Dopamine (moderate to high dose)

   Norepinephrine

FIGURE 9-25. Therapeutics for chronic heart failure. **A,** In patients with chronic congestive heart failure, optimization of standard therapy with angiotensin-converting enzyme inhibitors, β-blockers, diuretics, digoxin, and the judicious use of supplemental agents are often effective in averting clinical decompensation. *Asterisks* indicate drugs that are not yet approved for a heart failure indication by the Food and Drug Administration.

B, Once decompensation has occurred, parenteral agents are frequently necessary to regain clinical stability. The agents most commonly used to improve and stabilize severely decompensated chronic heart failure are shown. Dobutamine, dopamine, (low to moderate dose), or milrinone are particularly effective in acutely improving clinical and hemodynamic status and stabilizing the patient during a period of diuresis and readjustment of chronic therapy. Vasodilators are employed to improve hemodynamics and systemic perfusion in chronic heart failure patients with adequate to high systemic blood pressure, and vasopressors are used in conditions of marked hypotension or shock. The clinical application of these agents is similar to that discussed previously for the treatment of acute heart failure (see Figs. 9-6 to 9-8). IV—intravenous.

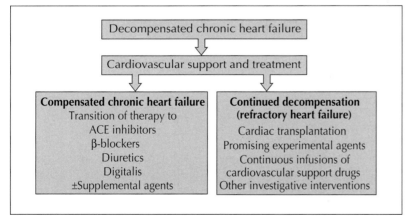

FIGURE 9-26. Course and treatment for postdecompensated chronic heart failure. With appropriate cardiovascular support and management, most patients with decompensated chronic heart failure can be converted to a state of clinical compensation. Other than cardiac transplantation, the management choices for patients who continue to have decompensated (refractory) chronic heart failure are limited to investigative approaches including experimental drugs, various surgical procedures (*eg*, modification of mitral valve), and/or continuous infusion of a cardiovascular support drug (*eg*, dobutamine, milrinone). ACE—angiotensin-converting enzyme.

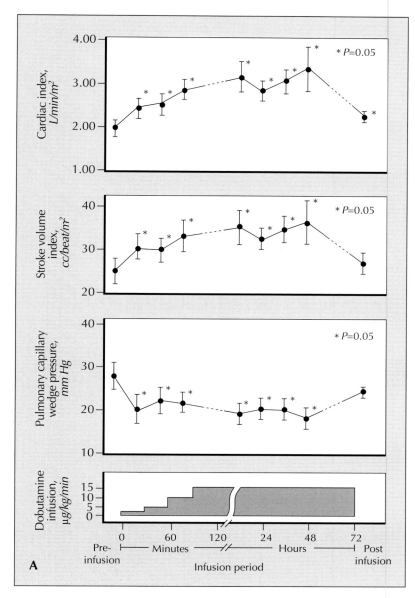

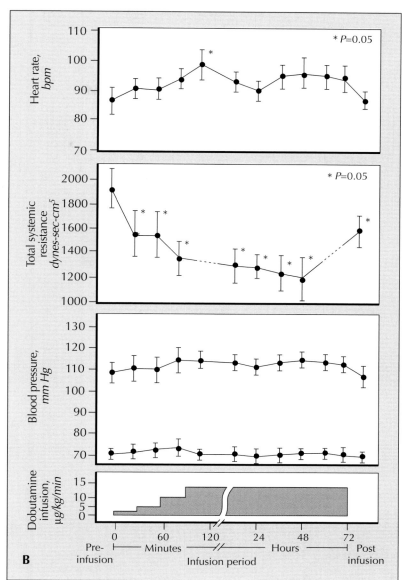

FIGURE 9-27. Hemodynamic dose-response (**A**) and continuous-infusion curves (**B**) for dobutamine in 25 patients with severe chronic congestive heart failure. Data are presented as ± SEM with $P<0.05$ versus baseline preinfusion value. (*Adapted from* Leier *et al.* [15].)

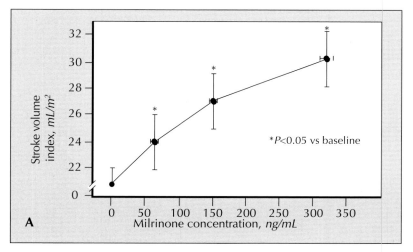

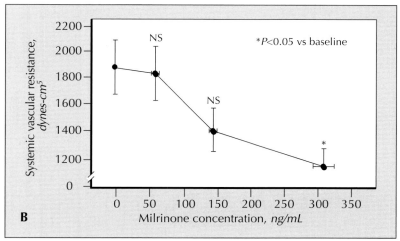

FIGURE 9-28. Dose-response of the hemodynamic effects to three doses (12.5, 25, and 50 µg/kg) of milrinone administered as an intravenous bolus over 15 to 60 seconds in 11 patients with moderate to severe congestive heart failure. The effects on stroke volume (**A**), systemic vascular resistance (**B**), LV+dP/dt (*continued*)

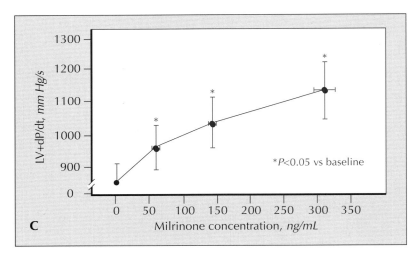

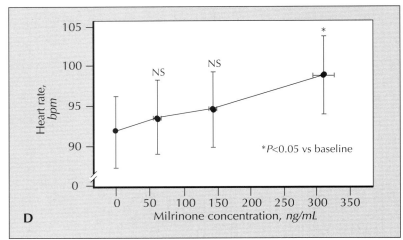

FIGURE 9-28. *(continued)* (**C**), and heart rate (**D**) are shown. NS—not significant. (*Adapted from* Jaski *et al.* [18].)

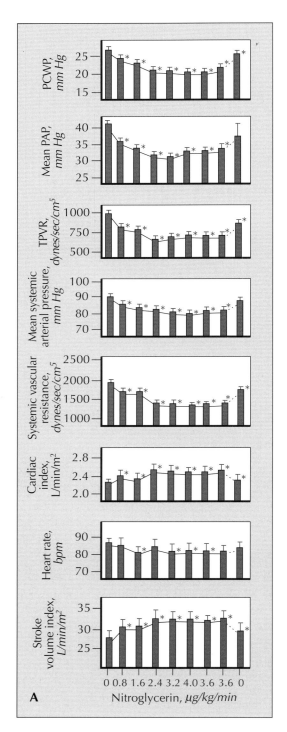

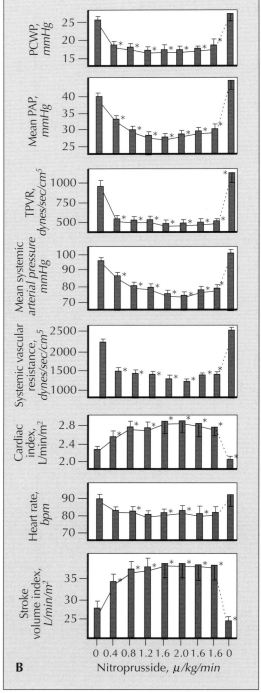

FIGURE 9-29. Hemodynamic responses to intravenously administered nitroglycerin (**A**) and nitroprusside (**B**) in patients with severe chronic congestive heart failure. Each drug was administered in five dose increments (30 minutes at each level) followed by the determined optimal maintenance dose. PAP —pulmonary artery pressure; PCWP —pulmonary capillary wedge pressure; TPVR —total pulmonary vascular resistance. (*Adapted from* Leier *et al.* [9].)

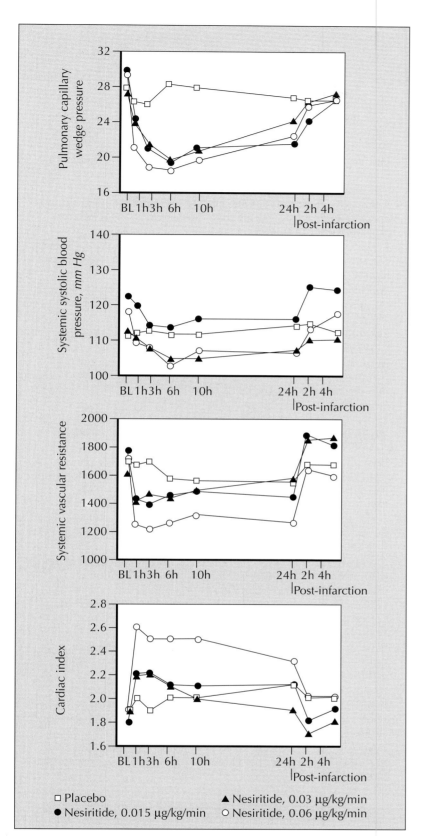

Figure 9-30. Hemodynamic effects of the commercially available β-natriuretic peptide, nesiritide, in patients with severe congestive heart failure. Each infusion of nesiritide was initiated with a bolus dose; 0.25 µg/kg bolus for the 0.015 µg/kg/min infusion dose, 0.50 µg/kg bolus for the 0.030 µg/kg/min infusion, and 1.0 µg/kg bolus for the 0.060 µg/kg/min infusion. The recommended infusion rates range from 0.010 to 0.030 µg/kg/min. (*Adapted from* Mills *et al.* [10].)

REFERENCES

1. Goldberger JJ, Peled HB, Stroh JA, *et al.*: Prognostic factors in acute pulmonary edema. *Arch Intern Med* 1986, 146:489–493.

2. Forrester JS, Diamond G, Chatterjee K, *et al.*: Medical therapy of acute myocardial infarction by application of hemodynamic subsets. *N Engl J Med* 1976, 295:1356–1362, 1404–1413.

3. Goldberg RJ, Yarzebski J, Lessard D, Gore JM: A two-decades (1975 to 1995) long experience in the incidence, in-hospital and long-term case fatality rates of acute myocardial infarction: a community-wide perspective. *J Am Coll Cardiol* 1999, 33:1533–1539.

4. Guidry UC, Evans JC, Larson MG, *et al.*: Temporal trends in event rates after Q wave myocardial infarction: the Framingham Heart Study. *Circulation* 1999, 100:2054–2059.

5. Gan SC, Beaver SK, Houck PM, *et al.*: Treatment of acute myocardial infarction and 30-day mortality among women and men. *N Engl J Med* 2000, 343:8–15.

6. Heart Failure Guidelines Committed of the American College of Cardiology/American Heart Association: Guidelines for the evaluation and management of heart failure. *J Am Coll Cardiol* 1995, 26:1376–1398.

7. Packer M, Cohn JN, Abraham WT, *et al.*: Consensus recommendations for the management of chronic heart failure. *Am J Cardiol* 1999, 83:1A–79A.

8. Franciosa JA, Guiha NH, Limas CL, *et al.*: Improved left ventricular function during nitroprusside infusion in acute myocardial infarction. *Lancet* 1972, 1:650–654.

9. Leier CV, Bambach D, Thompson MJ, *et al.*: Central and regional hemodynamic effects of intravenous isosorbide dinitrate, nitro-glycerin, and nitroprusside in patients with congestive heart failure. *Am J Cardiol* 1981, 48:1115–1123.

10. Mills RM, LeJeuntel TH, Horton DP, *et al.*: Sustained hemodynamic effects of nesiritide (human b-type natriuretic peptide) in heart failure: a randomized, double-blind, placebo-controlled clinical trial. *J Am Coll Cardiol* 1999, 34:155–162.

11. Colucci WS, Elkayan U, Horton DP, *et al.*: Intravenous nesiritide, a natriuretic peptide, in the treatment of decompensated heart failure. *N Engl J Med* 2000, 343:246–253.

12. Leier CV: Acute inotropic support: intravenously administered positive inotropic drugs. In *Cardiotonic Drugs*, edn 2. Edited by Leier CV. New York: Marcel Dekker; 1991:63–106.

13. Loeb HS, Winslow EBJ, Rahimtoola SH, *et al.*: Acute hemodynamic effects of dopamine in patients with shock. *Circulation* 1971, 44:163–173.

14. Holzer J, Karliner JS, O'Rourke RA, *et al.*: Effectiveness of dopamine in patients with cardiogenic shock. *Am J Cardiol* 1973, 32:79–84.

15. Leier CV, Webel J, Bush CA: The cardiovascular effects of the continuous infusion of dobutamine in patients with severe cardiac failure. *Circulation* 1977, 56:468–472.

16. Leier CV, Heban PT, Huss P, *et al.*: Comparative systemic and regional hemodynamic effects of dopamine and dobutamine in patients with heart failure. *Circulation* 1978, 58:466–475.

17. Francis GS, Sharma B, Hodges M: Comparative hemodynamic effects of dopamine and dobutamine in patients with acute cardiogenic circulatory collapse. *Am Heart J* 1982, 103:995–1000.

18. Jaski B, Fifer MA, Wright RF, *et al.*: Positive inotropic and vasodilator actions of milrinone in patients with severe congestive heart failure. *J Clin Invest* 1985, 75:643–649.

19. Sander CA, Buckley MJ, Leinbach RC, *et al.*: Mechanical circula-tory assistance: current status and experience with combining circulatory assistance, emergency coronary angiography, and acute myocardial revascularization. *Circulation* 1972, 45:1291–1313.

20. Bardet J, Masquet C, Kahn J-C, *et al.*: Clinical and hemodynamic results of intra-aortic balloon counterpulsation and surgery for cardiogenic shock. *Am Heart J* 1977, 93:280–288.

21. Johnson SA, Scanlon PJ, Loeb HS, *et al.*: Treatment of cardiogenic shock in myocardial infarction by intra-aortic balloon counter-pulsation and surgery. *Am J Med* 1977, 62:687–692.

22. Kovack PJ, Rasak MA, Bates ER, *et al.*: Thrombolysis plus aortic counterpulsation with and without reperfusion for myocardial infarction shock. *Circulation* 1980, 61:1105–1112.

23. Torchiana DF, Hirsch G, Buckley MJ, *et al.*: Intraaortic balloon pumping for cardiac support: trends in practice and outcome, 1968 to 1995. *J Thorac Cardiovasc Surg* 1997, 113:758.

24. Califf RM: Ten years of benefit from a one-hour intervention. *Circulation* 1998, 98:2649–2651.

25. Rothbaum DA, Linnemeier TJ, Landin RJ, *et al.*: Emergency percutaneous transluminal coronary angioplasty in acute myocardial infarction: a 3 year experience. *J Am Coll Cardiol* 1987, 10:264–272.

26. Lee L, Bates ER, Pitt B, *et al.*: Percutaneous transluminal coronary angioplasty improves survival in acute myocardial infarction complicated by cardiogenic shock. *Circulation* 1988, 78:1345–1351.

27. Ellis SG, O'Neill WW, Bates ER, *et al.*: Implications of patient triage from survival and left ventricular functional recovery analyses in 500 patients treated with coronary angioplasty for acute myocardial infarction. *J Am Coll Cardiol* 1989, 13:1251–1259.

28. Lee L, Erbel R, Brown TM, *et al.*: Multicenter registry of angioplasty therapy of cardiogenic shock: initial and long-term survival. *J Am Coll Cardiol* 1991, 17:599–603.

29. Hochman JS, Boland J, Sleeper LA, *et al.*: Current spectrum of cardiogenic shock and effect of early revascularization on mortality. *Circulation* 1995, 91:873–881.

30. Lamas GA, Glaker GA, Mitchell G, *et al.*: Effect of infarct artery patency on prognosis after acute myocardial infarction. *Circulation* 1995, 92:1101–1109.

31. Holmes DR Jr, Bates ER, Kleiman NS, *et al.*: Contemporary reperfusion therapy for cardiogenic shock: the Gusto-1 trial experience. *J Am Coll Cardiol* 1995, 26:668–674.

32. Berger PB, Holmes DR, Stebbins AL, *et al.* for the Gusto-1 Investigators: Impact of an aggressive invasive catheterization and revascularization strategy on mortality in patients with cardiogenic shock in the Gusto-1 trial. *Circulation* 1997, 96:122–127.

33. Dangas G, Stone GW: Primary mechanical reperfusion in acute myocardial infarction: the United States experience. *Semin Intervent Cardiol* 1999, 4:21–33.

34. Hochman JS, Sleeper LA, Webb JG, *et al.*: Early revascularization in acute myocardial infarction complicated by cardiogenic shock: should we emergently revascularize occluded coronaries for cardiogenic shock. *N Engl J Med* 1999, 341:625–634.

DIGITALIS AND DIURETICS

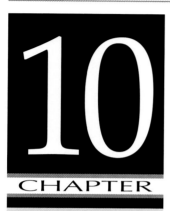

CHAPTER 10

D. Bradley S. Dyke and Robert J. Cody

Digitalis plays an important role in the treatment of patients in whom systolic dysfunction is a major component. Although its therapeutic benefits were demonstrated more than two centuries ago, the efficacy of digitalis in the treatment of patients in normal sinus rhythm with heart failure has remained controversial. Further, beneficial effects beyond a direct inotropic or hemodynamic benefit may account for much of the clinical outcome in humans. The absence of a significant reduction in mortality in a large prospective trial (Digitalis Investigation Group [DIG] trial) is balanced against the clinical benefit demonstrated in two independent digoxin withdrawal studies.

Diuretics are an effective and essential component of therapy for edema management in heart failure. In addition to their predictable effects on fluid and electrolyte balance, diuretics have a number of metabolic side effects. The value of diuretic therapy is enhanced by the thoughtful utilization of these agents. Earlier use of combined diuretic regimens, avoidance of excessive loop diuretic dosage, and identification of early stages of decompensation permit effective reduction of "congestive" symptoms and minimizes the requirement for hospitalization.

The triad of digoxin-diuretic-"vasodilator" therapy for heart failure was first established more than 25 years ago. This older, somewhat arbitrary, triad was subsequently challenged by the results of ACE inhibitor trials. As we begin the 21st century, a more rational algorithm for heart failure therapy must continue to evolve, encompassing primary disease management, targeted modification of secondary maladaptation, and more effective distribution of proven drug therapy.

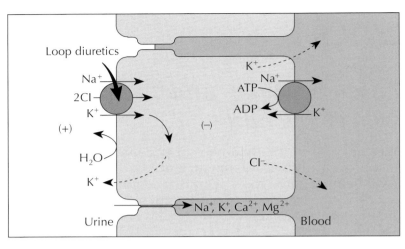

Figure 10-1. Loop diuretics in heart failure. The introduction in the 1960s of diuretics that act within the loop of Henle, so-called "high-ceiling" or "loop" diuretics, dramatically affected the ability of clinicians to improve symptoms of congestive heart failure with minimum toxicity and predictable efficacy compared with other drugs available at that time. These diuretics act on a specific transport protein, the $Na^+K^+/2Cl^-$ cotransporter, located on the apical membrane of renal epithelial cells in the ascending limb of Henle's loop. Ions transported into the cell are then transferred out of the cell by Na^+K^+-ATPase (the "sodium pump") on the basolateral membranes of these cells. Loop diuretics also decrease the absorption of Ca^{2+} and Mg^{2+} in this portion of the nephron, cations whose absorption is indirectly linked to NaCl uptake. Thus, hypocalcemia and hypomagnesia, as well as hypokalemia and volume depletion, may result from prolonged use of these drugs.

Loop diuretics also reduce the tonicity of the medullary interstitium by preventing the normal uptake of solute in the absence of water in the thick ascending limb of Henle's loop. This limits the kidney's ability to concentrate the urine and may contribute to the development of hyponatremia. The loop diuretics are clearly the most useful diuretics as single agents for patients with decompensated congestive failure, in large part because of the magnitude of the natriuresis that can be achieved over a short period, which can reach as high as 20% of the filtered load of sodium. Typically, the fraction of NaCl filtered at the glomerulus and reabsorbed in the ascending limb of the loop of Henle declines from about 20% to 13% with a loop diuretic, resulting in a 1% to 2% increase in the fractional excretion of sodium over 24 hours [1].

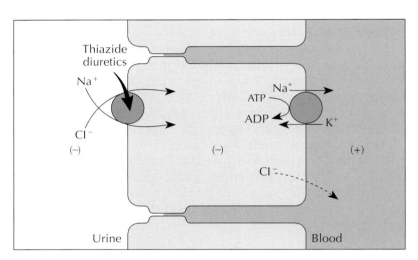

Figure 10-2. Thiazide diuretics. In general, the thiazide diuretics are not useful as single drugs for the therapy of volume retention in heart failure patients, largely because their site of action in the distal convoluted tubule permits rapid adjustment of water and solute absorption in other more proximal nephron segments. Interestingly, the target renal tubular protein of the thiazide class of diuretics, the electroneutral Na^+Cl^- cotransporter, has recently been cloned and sequenced. This is the last of the known diuretic-responsive renal epithelial cell transport proteins to be identified. Many other tissues also express this transport protein, which may have important implications for understanding the effectiveness of these drugs in the treatment of hypertension as well as their less desirable metabolic effects on lipid and glucose metabolism. Unlike loop diuretics, thiazides enhance calcium reabsorption but not that of magnesium, although magnesium wasting is much more pronounced with loop diuretics [1].

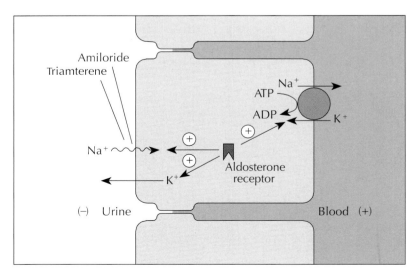

Figure 10-3. Potassium-sparing diuretics. The potassium-sparing diuretics fall into two categories: agents such as amiloride and triamterene, which reduce Na^+ conductance through an apical membrane sodium channel; and aldosterone antagonists, which, by inhibiting the actions of aldosterone at its intracellular receptor in renal epithelial cells of the distal collecting duct, reduce Na^+ uptake from the tubular lumen and decrease K^+ secretion by several mechanisms. Aldosterone antagonists also limit the kidney's ability to acidify the urine by inhibiting the action of aldosterone on a renal tubular proton pump. Although none of these diuretics is effective as a single agent in the treatment of heart failure, they play a useful role in diminishing renal K^+ wasting. When combined with loop or thiazide diuretics, the aldosterone antagonists also prevent Mg^{2+} depletion. Because ACE inhibitors increase the serum K^+ concentration, an effect that may be magnified by β-blockers and NSAIDS, potassium-sparing diuretics should be prescribed cautiously for patients who are already receiving vasodilators of this class [1].

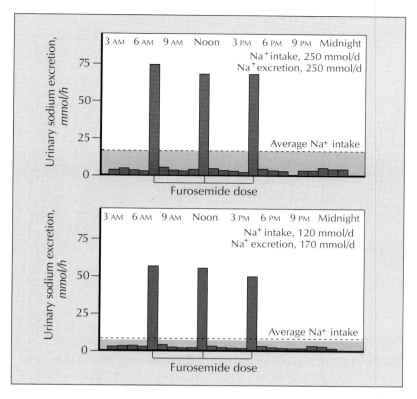

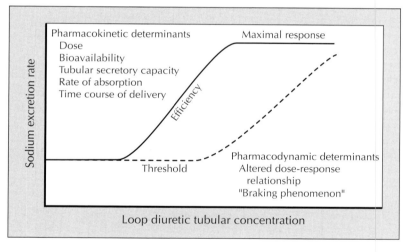

FIGURE 10-4. Importance of dietary salt intake on the renal response to loop diuretics. Because most loop diuretics are short-acting drugs, it is always more effective to give multiple daily doses rather than the same total amount as a single daily dose.

Avid sodium retention during the remainder of the day after a single dose tends to minimize the daily net loss of NaCl (*ie*, a negative sodium balance). Even multiple daily doses of a loop diuretic are ineffective unless the NaCl content in the diet is reduced concomitantly. The effect of three daily intravenous doses of furosemide (40 mg) on daily sodium balance is illustrated in patients on chronic diuretic therapy at two different levels of dietary sodium intake. In each panel, hourly sodium excretion is shown on the vertical axis of these histograms, and the result of the three daily doses is illustrated.

The *dashed horizontal lines* represent the daily sodium intake on each diet averaged over 24 hours. Negative Na^+ balance is shown above the dashed line, in *upper bars*, and positive balance (*ie*, sodium retention) appears below the dashed line. The small *lower bars* between furosemide doses reflect sodium excretion during each urinary collection period. Only urinary sodium excretion that represents a net negative sodium balance (*ie*, sodium loss greater than intake) is shown. For a daily net negative sodium balance to occur, the volume of all the bars must exceed the total area below the *dashed line* for a given diuretic and dietary sodium regimen. There was no net loss of sodium in these subjects on a high-sodium intake (250 mmol Na^+/d), whereas a moderate reduction in sodium intake to 120 mmoL/d (equivalent to a "no added salt" diet) resulted in a moderate negative sodium balance in each 24-hour period. A more severe dietary restriction (*eg*, to 20 mmoL/d) will lead to a marked negative sodium balance and weight loss but may be complicated by the development of excess volume depletion, hyponatremia and hypokalemia, and a hypochloremic metabolic alkalosis, unless the patient is carefully monitored. (*Adapted from* Wilcox *et al.* [2].)

FIGURE 10-5. Pharmacokinetic and pharmacodynamic determinants of loop diuretic response. Loop diuretics are delivered to the site of action, the lumen of the tubule, by organic anion transporters located in the proximal tubule. The *solid line* demonstrates several important points. There is a clear threshold concentration of the loop diuretic, below which there is no effective excretion of sodium or water above baseline. There is also a clear plateau concentration above which no further excretion of sodium and water occurs. The *dashed line* represents an altered dose-response relationship, as is frequently encountered in diuretic resistant states such as heart failure and renal disease. The "braking phenomenon" refers to a commonly seen physiologic response to diuretic therapy beyond the first dose. As the extracellular fluid volume decreases, a complex series of neuro-hormonal and hemodynamic and intrarenal changes occur that cause an avid state of postdiuretic sodium retention, which offsets the effectiveness of the initial diuresis. (*Adapted from* Sica and Deedwania [3].)

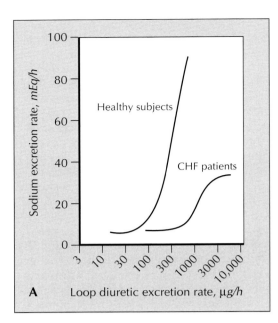

A

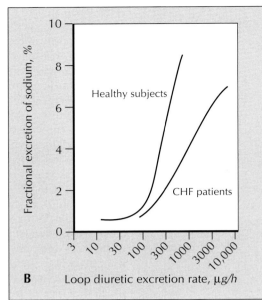

B

FIGURE 10-6. Loop diuretic–induced sodium excretion in healthy subjects versus patients with heart failure. Represented in these two graphs are the rightward and downward shift of loop diuretic effectiveness observed in patients with heart failure versus healthy individuals. Factors that are involved in this change in effectiveness include altered bioavailability (secondary to gut wall edema, reduced cardiac output, redirection of renal blood flow), nephron loss (secondary to concomitant diseases such as hypertension and diabetes), competition at the organic anion transporters (accumulated endogenous organic acids observed in patients with renal failure, probenecid), distal tubule hypertrophy (a compensatory reaction to chronic loop diuretic use), and the braking effect (see Fig. 10-5). (*Adapted from* Vargo *et al.* [4].)

DETERMINANTS OF DIURETIC RESPONSE

Pharmacokinetic factors
  Quantity of drug reaching the urine
    Dose administered
    Absolute bioavailability
    Tubular capacity for organic acid secretion
      Protein binding
      Renal blood flow
  Extrarenal diuretic clearance
  Time course of urinary drug delivery
    Rate of absorption
    Swift tubular secretory rate
Pharmacodynamic factors
  Dose-response relationship
    Underlying compensation state of disease
    Salt intake/intravascular volume
    Rebound sodium retention within a dosing interval
    Distal nephron hypertrophy
    Urinary diuretic binding as in nephrotic syndrome

FIGURE 10-7. Determinants of loop diuretic response. As defined previously, there is a clear dose-response curve associated with loop diuretic use. Bioavailability is influenced by route of administration—intravenous dosing allows for near complete bioavailability to the blood stream. Oral dosing bioavailability can vary from 20% to 80% depending on the drug used, the presence of gut wall edema, reduced gut blood flow secondary to low cardiac output states, and redirection of splanchnic blood flow. Even in the presence of optimal bioavailability, the time course of absorption can be altered. Tubular capacity for loop diuretic excretion is altered by the presence of endogenous organic acids, particularly in patients with accumulation of these acids secondary to renal failure, and the presence of drugs such as probenecid. Note that glomerular filtration itself is inconsequential, as loop diuretics are largely protein-bound and do not reach the site of action by filtration. Renal blood flow can be decreased secondary to low cardiac output, redirection of blood away from the renal vascular bed (which explains why diuretics are more effective if given to a supine patient), and renal artery stenosis. (*Adapted from* Sica and Deedwania [3].)

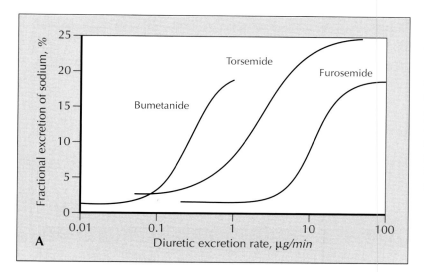

A

FIGURE 10-8. Pharmacodynamics and pharmacokinetics of diuretic drugs. **A,** Comparison of pharmacodynamic curves for bumetanide, furosemide, and torsemide. This graph demonstrates the difference in diuretic excretion rate, and hence tubular concentration, required for effective diuresis. Clinically, this is seen in the relative requirements of each diuretic in order to obtain comparable rates of sodium and water excretion. **B,** Pharmacokinetics of diuretic drugs, including oral bioavailability and elimination half-life. Of note, torsemide and bumetanide have an oral bioavailability that is consistently higher than that of furosemide, and with less variability. ND—not determined. (*Adapted from* Rudy *et al.* [5] and Brater [6].)

B. PHARMACOKINETICS OF DIURETIC DRUGS

DIURETIC		ELIMINATION HALF LIFE	
Loop	ORAL BIOAVAILABILITY, %	NORMAL SUBJECTS, %	PATIENTS WITH HEART FAILURE, N
Furosemide	10–100	1.5–2	2.7
Bumetanide	80–100	1	1.3
Torsemide	80–100	3–4	6
Thiazide			
Chlorothiazide	30–50	1.5	ND
Hydrochlorothiazide	65–75	2.5	ND
Distal			
Spironolactone	Conflicting data	1.5	ND
Active metabolites of spironolactone		>15	ND

LOOP DIURETICS IN HEART FAILURE WITH DIMINISHED INITIAL RESPONSE

FACTOR	HEART FAILURE WITH PRESERVED RENAL FUNCTION	HEART FAILURE WITH RENAL INSUFFICIENCY	
		MODERATE	SEVERE
Mechanism of diminished response	Diminished nephron response	Impaired delivery to site of action	
Therapeutic response	More frequent administration of effective dose	Administration of sufficiently high dose to attain effective amount of diuretic at the site of action	
Maximal intravenous dose, *mg*			
Furosemide	40–80	80–160	160–200
Bumetanide	1–2	4–8	8–10
Torsemide	10–20	20–50	50–100

FIGURE 10-9. Loop diuretics in heart failure with diminished initial response to therapy. This table demonstrates the mechanisms of diminished response, therapeutic approaches and maximal intravenous doses of commercially available loop diuretics for patients who have a less than adequate response to initial diuretic therapy. In summary, an adequate response can usually be obtained by increasing the dose of the loop diuretic until an effective diuresis is forced. The frequency of this dose is then increased in order to approximate a patient's daily fluid intake. This may vary from patient to patient depending on their ability to limit dietary sodium and fluid intake. (*Adapted from* Brater [6].)

DIURETIC	INTRAVENOUS LOADING DOSE, MG	INFUSION RATE*		
		CREATININE CLEARANCE < 26 ML/MIN (MG/H)	CREATININE CLEARANCE 25–75 ML/MIN (MG/H)	CREATININE CLEARANCE > 75 ML/MIN
Furosemide	40	20 then 40	10 then 20	10
Bumetanide	1	1 then 2	0.5 then 1	0.5
Torsemide	20	10 then 30	5 then 10	5

*Before the infusion rate is increased, the loading dose should be administered again.

FIGURE 10-10. Continuous intravenous infusion of loop diuretics. Circumstances occasionally require the use of a continuous loop diuretic infusion. Patients who have a relatively low response to maximal doses of bolus diuretic can have a more consistent output if the drug is maintained at the site of action. Continuous infusions allow the clinician to avoid the postdiuretic sodium retention that typically occurs between bolus doses. Another relative indication for a continuous infusion is that it may be easier for nursing staff than frequent administration of bolus doses. Of note, when initiating a continuous infusion of a loop diuretic, it is beneficial to give an initial loading dose in order to decrease the time needed to achieve therapeutic drug concentrations at the site of action. (*Adapted from* Brater [6].)

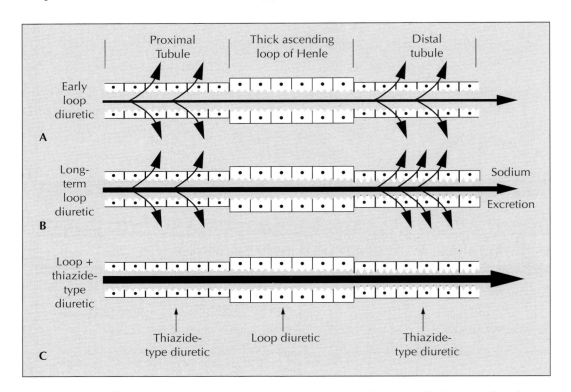

FIGURE 10-11. Three segments of the nephron: the proximal tubule, thick ascending loop of Henle, and distal tubule. Under normal conditions, sodium is reabsorbed along all three segments. This figure represents the condition in congestive heart failure in which many patients have a reduction in glomerular filtration rate and, therefore, increased proximal tubular sodium reabsorption. **A,** Early loop diuretic. Blockade of sodium reabsorption at the thick ascending loop of Henle is represented, also demonstrating that the loop diuretic has no appreciable effect on proximal or distal sodium reabsorption. **B,** Long-term loop diuretic. The adverse effect of distal tubular hypertrophy. Thus, an increased load of sodium continues to be avidly reabsorbed proximally. The loop diuretic blocks reabsorption at the thick ascending loop of Henle. However, in the presence of distal tubular hypertrophy, due to uncontrolled sodium intake and the effects of enhanced sodium delivery during loop diuretic therapy, there is additional avid sodium reabsorption in the distal tubule, resulting in a reduction of sodium excretion compared with earlier stages of loop diuretic therapy. **C,** Loop plus thiazide-type diuretic. Blockade of sodium reabsorption at both the proximal and distal tubule, combined with the effect of the loop diuretic, reestablishes enhanced sodium excretion. (*Adapted from* Cody and Pickworth [7].)

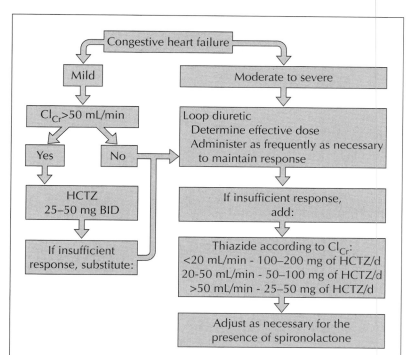

FIGURE 10-12. Algorithm for diuretic use in patients with heart failure. The treatment of edematous states in heart failure requires a flexible and dynamic approach to management. This frequently requires the use of combination therapy. Patients with mild heart failure and relatively preserved renal function can usually be treated with a thiazide-type diuretic alone. Patients with more severe heart failure, the presence of renal insufficiency, or both in combination, frequently need multiple daily dosing of a loop diuretic in combination with a thiazide-type diuretic in order to maintain an adequate diuresis. Of note, metolazone is also frequently used in the United States, but the practitioner should be cautioned that this agent has a more variable absorption and longer half-life than hydrochlorothiazide (HCTZ). Adequate attention needs to be given to patients receiving this combination, as intravascular volume and electrolyte changes can take several day to manifest.

Because of the recent finding that the use of spironolactone decreases mortality in patients with advanced heart failure, diuretic regimens should be tailored to include the diuretic effects, although somewhat minimal, of this drug. Particular attention should be paid to serum electrolytes. (*Adapted from* Brater [6].)

DIGOXIN

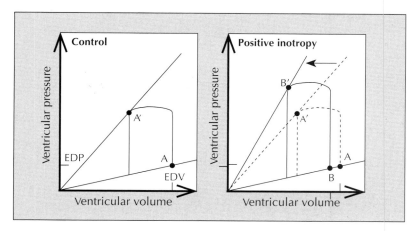

FIGURE 10-13. The positive inotropic effect of cardiac glycosides. Not until the 1920s was it understood that cardiac glycosides increase the force of contraction of cardiac muscle (*ie*, a positive inotropic effect), resulting in a shift upward and to the left of the ventricular function curve. The effect in the intact heart is illustrated by the two pressure-volume loops shown here, in which an increase in contractility due to digoxin results in a shift upward and to the left of the pressure-volume relation at the end of systole (A'–B'). When stroke volume remains constant, as shown here, or increases, as is often the case clinically in patients with heart failure, the end-diastolic pressure (EDP) and volume (EDV) also decline (A-B). This results in decreased congestive symptoms and increased cardiac output. As predicted by the Laplace relationship, the resulting decrease in ventricular chamber dimensions also reduces wall tension, a major determinant in myocardial oxygen consumption. Therefore, although the initial increase in myocardial contractility necessarily results in an increase in cardiac muscle cell ATP (and oxygen) consumption, the final net effect of the drug may be to lower cardiac oxygen consumption [1].

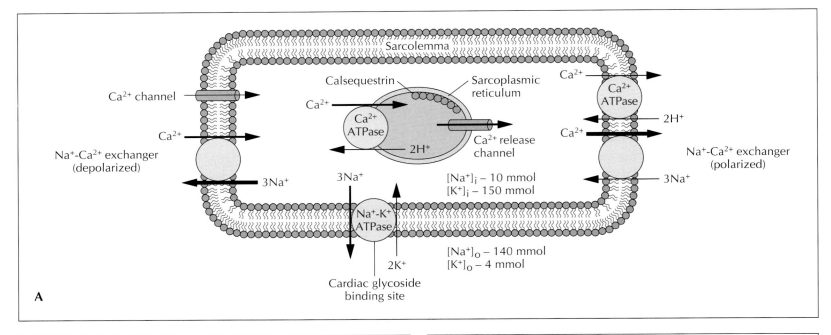

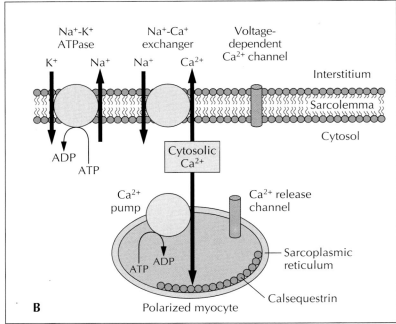

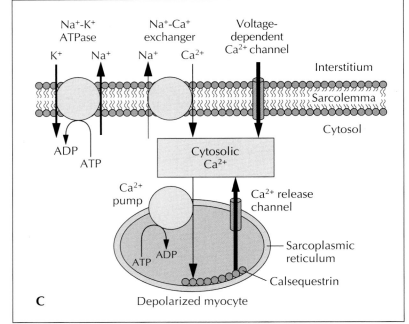

FIGURE 10-14. Sodium pump inhibition by cardiac glycosides. The present understanding of the mechanism by which the cardiac glycosides induce a positive inotropic effect in cardiac muscle is based on the specificity of these drugs for Na^+K^+-ATPase (or the "sodium pump"), a cell membrane protein responsible for the active (*ie*, ATP-consuming) transport of the monovalent cations Na^+ and K^+.

A, Both Na^+ and Ca^{2+} ions enter cardiac muscle cells during each cycle of depolarization, contraction, and repolarization. Ca^{2+} is also released from internal stores in an intracellular compartment called the sarcoplasmic reticulum (SR), where it is bound to the protein calsequestrin. During cellular repolarization, Na^+ is actively extruded by Na^+K^+-ATPase, whereas Ca^{2+} is

either pumped back into the SR by a Ca^{2+}-ATPase or is removed from the cell by a cell membrane transport protein that exchanges Na^+ for Ca^{2+}. This Na^+ for Ca^{2+} exchanger transports three Na^+ ions in for every Ca^{2+} ion out when the cell is polarized, using the favorable chemical and electrical potential of Na^+ to drive the exchange reaction. **B,** The direction and magnitude of Na^+ and Ca^{2+} transport during diastole (polarized myocyte).

C, The direction and magnitude of Na^+ and Ca^{2+} transport during systole (depolarized myocyte). Note that the exchanger may briefly run in reverse during cell depolarization when the electrical gradient across the plasma membrane is transiently reversed. The capacity of the exchanger to extrude Ca^{2+} from the cell depends critically on the intracellular Na^+ concentrations [1].

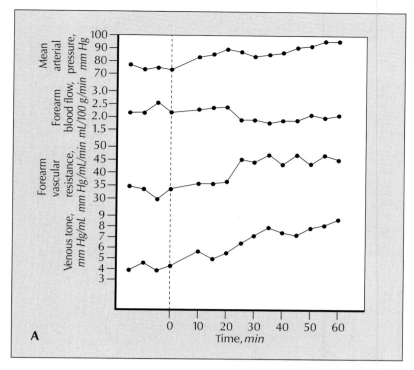

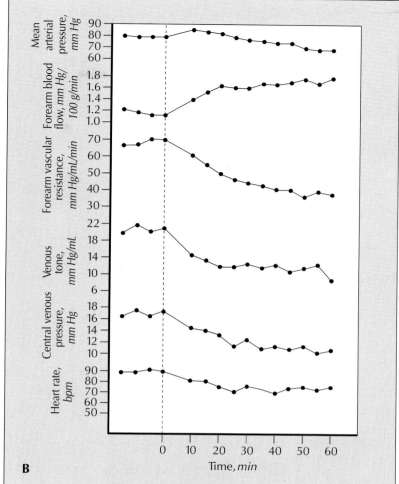

FIGURE 10-15. Cardiac glycosides and peripheral vascular resistance in heart failure. Cardiac glycosides have been known for over 30 years to affect peripheral venous and arterial tone.

A, In a series of pioneering studies, Mason *et al.* [8] noted that a 10-minute intravenous infusion of 8.5 µg/kg ouabain in normal subjects increased mean arterial pressure as well as forearm vascular resistance and venous tone.

B, In marked contrast, forearm vascular resistance and venous tone decreased in patients with New York Heart Association (NYHA) class III or IV heart failure symptoms after an intravenous dose of ouabain, as shown by the data from a representative patient. Whereas the response in normal subjects is due in part to a direct effect of cardiac glycosides on peripheral vascular tone, the opposite and rapid hemodynamic response to ouabain observed in heart failure patients is now believed to be due in part to a decrease in sympathetic nervous system activity mediated by enhanced sensitivity of the baroreflex response. (*Adapted from* Mason *et al.* [8].)

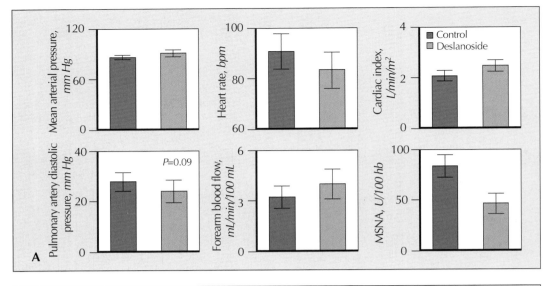

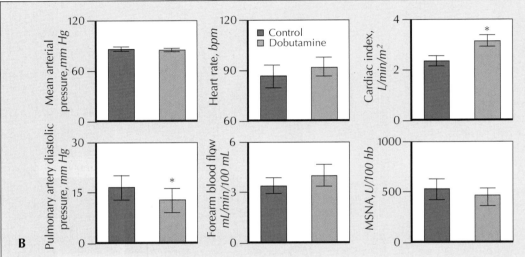

FIGURE 10-16. Sympathetic nervous system activity in heart failure: response to digitalis versus dobutamine. Ferguson *et al.* [9] noted that although infusion of the cardiac glycoside deslanoside was associated with increased forearm blood flow and cardiac index was increased, muscle sympathetic nerve activity (MSNA) was markedly decreased in patients with NYHA class III and IV heart failure (*n*=8; mean ± SEM).

B, To determine whether these changes could be ascribed to an increase in cardiac output per se, Ferguson *et al.* also examined the response of a similar group of heart failure patients to dobutamine, titrated to achieve the same increase in pulmonary artery O$_2$ saturation as was achieved by infusion of deslanoside. Although cardiac index increased and pulmonary artery pressure declined significantly, as expected, there were no significant changes in heart rate, forearm blood flow, or MSNA in these patients (*n*=8). *Asterisk* indicates *P*<0.05. hb—heartbeat. (*Adapted from* Ferguson *et al.* [9].)

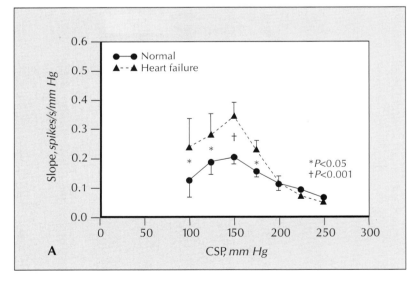

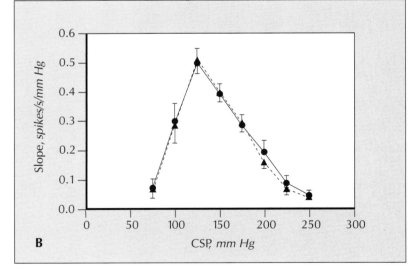

FIGURE 10-17. Improved carotid baroreflex responsiveness after cardiac glycosides. **A,** Direct infusions of ouabain into the arterial supply of isolated carotid sinus preparations (CSP) from a dog model of heart failure with a documented desensitization of the baroreflex response restored the responsiveness of the isolated baroreceptor to increases in CSP toward normal. **B,** No change was observed after ouabain in isolated CSPs from normal dogs. These and other experimental data reinforce data from patients that cardiac glycosides act directly to reset arterial baroreflex sensitivity in heart failure. (*Adapted from* Wang *et al.* [10].)

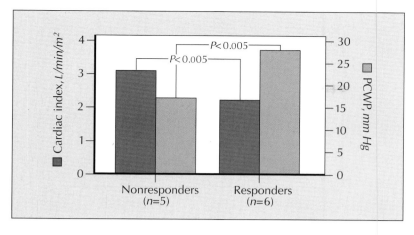

FIGURE 10-18. Digoxin in hospitalized heart failure patients. Gheorghiade *et al.* [11] carried out a small, prospective trial of intravenous digoxin administration to hospitalized patients who had severe (NYHA class IV) symptoms and who had been medically stabilized with diuretics and vasodilators. Approximately half of the patients (six of 11) experienced a significant hemodynamic improvement after receiving 1.0 mg of intravenous digoxin, as judged by a decrease in pulmonary capillary wedge pressure (PCWP) of 5 mm Hg and/or an increase in cardiac index of 0.5 L/min/m². There were important baseline hemodynamic differences between digoxin responders and nonresponders, as shown in this figure, although reportedly there were no other significant differences in the etiology of the heart failure in each patient's heart failure score or in left ventricular ejection fraction. Although all patients had class IV symptoms on admission to hospital, those with markedly abnormal hemodynamics after initiation of optimal medical management with diuretics and vasodilators were more likely to exhibit a favorable hemodynamic response. (*Adapted from* Gheorghiade *et al.* [11].)

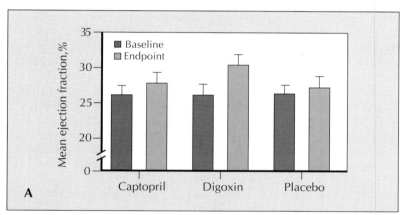

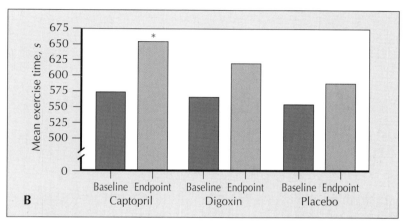

FIGURE 10-19. Captopril-Digoxin Multicenter Research Group trial. **A,** In the Captopril-Digoxin Multicenter Research Group trials [12], 300 patients with generally mild to moderate (NYHA classes II and III) heart failure symptoms were randomly assigned to receive captopril, digoxin, or placebo, with diuretics administered as necessary. Both captopril and digoxin significantly reduced morbidity, as judged by the need for increasing doses of diuretics, emergency room visits, or hospitalization, compared with placebo. This figure illustrates the change in left ventricular ejection fraction from baseline for patients assigned to captopril, digoxin, or placebo. Only patients who received digoxin exhibited a significant increase in ejection fraction (*P*<0.05) during the trial. An important caveat in interpreting the results of this trial is that during the pretrial patient evaluation period, any patient who did not tolerate withdrawal from standard (*ie*, digoxin) therapy was

not randomly assigned or entered into the study, thereby excluding a number of patients who, by definition, would probably have been digoxin responders. **B,** All patients in this study were receiving background diuretic therapy. Captopril was associated with a significant increase in exercise performance compared with placebo. The digoxin treatment group showed a small trend toward improvement of exercise tolerance. The digoxin group demonstrated a small but significant increase of ejection fraction. *Asterisk* indicates a significantly greater increase of exercise duration from baseline compared with the placebo response (*P*<0.05). There were greater requirements for diuretic supplementation, more frequent emergency room visits, and a greater need for hospitalization in the placebo group, who were receiving only diuretic therapy. (*Adapted from* the Captopril-Digoxin Multicenter Research Group [12].)

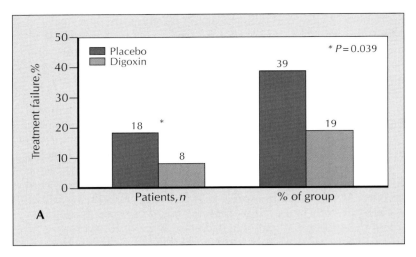

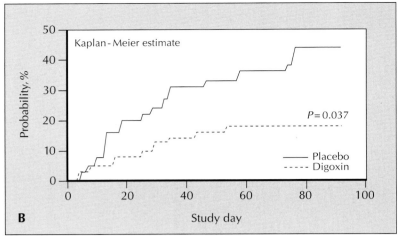

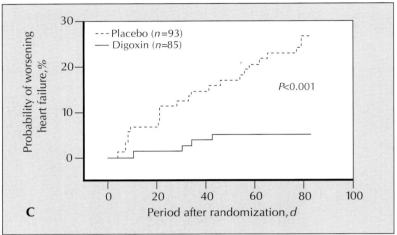

significantly higher in the placebo group compared with the digoxin-treated group. **C,** Digoxin in heart failure: the RADIANCE (Randomized Assessment [of the effect of] Digoxin and Inhibitors of the Angiotensin Converting Enzyme [ACE]) trial. The RADIANCE trial design was essentially identical to that shown in **A** for the PROVED trial, except that patients were receiving either captopril or enalapril, in addition to digoxin and diuretics, before randomization [14]. Study investigators were asked to achieve optimal fluid balance on diuretics during the stabilization period, and a captopril or enalapril dose of at least 25 mg or 5 mg/d, respectively (average dose, 73 and 13 mg/d in the placebo group, 77 and 17 mg/d in the digoxin group). As in PROVED, the target serum digoxin concentration was between 0.9 and 2.0 ng/mL, and the average serum concentration of digoxin was about 1.2 ng/mL on an average dose of 0.38 mg/d. Of the 178 patients randomized, all were in NYHA class II or III. No patients with severe heart failure (NYHA class IV) were studied, largely because digoxin's efficacy was already considered established for this group of patients. Nevertheless, the proportion of patients in class III heart failure was somewhat higher (about 35% of the total) than in PROVED (about 19%).

There were highly significant differences in both primary and secondary endpoints between patients receiving optimal ACE inhibitor and diuretic therapy who were randomized to continue receiving digoxin compared with those who were switched to placebo. There was a significant increase in the cumulative probability of worsening heart failure (defined as in PROVED) in this Kaplan-Meier analysis over the duration of the study. This amounts to a 20% absolute risk reduction for patients who continued to receive digoxin. (parts A and B *adapted from* Uretsky *et al.* [13]; part C *adapted from* Packer *et al.* [14].)

FIGURE 10-20. Digoxin in heart failure: the PROVED (Prospective Randomized Study of Ventricular Failure and the Efficacy of Digoxin) trial. To evaluate prospectively whether patients with well-compensated heart failure symptoms in sinus rhythm who were already receiving digoxin, with or without a diuretic, would tolerate withdrawal from the cardiac glycoside, 88 patients with mild to moderate heart failure (NYHA class II predominantly), who were not receiving a vasodilator, were randomly assigned either to continue on active drug or to receive a placebo in the PROVED trial [13]. **A,** Treatment failure, defined as number of patients and percentage of treatment group demonstrating a statistically greater occurrence of failure in patients withdrawn from digoxin treatment. **B,** The time to treatment failure, or a hospital evaluation or admission for heart failure symptoms, was

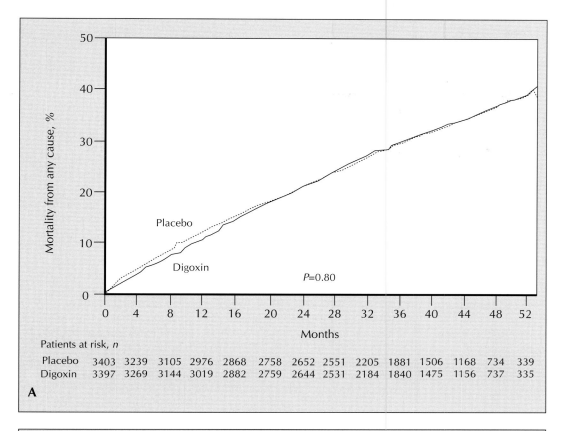

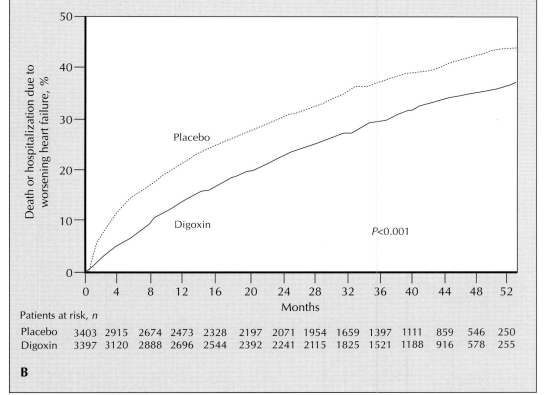

FIGURE 10-21. The Digitalis Investigation Group (DIG) trial evaluated the effects of digoxin on survival in 6800 patients. The average follow-up was 37 months. Digoxin did not increase or decrease overall mortality (**A**). However, digoxin-treated patients had a reduction in the overall rate of hospitalization and also the rate of hospitalization for worsening heart failure (**B**). There was no increased risk of ventricular arrhythmias in the digoxin-treated group. (*Adapted from* Digitalis Investigation Group report [15].)

REFERENCES

1. Kelly RA, Smith TW: Treatment of stable heart failure: digitalis and diuretics. In *Atlas of Heart Diseases, vol IV: Heart Failure: Cardiac Function and Dysfunction.* Edited by Colucci WS, Braunwald E. Philadelphia: Current Medicine; 1995:10.1–10.16.

2. Wilcox CS, Mitch WE, Kelly RA, *et al.*: Response to furosemide: I. Effect of salt intake and renal compensation. *J Lab Clin Med* 1983, 102:450–458.

3. Sica DA, Deedwania P: Pharmacotherapy in congestive heart failure: principles of combination diuretic therapy in congestive heart failure. *Congestive Heart Failure* 1997, 3:29–38.

4 Vargo D, Kramer WG, Black PK, *et al.*: The pharmacodynamics of torsemide in patients with congestive heart failure. *Clin Pharmacol Ther* 1994, 56:48–54.

5. Rudy DW, Gehr TWB, Matzke G, *et al.*: The pharmacodynamics of intravenous and oral torsemide in patients with chronic renal insufficiency. *Clin Pharmacol Ther* 1994, 56:39–47.

6. Brater DC: Diuretic therapy. *N Engl J Med* 1998, 339:387–395.

7. Cody RJ, Pickworth KK: Approaches to diuretic therapy and electrolyte imbalance in congestive heart failure. In *Update in Congestive Heart Failure: Cardiology Clinics,* vol 12. Edited by Deedwania PC. Philadelphia: WB Saunders; 1994:37–50.

8. Mason DT, Braunwald E, Karsh RB, *et al.*: Studies on Digitalis: X. Effects of ouabain on forearm vascular resistance and venous tone in normal subjects and in patients in heart failure. *J Clin Invest* 1964, 43:532–543.

9. Ferguson DW, Berg WJ, Sanders JS, *et al.*: Sympathoinhibitory responses to digitalis glycosides in heart failure patients: direct evidence from sympathetic neural recordings. *Circulation* 1989, 80:65–77.

10. Wang W, Chen J-S, Zucker IH: Carotid sinus baroreceptor sensitivity in experimental heart failure. *Circulation* 1990, 81:1959–1966.

11. Gheorghiade M, St Clair J, St Clair C, *et al.*: Hemodynamic effects of intravenous digoxin in patients with severe heart failure initially treated with diuretics and vasodilators. *J Am Coll Cardiol* 1987, 9:849–857.

12. Captopril-Digoxin Multicenter Research Group: Comparative effects of therapy with captopril and digoxin in patients with mild to moderate heart failure. *JAMA* 1988, 259:539–544.

13. Uretsky BF, Young JB, Shahidi FE, *et al.*: Randomized study assessing the effect of digoxin withdrawal in patients with mild to moderate chronic congestive heart failure: results of the PROVED trial. *J Am Coll Cardiol* 1993, 22:955–962.

14. Packer M, Gheorghiade M, Young JB, *et al.*: Withdrawal of digoxin from patients with chronic heart failure treated with angiotensin-converting-enzyme inhibitors. *N Engl J Med* 1997, 329:1–7.

15. Digitalis Investigation Group: The effect of digoxin on mortality and morbidity in patients with heart failure. The Digitalis Investigation Group (DIG) Trial. *N Engl J Med* 1997, 336:525–533.

Angiotensin-converting Enzyme Inhibition and Angiotensin Receptor Blockade

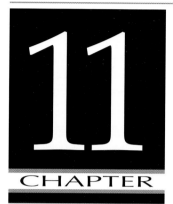

11

CHAPTER

Todd M. Koelling and Robert J. Cody

Activation of the renin-angiotensin-aldosterone system is one of the predominant abnormalities of heart failure. The degree of increase in plasma renin activity provides an indicator for prognosis in heart failure patients [1]. Patients with mild and asymptomatic heart failure demonstrate relatively less activation, but even these values are increased compared with normal. The degree of renin activity is intensified in the presence of diuretic therapy. Angiotensin II causes constriction of the systemic vasculature and causes vasoconstriction of both the afferent and efferent renal arterioles. In some patients with severe heart failure, treatment with angiotensin-converting enzyme (ACE) inhibitors may cause a deterioration of renal function. This may be related to fixed renal artery disease, or alternatively from selective blocking of the constrictor action of angiotensin II on the efferent arteriole [2]. Renin system components have been identified in the myocardium and vasculature, where they adversely affect fibrosis and remodeling, as well as cellular dysfunction. These findings suggest that the renin-angiotensin-aldosterone system has effects on cardiac function beyond altering sodium excretion and cardiac afterload. Not only is angiotensin II a potent vasoconstrictor, but it causes a direct effect on hypertrophy of myocytes, and may lead to energy supply mismatch as the capillary bed perfuses a larger bed [3].

In addition to vasoconstriction, angiotensin II stimulates aldosterone secretion by the adrenal gland, producing sodium retention and potassium excretion at the distal nephron. Elevations in the activity of aldosterone leads to a sodium retentive state found in heart failure patients. It has been shown previously that although ACE inhibition continues to suppress angiotensin II levels over the course of 1 year, levels of aldosterone are initially suppressed during the first 1 to 3 months of therapy, but fail to be suppressed beyond 6 months of therapy [4,5]. This is thought to occur because stimuli in the form of glucocorticoids, hyperkalemia, hypermagnesemia, melanocyte-stimulating hormone, and endothelin continue to increase aldosterone secretion when angiotensin II levels are low [6]. Analysis of the Cooperative North Scandinavian Enalapril Survival Study (CONSENSUS) revealed that elevated levels of aldosterone were associated with the lowest survival, and a reduction in plasma aldosterone during the course of therapy was associated with a favorable impact on survival [7]. Although elevated aldosterone levels may track the clinical state of patients with congestive heart failure, they may also be responsible in part for progression of myocardial dysfunction through mechanisms that lead to abnormal accumulation of collagen, surrounding and encasing myocytes, resulting in diastolic and systolic ventricular dysfunction [8]. Such deposition of collagen may lead to pathologic hypertrophy of the myocardium [9,10] and has been shown to be prevented by spironolactone in a rat model of arterial hypertension [11].

Angiotensin-converting enzyme inhibitors, in contrast to direct-acting vasodilators, have been highly successful in all stages of congestive heart failure. Although ACE inhibitors have vasodilator properties, their mechanism of action extends to other effects of suppressing angiotensin II, and modulation of additional vasoactive substances. ACE serves to catalyze the conversion of angiotensin I to angiotensin II, a potent vasoconstrictor and stimulant for aldosterone release. The ACE also acts as a kininase, and inhibition of this enzyme leads to decreased breakdown of bradykinin [12] in the kininase activity that may explain the advantage of ACE inhibitors over angiotensin receptor blockers [13].

Although ACE inhibitors have been shown to improve heart failure symptoms and reduce mortality in multiple studies, additional therapies are being sought for patients intolerant to ACE inhibitors and for patients with residual production of angiotensin II despite maximally recommended doses of ACE inhibitors. Because angiotensin II antagonists directly block angiotensin II at the AT1 receptor without blocking the breakdown of bradykinin, many investigators have felt that these agents would be better tolerated by patients and would provide similar or greater efficacy. The clinical ramifications of blocking AT1 receptors, allowing unopposed stimulation of AT2 receptors, have not been fully elucidated.

ANGIOTENSIN-CONVERTING ENZYME INHIBITORS

POTENTIAL MECHANISMS FOR ACE INHIBITOR BENEFIT

Neurohumoral and paracrine effects
  Diminished circulating and tissue effects of angiotensin II
  Diminished aldosterone
  Prevention of sodium retention
  Reduction of circulating catecholamines
  Improved baroreceptor function
  Restoration of sympathetic-parasympathetic balance
  Diminished bradykinin breakdown
Left ventricular structural and functional effects
  Decreased transmural wall stress
  Reduction of compensatory ventricular dilatation
  Improved coronary flow
Hemodynamic effects
  Reduction of vascular resistance
  Absence of chronotropic stimulation
  Reduction of inotropic stimulation
Other effects
  Blockade of cell growth effects of angiotensin II
  Potential direct cellular effects of ACE (carboxypeptidase)
  Inhibition or reversal of adverse collagen remodeling

FIGURE 11-1. Potential mechanisms for angiotensin-converting enzyme (ACE) inhibitor benefit. ACE inhibitors have demonstrated clinical benefit in all stages of heart failure. It is now apparent from many studies that the short- and long-term benefits of ACE inhibitors go beyond their vasodilating properties. The primary mechanism of action of this class of agents is blockade of angiotensin II formation, which inhibits endocrine, paracrine, and cellular growth effects of angiotensin II. Among beneficial outcomes are reversal of vasoconstriction and suppression of aldosterone synthesis, which thereby limits aldosterone mediated sodium retention and potassium loss. Cellular effects include inhibition of angiotensin II–mediated hypertrophy, and it has been proposed that reversal of collagen matrix deposition, mediated by angiotensin II or aldosterone, is of clinical relevance.

Additional contributing effects that are difficult to quantify include inhibition of bradykinin degradation and promotion of prostaglandin synthesis. The former may be important at a cellular level by enhancing the vasorelaxant effects of endothelium-derived relaxing factor, and the latter may be important in terms of improving regional blood flow, particularly within the kidney. Finally, a pure hemodynamic effect regardless of the mechanisms that produce it could contribute to the beneficial effects of ACE inhibitors. However, on the basis of findings with other pure vasodilators, it is unlikely to be the only mechanism [14].

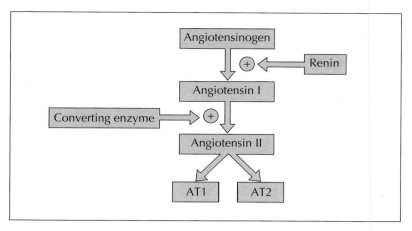

FIGURE 11-2. Cascade of events in the production of angiotensin II presented by the syndrome of congestive heart failure. Reduced cardiac output, reduced arterial pressure, and reduced renal blood flow contribute to the release of renin within the kidney. Elevations and levels of circulating renin lead to conversion of angiotensinogen to angiotensin I. Angiotensin-converting enzyme then catalyzes the conversion of angiotensin I to angiotensin II. Angiotensin II exerts its effects through the binding of the angiotensin II receptors AT1 and AT2. Binding of these receptors has been shown to lead to vasoconstriction and release of aldosterone [15].

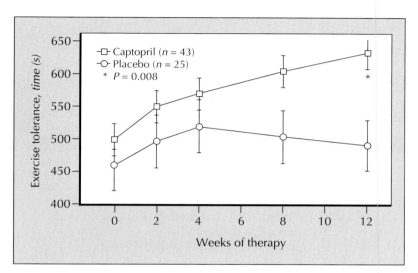

FIGURE 11-3. Findings from the Captopril MultiCenter Research Group. This group conducted the first placebo-controlled exercise study in heart failure patients, evaluating the response to captopril versus placebo. This figure demonstrates the importance of frequent baseline exercise tests and the need for longer term follow up evaluation in clinical drug trials. An increase in exercise performance in the placebo group was evident in the first 4 weeks of the study, and paralleled the improvement in the captopril group. However, the exercise response in the placebo group showed a plateau after 4 weeks of therapy and by 12 weeks had fallen back near to baseline levels. The captopril-treated group continued to demonstrate a progressive increase in exercise time. This study demonstrated the clinical efficacy of captopril in improving functional performance [16].

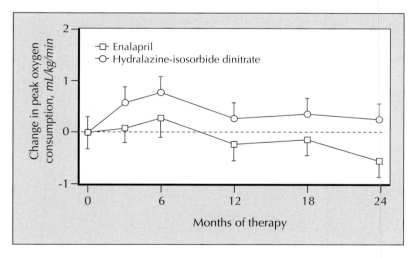

FIGURE 11-4. Changes in peak oxygen consumption measured during cardiopulmonary exercise testing with enalapril versus changes with hydralazine-isosorbide dinitrate in the Vasodilator-Heart Failure Trial II (V-HeFT II) study. Systemic oxygen consumption at peak exercise was measured after randomization, at 3 months, at 6 months, and subsequently at 6-month intervals. Oxygen consumption was increased significantly by hydralazine-isosorbide dinitrate at the 3-month time point and at subsequent time points after the 6-month time period. Peak oxygen consumption did not change significantly in those patients treated with enalapril. Improvements in exercise with hydralazine-isosorbide dinitrate combinations may be expected, given increases in heart rate and sympathetic tone observed with this combination [17].

EFFECT OF ANGIOTENSIN-CONVERTING ENZYME INHIBITORS ON MORTALITY IN HEART FAILURE

PLACEBO-CONTROLLED STUDIES

TRIAL (PATIENTS, N)	NYHA	AGENT	MEAN FOLLOW-UP	PLACEBO, %	ACE-I, %	RISK REDUCTION, %	P VALUE
Largely asymptomatic							
SOLVD-P (4228)	I–II	Enalapril	37 mo	15.8	14.8	8.0	0.3
Munich Trial (170)	I–III	Captopril	30 mo	25.3	26.5	-4.7	NS
Captopril-Digoxin (300)	I–III	Captopril	6 mo	6.0	7.7	-28.0	NS
Moderate symptoms							
SOLVD-T (2569)	I–III	Enalapril	41 mo	39.7	35.2	16.0	0.0036
CMRG (92)	II–III	Captopril	12 wk	9.5	0.0	100.0	NS
Severe symptoms							
CONSENSUS (253)	IV	Enalapril	6 mo	54.0	39.0	27.0	0.003

HYDRALAZINE/NITRATE-CONTROLLED STUDIES

TRIAL (PATIENTS, N)	NYHA	AGENT	MEAN FOLLOW-UP, MO	HYD/N, %	ACE-I, %	RISK REDUCTION, %	P VALUE
V-HeFT II (804)	II–III	Enalapril	24	25.0	18.0	28.0	0.016
Hy-C (104)	III–IV	Captopril	8	49.0	19.0	61.0	0.05

FIGURE 11-5. Effective angiotensin-converting enzyme (ACE) inhibitors on mortality in heart failure. Placebo-controlled studies of the use of ACE inhibitors in heart failure patients have assessed mortality endpoints in mild, moderate, and severe heart failure. Trials performed in patients largely asymptomatic, such as Studies of Left Ventricular Dysfunction–Treatment (SOLVD-T), the Munich trial, and the Captopril-Digoxin Trial, have not demonstrated an improvement in survival in these patients. The SOLVD-T trial performed largely in patients with New York Heart Association class II and III symptoms showed a 16% reduction in all-cause mortality using enalapril. A 27% reduction in all-cause mortality was observed in the CONSENSUS trial. This study was performed in patients with severe heart failure. ACE inhibitors have also been shown to improve survival when compared with the combination of hydralazine and dinitrate (Hyd/N) preparations. The V-HeFT II study showed a 28% reduction in all-cause mortality using enalapril versus hydralazine isosorbide dinitrate in patients with New York Heart Association class II and III symptoms. A 61% reduction in mortality was observed in the Hydralazine plus Isosorbide Dinitrate versus Captopril (HY-C) trial, a study of 104 patients with moderate to severe heart failure symptoms [17–22].

EFFECT OF ACE INHIBITORS ON MORBIDITY IN HEART FAILURE

PLACEBO-CONTROLLED STUDIES

TRIAL	ENDPOINT	PLACEBO, %	ACE-I, %	RISK REDUCTION, %	P VALUE
Largely asymptomatic					
SOLVD-P	HF hospitalization	12.9	8.7	32.6	<0.001
Munich trial	Severe HF	26.4	10.8	59.0	0.01
Captopril-Digoxin	HF hospitalization	29.0	16.0	45.0	<0.05
Moderate symptoms					
CMRG	Symptom improvement	68.0	36.0	47.0	0.04
SOLVD-T	HF hospitalization	36.6	25.8	29.5	<0.001
Severe symptoms					
CONSENSUS	NYHA IV	24.0	16.5	31.0	0.001

HYDRALAZINE/NITRATE-CONTROLLED STUDIES

TRIAL	ENDPOINT	PLACEBO, %	ACE-I, %	RISK REDUCTION, %	P VALUE
VHeFT II	HF hospitalization	18.4	18.9	2.7	NS

FIGURE 11-6. The effect of angiotensin-converting enzyme (ACE) inhibitors on heart failure endpoints in patients with left ventricular dysfunction. Randomized controlled trials have been consistent in their observation that ACE inhibitors reduce heart failure hospitalization or the development of severe congestive heart failure symptoms. ACE inhibitors have been shown to reduce the risk of heart failure hospitalizations or development of severe heart failure by 32.6% to 59.0% in patients with mild heart failure in the SOLVD-P (Prevention) trial, the MUNICH trial, and the Captopril-Digoxin trial. A similar reduction in heart failure hospitalization, in symptomatic improvement of heart failure symptoms, has been shown in trials of patients with moderate heart failure symptoms. These include the Captopril MultiCenter Research Group Study as well as the SOLVD-T trial. The CONSESUS study observed a 31% reduction in the percentage of patients who remained with New York Heart Association class IV symptoms at the conclusion of follow-up [16,18–21,23].

EFFECT OF ACE INHIBITORS ON MORTALITY AFTER MYOCARDIAL INFARCTION

PLACEBO-CONTROLLED STUDIES

TRIAL (PATIENTS, N)	TIMING	AGENT	MEAN FU	PLACEBO, %	ACE-I, %	RISK REDUCTION, %	P VALUE
Largely no symptoms							
SMILE (1556)	<24 h	Zofenopril	6 wk	6.5	4.9	25.0	0.19
CATS (298)	<6 h	Captopril	3 mo	4.0	6.0	-50.0	NS
CONSENSUS II (6090)	<24 h	Enalaprilat/enalapril	6 mo	9.4	10.2	-10.0	0.26
ISIS-4 (58050)	<24 h	Captopril	35 d	7.7	7.2	7.0	0.02
GISSI-3 (19394)	<24 h	Lisinopril	6 wk	7.1	6.3	12.0	0.03
LV dysfunction							
SAVE (2231)	3–16 d	Captopril	42 mo	25.0	20.0	19.0	0.019
LV dysfunction with symptoms							
TRACE (6676)	3–7 d	Trandolipril	36 mo	42.3	34.7	22.0	0.001
AIRE (2006)	3–10 d	Ramipril	15 mo	23.0	17.0	27.0	0.002

FIGURE 11-7. The effect of angiotensin-converting enzyme (ACE) inhibitors on mortality in patients suffering myocardial infarction. Although the pathophysiology of infarct healing is complex, there are several potential mechanisms by which ACE inhibitors may favorably improve left ventricular remodeling. Angiotensin II is a potent vasoconstrictor and is up regulated in the postinfarction period. This will lead to increased wall stress leading to regional hypertrophy and infarct expansion. Inhibiting the effects of angiotensin II in the postinfarction period may prevent the development of progressive heart failure. Placebo-controlled studies have been performed in patients suffering myocardial infarction with left ventricular dysfunction with or without symptoms of heart failure. In studies that included patients without left ventricular dysfunction or heart failure symptoms, a mortality benefit was not observed in the CONSENSUS II trial. No benefit on mortality was seen in the Survival of Myocardial Infarction Long-term Evaluation (SMILE) study, which followed up 1556 patients using oral zofenopril. Much larger studies of patients in the postinfarction period were performed in Italy, including the fourth International Study of Infarct Survival (ISIS-4) study and the Gruppo Italiano per lo Studio della Soprawivenza nell'Infarcto (GISSI)-3 Study. These studies showed a reduction in the risk of mortality of 7% and 12%, respectively. The effect of ACE inhibitors on mortality after myocardial infarction has been more consistent in patents with documented left ventricular dysfunction. The Survival and Ventricular Enlargement (SAVE) study showed a 19% reduction in all-cause mortality using captopril. The Trandolapril Cardiac Evaluation (TRACE) and Acute Infarction Ramipril Efficacy (AIRE) studies showed a 22% and 27% reduction in the risk of mortality after myocardial infarction, respectively [24–29].

EFFECT OF ACE INHIBITORS ON MORBIDITY AFTER MYOCARDIAL INFARCTION (PLACEBO-CONTROLLED STUDIES)					
TRIAL	ENDPOINT	PLACEBO, %	ACE-I, %	RELATIVE RISK, %	P VALUE
Largely no symptoms					
SMILE	Worsened HF	4.1	2.2	46.0	0.018
CATS	Worsened HF	28.0	18.8	34.0	0.05
CONSENSUS II	HF hospitalization	6.0	4.0	50.0	NS
ISIS-4	Worsened HF	7.2	6.9	4.0	NS
GISSI-3	Worsened HF	3.7	3.9	5.0	NS
LV dysfunction					
SAVE	HF hospitalization	17.0	14.0	22.0	0.019
LV dysfunction					
TRACE	Worsened HF	29.0	23.0	29.0	0.003
AIRE	Worsened HF	18.0	14.0	19.0	0.008

FIGURE 11-8. The effect of angiotensin-converting enzyme (ACE) inhibitors on heart failure endpoints in patients suffering myocardial infarction. Despite enrolling patients without heart failure symptoms and without documentation of left ventricular dysfunction, both the SMILE and Captopril and Thrombolysis Study (CATS) trials have shown a significant reduction in the incidence or worsening heart failure in the postinfarction period. Studies of patients with documented left ventricular dysfunction have been more consistent in showing reduction in heart failure endpoints in the postinfarction populations. The SAVE study showed a 22% reduction in heart failure hospitalizations in a study of Captopril with a 42-month median follow up. The reduction in the incidence of worsened heart failure was similar in the TRACE Study (29% reduction) and the AIRE trial (19% reduction) [24,26,30–32].

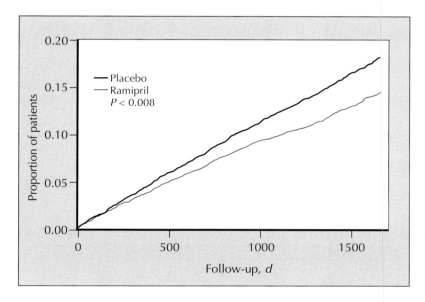

FIGURE 11-9. The effect of ramipril on composite outcome of myocardial infarction stroke or death in high-risk patients. In addition to those studies using angiotensin-converting enzyme (ACE) inhibitors in patients who have suffered myocardial infarctions, the Heart Outcomes Prevention Evaluation (HOPE) study assessed the role of ramipril in patients who were at high risk of cardiovascular events but who did not have left ventricular dysfunction or heart failure. This study showed a 22% reduction in the risk of reaching the primary endpoint (death, myocardial infarction, or stroke) compared with placebo. In this study, death from any cause was reduced from 12.2% in the placebo group to 10.4% in the ramipril group for an overall 16% reduction. (P=0.005). Patients enrolled into this study were at least 55 years of age and had a history of either coronary artery disease, stroke, peripheral vascular disease, or diabetes, and had at least one other risk factor among hypertension, elevated total cholesterol level, low high-density lipoprotein cholesterol level, cigarette smoking, or documented albuminuria [32].

EFFECT OF RAMIPRIL ON CARDIOVASCULAR EVENTS IN HIGH-RISK PATIENTS

SECONDARY ENDPOINTS	PLACEBO,	RAMIPRIL	RELATIVE RISK, (CI)	P VALUE
Patients, n	4652	4645		
Revascularization	18.3%	16.0%	0.85 (0.77–0.94)	0.002
Diabetic complications	7.6%	6.4%	0.84 (0.72–0.98)	0.03
Heart failure hospitalizations	3.4%	3.0%	0.88 (0.70–1.10)	0.25
All heart failure	11.5%	9.0%	0.77 (0.67–0.87)	<0.001
Cardiac arrest	1.3%	0.8%	0.62 (0.41–0.94)	0.02
Worsening of angina	26.2%	23.8%	0.89 (0.82–0.96)	0.004
New diagnosis of diabetes	5.4%	3.6%	0.66 (0.51–0.85)	<0.001

FIGURE 11-10. Effect of ramipril on cardiovascular events in high-risk patients. In the HOPE trial, significantly fewer patients in the ramipril group than the placebo group underwent revascularization, and there was a trend toward fewer hospitalizations for heart failure in the ramipril group. Additionally, ramipril was shown to have a significant affect on the reduction in the development of heart failure, cardiac arrest, worsening angina, and new diagnoses of diabetes mellitus. The findings from the HOPE trial suggest that the spectrum of patients who had benefited from treatment with an angiotensin-converting enzyme inhibitor should not be restricted to those patients with left ventricular systolic dysfunction or with heart failure symptoms. It has been suggested that only a small part of the benefit of ramipril in this study could be attributed to a reduction in blood pressure because the majority of the patients did not have hypertension at baseline and the mean reduction in blood pressure with treatment was extremely small (3/2 mm Hg). It is likely that angiotensin-converting enzyme inhibitors exert additional direct mechanisms on the heart or the vasculature. These may include antagonizing the direct effect of angiotensin II on vasoconstriction, the proliferation of vascular smooth muscle cells, the rupture of plaques, vascular endothelial function, myocyte hypertrophy, and intrinsic fibrinolysis [33].

EFFECT OF LOW- AND HIGH-DOSE ACE INHIBITORS IN HEART FAILURE PATIENTS

ATLAS TRIAL

VARIABLE	LOW-DOSE (2.5–5 MG/D)	HIGH-DOSE (32.5–35 MG/D)	HR, CI	P VALUE
Patients, n	1596	1568		
All-cause mortality	717 (44.9%)	666 (42.5%)	0.92 (0.82–1.03)	0.128
Cardiovascular mortality	641 (40.2%)	583 (37.2%)	0.90 (0.81–1.01)	0.073
All-cause mortality + hospitalization	1338 (83.8%)	1250 (79.7%)	0.88 (0.82–0.96)	0.002

HIGH-DOSE ENALAPRIL STUDY

VARIABLE	MEDIUM-DOSE (20 MG/D)	HIGH DOSE (60 MG/D)	HR, CI	P VALUE
Patients, n	122	126	-	
All-cause mortality	18.0%	18.2%	0%	0.995
All-cause mortality + hospitalizations	30%	32%	-6%	0.645

FIGURE 11-11. The effect of low- and high-dose angiotensin-converting enzyme (ACE) inhibitors in heart failure patients. Because of observations showing residual angiotensin II production in patients receiving recommended doses of ACE inhibitors, trials have been performed to compare low dose to high dose inhibitor strategies as well as medium dose to high dose ACE inhibitor strategies. In the Assessment of Treatment with Lisinopril and Survival (ATLAS) trial, low-dose lisinopril (2.5 to 5 mg/d) was compared to high-dose lisinopril (32.5 to 35 mg/d). This study showed a nonsignificant trend toward reduction in all- cause mortality, the primary endpoint of the trial. An 8% reduction in all-cause mortality was observed, however (P=0.128). The secondary endpoint included all-cause mortality and hospitalizations. Using this endpoint, a 12% reduction in this composite endpoint was observed (P=0.002). The relevance of this finding has been disputed due to the inclusion of the low-dose group rather than the control group being a dose that has been previously shown to be effective. The High-Dose Enalapril Study compared clinical outcomes in medium-dose enalapril (20 mg/d) versus high-dose enalapril (60 mg/d). This study was relatively small, enrolling 248 patients. This study failed to show any difference in clinical outcomes using these two dosing strategies [36,37].

HAZARD RATIOS OF MORTALITY AND MORBIDITY IN ANTIPLATELET USERS VERSUS ANTIPLATELET NONUSERS IN THE SOLVD STUDIES GROUPED BY DRUG RANDOMIZATION

END POINT	ENALAPRIL-ADJUSTED HR	PLACEBO-ADJUSTED HR	P VALUE (INTERACTION)
All-cause mortality	1.00 (0.85–1.17)	0.68 (0.58–0.80)	0.0005
Death + HF hospitalization	0.88 (0.76–1.01)	0.77 (0.68–0.87)	0.09

HAZARD RATIOS OF MORTALITY AND MORBIDITY IN PATIENTS RANDOMIZED TO ENALAPRIL VS PLACEBO IN THE SOLVD STUDIES GROUPED BY ANTIPLATELET USE

END POINT	APA USERS-ADJUSTED HR	APA NONUSERS-ADJUSTED HR	P VALUE (INTERACTION)
All-cause mortality	1.10 (0.93–1.30)	0.77 (0.67–0.87)	0.0005
Death + HF hospitalization	0.81 (0.70–0.93)	0.71 (0.64–0.79)	0.09

FIGURE 11-12. Interaction between aspirin and angiotensin-converting enzyme (ACE) inhibitors in the SOLVD studies. A, Hazard ratios of mortality and morbidity in antiplatelet users versus antiplatelet nonusers grouped by drug randomization. B, Hazard ratios of mortality and morbidity in patients randomly assigned to enalapril versus placebo grouped by antiplatelet use. Because coronary artery disease is the leading cause of heart failure, it is common for patients to be receiving both aspirin and ACE inhibitors. Although aspirin therapy may prevent further ischemic incidence in patients with ischemic cardiomyopathy, its effects on prostaglandins may adversely effect hemodynamic function. Aspirin antagonizes the beneficial effects of antihypertensive therapy, and may reduce systemic vasodilatory reserve. Aspirin has also been observed to decrease glomerular filtration rate and has been shown to blunt the effects of diuretic drugs by reducing sodium and water excretion. Investigators reviewed data on antiplatelet agent use in 6797 patients enrolled into the studies of left ventricular dysfunction (SOLVD) trial and analyzed their relation between their use and all-cause mortality as well as the combined endpoint of death or hospital admission for heart failure. A Cox model was used to adjust for differences in baseline characteristics and to test for interaction for antiplatelet agent use and selected patient variables in relation to outcome. Hazard ratios of mortality in antiplatelet users versus antiplatelet nonusers when the study patients are grouped by drug randomization shows that the benefit of antiplatelet use with respect to mortality is primarily in patients randomly assigned to the placebo arm. Antiplatelet agent use was not associated with an improvement in survival in patients randomly assigned to enalapril. The analysis for interaction between these two medications was highly significant ($P=0.0005$). When the combined endpoint of death or heart failure hospitalization was analyzed, antiplatelet use was associated with an improved survival in the enalapril but not as favorable as those patients randomly assigned to placebo. When the hazard ratios of mortality and morbidity in patients randomly assigned to enalapril versus placebo with respect to antiplatelet use, the mortality benefit with enalapril was observed only in those patients not receiving an antiplatelet agent. The combined endpoint of death and heart failure hospitalization was reduced with the use of enalapril in both antiplatelet users and nonusers. These data suggest that the beneficial effects of enalapril are attenuated by the use of antiplatelet agents but are not entirely eradicated [41].

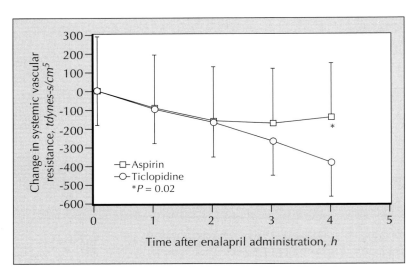

FIGURE 11-13. Interaction between aspirin, ticlopidine, and angiotensin-converting enzyme (ACE) inhibitors. ACE inhibitors are effective drugs that have been shown to lower morbidity and mortality rates in heart failure. Coronary artery disease is the

most common cause of heart failure. Aspirin can improve both short- and long-term prognosis for patients with coronary artery disease. The combination of aspirin and ACE inhibitors is therefore common in clinical practice; however, aspirin has been found to attenuate the acute vasodilator effect of ACE inhibitors. The mechanism for aspirin–ACE inhibitor interaction involves prostaglandin synthesis as ACE inhibitors impede the degradation of bradykinin, which stimulates the synthesis of prostaglandins. Aspirin inhibits cyclooxygenase, reducing the production of vasodilating prostaglandins. To verify this hypothesis, investigators compared the hemodynamic effects of enalapril in 20 patients with severe heart failure. Twelve of these patients were treated with ticlopidine and eight patients were treated with aspirin. Hemodynamic evaluation was performed after 7 days of antiplatelet agent treatment. Significant reductions and systemic vascular resistance were observed in the ticlopidine group, in contrast to no significant decrease in the aspirin group. A significant ($P=0.03$) time by treatment interaction indicated significant enalapril-aspirin drug interactions. Ticlopidine inhibits ADP-mediated platelet adhesion, and has not been found to have interactions with ACE inhibitor therapy [42].

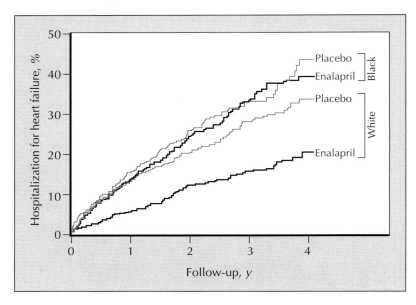

FIGURE 11-14. Effect of angiotensin-converting enzyme (ACE) inhibitors on both black and white patients. Although large-scale trials of therapy for heart failure have shown improvement in outcome with ACE inhibitors, these benefits have not been demonstrated in black patients. Black patients with heart failure

have a poorer prognosis than white patients, a difference that has not been adequately explained. To assess this question, investigators pooled and analyzed data from the SOLVD Prevention and Treatment Trials, comparing enalapril with placebo in patients with left ventricular dysfunction. In this analysis, 1196 white patients were matched with 800 black patients. Approximately half of each population was derived from the treatment trial and half from the prevention trial. Black patients were noted to have higher rates of death from any cause (12.2% vs 9.7%), as well as higher rates of hospitalization for heart failure (13.2% vs 7.7%). Enalapril therapy, as compared with placebo, was associated with a 44% reduction in the risk of hospitalization for heart failure among white patients ($P<0.001$) but no significant reduction was observed among black patients ($P=0.74$). The mechanism for this difference in response to ACE inhibitor is not well understood; however, it was observed in this study as well as the V-HeFT II trial that reductions in blood pressure did not occur in black patients. This provides evidence that some of the difference in benefit may be due to a difference in response to the ACE inhibitor therapy. Black patients with hypertension had been previously noted to have lower plasma renin activity than white patients. Even so, renin activity has not been found to be a useful marker for the long-term effects of ACE inhibitor therapy in heart failure trials. Clinical trials in black patients that are designed prospectively to evaluate therapeutic responses are warranted [43].

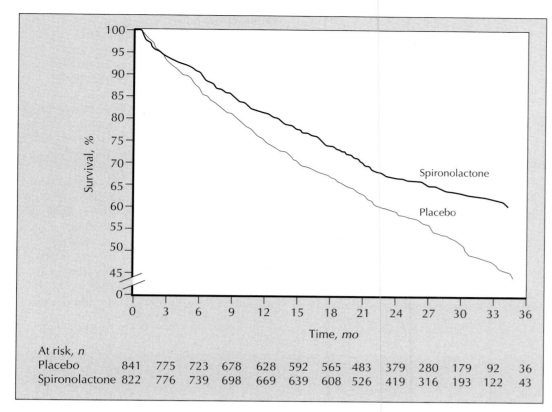

At risk, n													
Placebo	841	775	723	678	628	592	565	483	379	280	179	92	36
Spironolactone	822	776	739	698	669	639	608	526	419	316	193	122	43

FIGURE 11-15. Effect of spironolactone on survival in patients with severe heart failure. Patients with severe heart failure have been shown to have elevated levels of aldosterone compared with that of normal subjects. Treatment with angiotensin-converting enzyme (ACE) inhibitors reduces aldosterone release by limiting the production of angiotensin II. Due to non-ACE–dependent production of angiotensin II (serine protease pathways), aldosterone levels have been shown to rise over time in patients treated with recommended doses of ACE inhibitor. Aldosterone has direct effects on the kidney, leading to sodium retention and reduction in serum potassium concentration. Additionally, animal models of heart failure have shown that aldosterone may be responsible for myocardial fibrosis and myocyte hypertrophy seen with chronic heart failure. The Randomized Aldactone Evaluation Study (RALES) was performed in 1663 patients with ejection fraction of 35% or lower and New York Heart Association (NYHA) IV symptoms, or NYHA III symptoms who had experienced NYHA IV symptoms within the past 6 months. Patients were randomly assigned to receive 25 to 50 mg of spironolactone daily versus placebo, delivered in a double-blind fashion. The survival plot demonstrates the effect of spironolactone on all-cause mortality, with a reduction of 30% compared with placebo. This reduction in the risk of death among patients in the spironolactone group was attributed to a lower risk of both death from progressive heart failure and sudden death from cardiac causes. The frequency of hospitalization for worsening heart failure was 35% lower in the spironolactone group than in the placebo group. Patients receiving spironolactone treatment should have close monitoring of the serum potassium level, particularly in the first month of therapy [44].

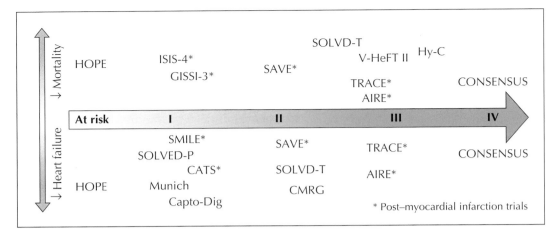

FIGURE 11-16. The relationship between disease severity and outcomes from clinical trials using angiotensin-converting enzyme (ACE) inhibitors. The relationship of positive or favorable clinical trials with ACE inhibitors can be shown in relation to the severity of congestive heart failure. The *horizontal arrow* depicts the progression from patients at risk for heart disease through asymptomatic left ventricular dysfunction to severe heart failure corresponding to New York Heart Association functional classification. Trials listed above the horizontal arrow have shown that treatment with ACE inhibitors results in a reduction in mortality of these patients. In all stages of heart disease and congestive heart failure, ACE inhibitors have been shown to reduce mortality. These studies include the HOPE trial in patients at high risk for cardiovascular events as well as the CONSENSUS study performed in patients with advanced heart failure. The study acronyms shown *below the horizontal arrow* have shown to reduce the incidence of worsened heart failure and/or heart failure hospitalizations. In all stages of heart failure, including those patients at risk for cardiac disease, studies using ACE inhibitors have shown a reduction in heart failure morbidity endpoints.

ANGIOTENSIN RECEPTOR BLOCKERS

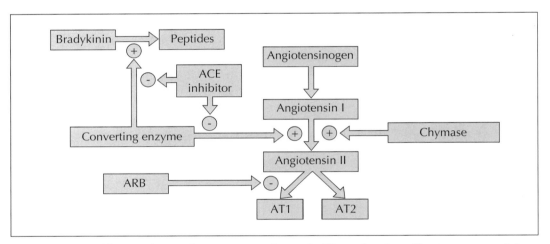

FIGURE 11-17. Alternative pathways to angiotensin II production. Controversy exists regarding the rule of angiotensin-receptor blockade (ARB) in the activation of the renin-angiotensin system. Several nonenzymatic pathways independent of angiotensin-converting enzyme (ACE) exist for the conversion of angiotensin I to angiotensin II and may contribute to persistent availability of both circulating and tissue angiotensin II despite treatment with ACE inhibitors. These alternative pathways invoke serine-protease inhibitors such as chymase, which have been shown in vivo to convert angiotensin I to angiotensin II. Because ACEs also act to break down products such as bradykinin, a factor with prominent vasodilatory properties, ACE inhibitors lead to higher levels of circulating bradykinin. The clinical relevance of this difference between the effects of ACE inhibitors and angiotensin-receptor blockers has not been fully elucidated [34].

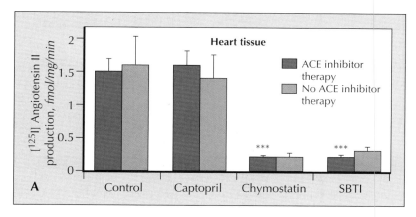

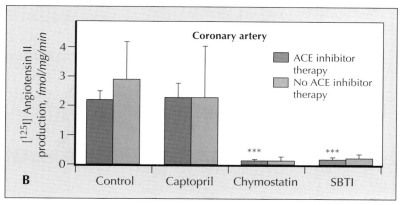

FIGURE 11-18. Effect of protease inhibitors on angiotensin I processing. Blockade of the renin-angiotensin system by inhibition of angiotensin-converting enzyme is beneficial for the treatment of heart failure patients. It is unclear, however, how complete the blockade of ACE inhibitors is and if there is continuing angiotensin II formation during chronic treatment with ACE inhibitors. Chymase has been shown to be present in the human heart and is able to form angiotensin II from angiotensin I. This study shows the effects of two protease inhibitors, chymostatin, and soy bean trypsin inhibitor (SBTI) on angiotensin II production in left ventricular tissue (**A**) and coronary artery tissue (**B**) incubated with 1 nmol/L angiotensin I in the presence of the ACE

inhibitor captopril. In the absence of a protease inhibitor, angiotensin II formation in ventricular tissue exposed to prior ACE inhibitor therapy could not be significantly inhibited by captopril in this assay. Only the two serine-protease inhibitors significantly inhibited angiotensin II formation. Likewise, the tissue from four hearts with no history of ACE inhibitor therapy had similar results. This study suggests that the majority of angiotensin II formation occurs through the chymase pathways, at least in this in vivo preparation. Thus, drugs such as renin inhibitors and angiotensin II receptor blockers might be able to induce a more complete blockade of the renin-angiotensin system, providing more efficacious therapy [34].

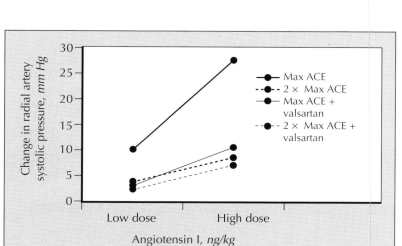

FIGURE 11-19. Comparison of supplemental angiotensin-converting enzyme (ACE) inhibitor versus addition of angiotensin receptor blocker on the blood pressure response to angiotensin I. The possibility of a clinically relevant alternative pathway to angiotensin II production has led investigators to compare the hemodynamic effects of angiotensin II receptor blockers to administering doses of ACE inhibitors above the maximally recommended doses. This study was performed in 42 patients with congestive heart failure who had been receiving maximally recommended doses of ACE inhibitors for greater than 3 months. The difference between the change in radial artery systolic pressure with low-dose and high-dose angiotensin I was 28 mm Hg in patients on maximal recommended doses of ACE inhibitors. This would indicate that a significant amount of angiotensin II is can be produced despite these doses of ACE inhibitors. The addition of valsartan and angiotensin receptor blocker significantly reduces the difference between the low- and high-dose angiotensin I administration. This effect, however, is nearly replicated by doubling the dose of angiotensin converting enzyme inhibitor. Further, the addition of valsartan to the double dose of ACE inhibitor has only a small and insignificant reduction in these measured blood pressure changes. These results suggest that residual angiotensin II production on recommended doses of ACE inhibitors can be attributed to the angiotensin-converting enzyme, rather than the chymase pathway [35].

RESULTS OF TRIALS USING AN ARB IN ACE INHIBITOR NAIVE AND INTOLERANT PATIENTS

TRIAL (PATIENTS, N)	SEVERITY	AGENTS	MEAN FU	CONTROL, %	ARB, %	RISK REDUCTION, %	P VALUE
ELITE II (3152)	NYHA II–IV	Losartan vs captopril	18 mo	15.9	17.7	-13.0%	0.16
RESOLVD (768)	NYHA II–IV	Candesartan vs enalapril	43 wk	6.4	13.1	-105.0%	0.09
SPICE (270)	NYHA II–III	Candesartan vs placebo	12 wk	3.3	3.4	-4%	NS

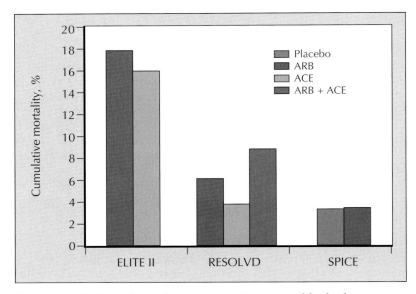

FIGURE 11-20. The effect of angiotensin II receptor blockade on mortality. **A,** Results of trials using angiotensin-converting enzyme (ACE) inhibitor naïve and intolerant patients. The Evaluation of Losartan In The Elderly (ELITE) study randomly selected 722

patients of 65 years of age or older with symptomatic left ventricular failure to receive 50 mg of losartan or captopril titrated to 50 mg three times per day. The primary endpoint of this initial study was an increase in serum creatinine. There were no differences seen with the incidence of rising creatinine. **B,** However, an unexpected 46% decrease in all-cause mortality was observed with losartan. Because of the limited power of this study to demonstrate this difference, a follow-up study was performed (ELITE-II). The ELITE-II trial was performed in 3152 patients with New York Heart Association class II to IV symptoms. This study failed to show any significant difference in all-cause mortality between losartan and captopril. There was a nonsignificant trend (P=0.16) favoring captopril in this analysis. The Randomized Evaluation of Strategies for Left Ventricular Dysfunction (RESOLVD) trial enrolled 768 patients in one of three arms, which included candesartan, enalapril, and the combination of candesartan and enalapril. This study also showed a nonsignificant trend toward worsened survival in the candesartan arms. Finally, the Study of Patients Intolerant of Converting Enzyme Inhibition (SPICE) trial studied 270 patients who were previously found to be ACE inhibitor intolerant. This study followed patients over 12 weeks who had received either candesartan or placebo. There was no significant difference in mortality in this relatively low-risk population [13,38–40].

EFFECT OF ANGIOTENSIN I RECEPTOR BLOCKADE ON MORBIDITY/MORTALITY IN ADDITION TO STANDARD HEART FAILURE MEDICATIONS

PRIMARY ENDPOINTS

VARIABLE	PLACEBO	VALSARTAN	RR, CI	P VALUE
Patients, n	2499	2511		
All-cause mortality, n (%)	484 (19.4%)	495 (19.7%)	1.02 (0.90–1.15)	0.80
Mortality + hospitalization + sudden death + inotrope need, n (%)	801 (32.1%)	723 (28.8%)	0.87 (0.79–0.96)	0.009

SECONDARY ENDPOINT

VARIABLE	PLACEBO	VALSARTAN	RR, CI	P VALUE
Heart failure hospitalizations, n (%)	463 (18.5%)	349 (13.9%)	0.73 (0.63–0.83)	0.00001

FIGURE 11-21. The effect of angiotensin receptor blockade on morbidity and mortality in the Valsartan in Heart Failure Trial (Val-HeFT) study. This trial studied the clinical effect of the addition of valsartan to standard heart failure care that included angiotensin-converting enzyme inhibitor therapy. This study enrolled 5010 patients and included two primary endpoints, all-cause mortality, and the composite endpoint of mortality, hospitalization, the need for defibrillation for sudden cardiac death, and the need for intravenous inotropes for greater than 4 hours. The

addition of valsartan to standard heart failure care resulted in no improvement in all-cause mortality. However, the risk of reaching the composite endpoint was reduced by 13% with valsartan. The vast majority of the benefit found in this composite endpoint was through reduction in heart failure hospitalizations. Hospitalizations were reduced by 27% with the addition of valsartan, with a highly significant P value of 0.0001. (Data presented by Cohn at the American Heart Association Scientific Sessions, 2000.)

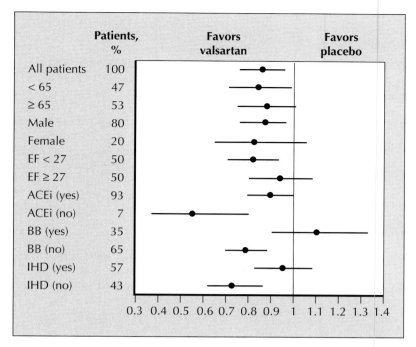

FIGURE 11-22. Effective angiotensin receptor blockade on morbidity and mortality: subgroup analysis (Val-HeFT). Analysis of subgroups within the Val-Heft trial showed that these benefits applied nearly equally with patients, with older and younger patients, as well as males and females. Patients with lower left ventricular ejection fractions seemed to benefit more with the addition of valsartan. Although the percentage of patients not receiving ACE inhibitors in this study was rather small (7%), these patients were observed to have a marked reduction in their composite endpoint with a relative risk of 0.55. Interestingly, patients receiving β-blocker therapy (comprising 35% of the patient population) were observed to reach fewer endpoints if on placebo. Finally, patients without ischemic heart disease had a more pronounced benefit with the addition of valsartan than those patients with ischemic heart disease. (Data presented by Cohn at the American Heart Association Scientific Sessions, 2000.)

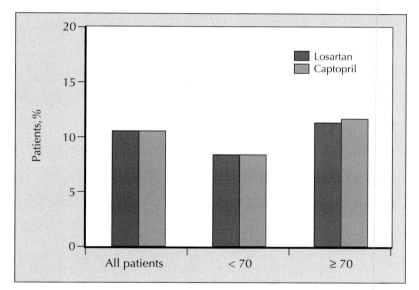

FIGURE 11-23. Comparison of increases in serum creatinine with angiotensin receptor blockers versus angiotensin-converting enzyme (ACE) inhibitors. Initial interest in angiotensin receptor blockers was also driven by the hypothesis that these agents may be less prone to cause renal insufficiency, particularly in elderly patients. The ELITE trial studied this effect in 722 ACE inhibitor–naive patients 65 years of age or older. The incidence of a rise in creatinine (defined as a rise of 0.3 or greater mg/dL) was 10% in the captopril arm of this study. There was no significant difference in the incidence of increase in creatinine with losartan therapy. The results were similar for younger as well as older patients [38].

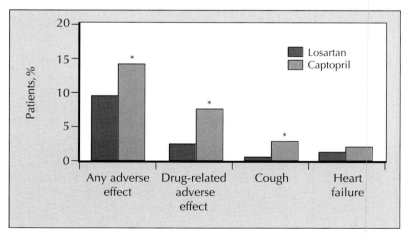

FIGURE 11-24. Comparison of withdrawals for adverse effects. Investigators in the ELITE-II observed that significantly fewer patients taking losartan discontinued treatment because of adverse effects. Nearly 15% of patients taking captopril in this study were unable to continue the study drug throughout the follow-up period. Over 90% of patients assigned to the losartan treatment arm were able to continue study drug throughout the follow-up period. Approximately 8% of patients assigned to the captopril treatment arm stopped the study drug due to a drug-related adverse effect. Less than half of these patients stopped due to an intolerable cough, a side effect seen infrequently in patients assigned to the losartan arm. Presumably, the majority of the remaining drug-related adverse effects were caused by symptomatic hypotension. This difference may have been expected when comparing captopril and losartan given the difference in pharmacokinetics between these two agents [13].

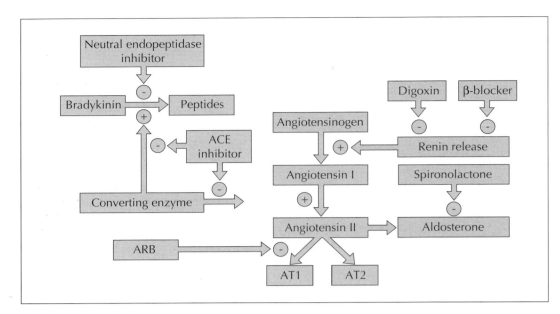

diversity in their therapeutic effects, have been shown to inhibit the renin-angiotensin-aldosterone system to varying degrees. Digoxin blocks release of renin from the juxtaglomerular cells of the kidney. Sympatholytic agents, or β-blockers, inhibit the sympathetic stimulus for renin release, which is a prominent feature for renin release in heart failure. Both converting inhibitors and angiotensin receptor antagonists have hemodynamic properties that would be considered "vasodilator" in overall action. Whereas converting enzyme inhibitors prevent the generation of angiotensin II, the receptor antagonists block the effects of circulating angiotensin II at multiple target organ sites. Finally, angiotensin II upregulation leads to release to aldosterone. Aldosterone has been shown to lead to myocyte hypertrophy as well as fibrosis of the myocardium. Spironolactone is a competitive inhibitor to aldosterone and has been shown to reduce mortality in patients with advanced heart failure.

FIGURE 11-25. New paradigm to attenuate the renin-angiotensin-aldosterone system. Although the angiotensin-converting enzyme (ACE) inhibitors are considered to be the standard approach for inhibition of the renin-angiotensin-aldosterone system, a review of the literature clearly demonstrates that many pharmacologic classes, despite a broad

REFERENCES

1. Francis GS, Cohn JN, Johnson G, *et al.*: Plasma norepinephrine, plasma renin activity, and congestive heart failure: relations to survival and the effects of therapy in V-HeFT II. The V-HeFT VA Cooperative Studies Group. *Circulation* 1993, 87:VI40–V148.

2. Schrier RW, Abraham WT: Hormones and hemodynamics in heart failure. *N Engl J Med* 1999, 341:577–585.

3. Rakusan K, Flanagan M, Geva T, *et al.*: Morphometry of human coronary capillaries during normal growth and the effect of age in left ventricular pressure-overload hypertrophy. *Circulation* 1992, 86:38–46.

4. Myers B, Deen W, Brenner B: Effects of norepinephrine and angiotensin II on the determinants of glomerular ultrafiltration and proximal tubule fluid reabsorption in the rat. *Circ Res* 1983, 37:101–110.

5. Staessen J, Lijnen P, Fagard R, *et al.*: Rise in plasma concentration of aldosterone during long-term angiotensin II suppression. *J Endocrinol* 1981, 91:457–465.

6. Weber K, Villarreal D: Aldosterone and antialdosterone therapy in congestive heart failure. *Am J Cardiol* 1993, 771:3A–11A.

7. Swedberg K, Eneroth P, Kjekshus J, *et al.*: Hormones regulating cardiovascular function in patients with severe congestive heart failure and their relation to mortality: CONSENSUS Trial Study Group. *Circulation* 1990, 82:1730–1736.

8. Brilla C, Maisch B, Weber K: Myocardial collagen matrix remodeling in arterial hypertension. *Eur Heart J* 1992, 13(suppl D):24–32.

9. Weber K, Brilla C: Pathological hypertrophy and cardiac interstitium: fibrosis and renin-angiotensin-aldosterone system. *Circulation* 1991, 83:1849–1865.

10. Duprez D, Bauwens F, De Buyzere M, *et al.*: Influence of arterial blood pressure and aldosterone on left ventricular hypertrophy in moderate essential hypertension. *Am J Cardiol* 1993, 71:17A–20A.

11. Brilla C, Matsubara L, Weber K: Antifibrotic effects of spironolactone in preventing myocardial fibrosis in systemic arterial hypertension. *Am J Cardiol* 1993, 71:12A–16A.

12. Davis R, Ribner HS, Keung E, *et al.*: Treatment of chronic congestive heart failure with captopril, an oral inhibitor of angiotensin-converting enzyme. *N Engl J Med* 1979, 301:117–121.

13. Pitt B, Poole-Wilson PA, Segal R, *et al.*: Effect of losartan compared with captopril on mortality in patients with symptomatic heart failure: randomised trial. The losartan heart failure survival study ELITE II. *Lancet* 2000, 355:1582–1587.

14. Cody R: ACE inhibitors: mechanisms, pharmacodynamics, and clinical trials in heart failure. *Cardiology in Review* 1994, 3:145–146.

15. Cody R, Laragh J: The renin-angiotensin-aldosterone system in chronic congestive heart failure: pathophysiology and implications for treatment. In *Drug Treatment of Heart Failure*. Edited by Cohn J. Secaucus, NJ: Advanced Therapeutics Communications International; 1988:109–104.

16. Captopril Multi-Center Research Group: A placebo controlled trial with captopril in refractory heart failure. *J Am Coll Cardiol* 1983, 2:755–763.

17. Cohn J, Johnson G, Ziesche S: A comparison of enalapril with hydralazine-isosorbide dinitrate in the treatment of chronic congestive heart failure. *N Engl J Med* 1991, 325:303–310.

18. The SOLVD Investigators: Effect of enalapril on survival in patients with reduced left ventricular ejection fractions and congestive heart failure. *N Engl J Med* 1991, 325:293–302.

19. Kleber F, Niemoller L, Doering W: Impact of converting enzyme inhibition on progression of chronic heart failure: results of the Munich Mild Heart Failure Trial. *Br Heart J* 1992, 67:289–296.

20. Gradman A, Deedwania P, Cody R, *et al.*: Predictors of total mortality and sudden death in mild to moderate heart failure: Captopril-digoxin study group. *J Am Coll Cardiol* 1989, 14:564–572.

21. The CONSENSUS Trial Study Group: Effects of enalapril on mortality in severe congestive heart failure: results of the Cooperative North Scandinavian Enalapril Survival Study (CONSENSUS). *N Engl J Med* 1987, 316:1429–1435.

22. Fonarow G, Chelimsky-Fallick C, Stevenson L: Effect of direct vasodilation with hydralazine versus angiotensin-converting enzyme inhibition with captopril on mortality in advanced heart failure: the Hy-C trial. *J Am Coll Cardiol* 1992, 19:842–850.

23. The SOLVD Investigators: Effect of enalapril on mortality and the development of heart failure in asymptomatic patients with reduced left ventricular ejection fractions. *N Engl J Med* 1992, 327:685–691.

24. Ambrosioni E, Borghi C, Magnani B: The effect of the angiotensin-converting-enzyme inhibitor zofenopril on mortality and morbidity after anterior myocardial infarction: the survival of myocardial infarction long-term evaluation (SMILE) study. *N Engl J Med* 1995, 332:80–85.

25. Swedberg K, Held P, Kjekshus J, *et al.*: Effects of the early administration of enalapril on mortality in patients with acute myocardial infarction: results of the cooperative new scandinavian enalapril survival study II (CONSENSUS II). *N Engl J Med* 1992, 327:678–684.

26. Cody R: ACE inhibitors: mechanisms, pharmacodynamics, and clinical trials in heart failure. *Cardiology in Review* 1994, 3:145–146.

27. Pfeffer MA, Braunwald E, Moye LA, *et al.*: Effect of captopril on mortality and morbidity in patients with left ventricular dysfunction after myocardial infarction: results of the survival and ventricular enlargement trial. The SAVE investigators. *N Engl J Med* 1992, 327:669–677.

28. ISIS-4 (Fourth International Study of Infarct Survival) Collaborative Group: Isis-4: a randomised factorial trial assessing early oral captopril, oral mononitrate, and intravenous magnesium sulphate in 58,050 patients with suspected acute myocardial infarction. *Lancet* 1995, 345:669–685.

29. Gruppo Italiano per lo Studio della Soprawivenza Nell'infarto Miocardico: Six-month effects of early treatment with lisinopril and transdermal glyceryl trinitrate singly and together withdrawn six weeks after acute myocardial infarction: the GISSI-3 trial. *J Am Coll Cardiol* 1996, 27:337–344.

30. Kingma JH, van Gilst WH, Peels CH, *et al.*: Acute intervention with captopril during thrombolysis in patients with first anterior myocardial infarction: results from the captopril and thrombolysis study (CATS). *Eur Heart J* 1994, 15:898–907.

31. Kober L, Torp-Pedersen C, Carlsen JE, *et al.*: A clinical trial of the angiotensin-converting-enzyme inhibitor trandolapril in patients with left ventricular dysfunction after myocardial infarction: Trandolapril Cardiac Evaluation (TRACE) study group. *N Engl J Med* 1995, 333:1670–1676.

32. The Acute Infarction Ramipril Efficacy (AIRE) Study Investigators: Effect of ramipril on mortality and morbidity of survivors of acute myocardial infarction with clinical evidence of heart failure. *Lancet* 1993, 342:821–828.

33. Yusuf S, Sleight P, Pogue J, *et al.*: Effects of an angiotensin-converting-enzyme inhibitor, ramipril, on cardiovascular events in high-risk patients: the heart outcomes prevention evaluation study investigators. *N Engl J Med* 2000, 342:145–153.

34. Wolny A, Clozel J, Rein J, *et al.*: Functional and biochemical analysis of angiotensin II forming pathways in the human heart. *Circ Res* 1997, 80:219–227.

35. Jorde UP, Ennezat PV, Lisker J, *et al.*: Maximally recommended doses of angiotensin-converting enzyme (ACE) inhibitors do not completely prevent ace-mediated formation of angiotensin ii in chronic heart failure. *Circulation* 2000, 101:844–846.

36. Packer M, Poole-Wilson PA, Armstrong PW, *et al.*: Comparative effects of low and high doses of the angiotensin-converting enzyme inhibitor, lisinopril, on morbidity and mortality in chronic heart failure: ATLAS study group. *Circulation* 1999, 100:2312–2318.

37. Nanas JN, Alexopoulos G, Anastasiou-Nana MI, *et al.*: Outcome of patients with congestive heart failure treated with standard versus high doses of enalapril: a multicenter study. High enalapril dose study group. *J Am Coll Cardiol* 2000, 36:2090–2095.

38. Pitt B, Segal R, Martinez FA, *et al.*: Randomised trial of losartan versus captopril in patients over 65 with heart failure (Evaluation of Losartan in the Elderly Study, ELITE). *Lancet* 1997, 349:747–752.

39. McKelvie RS, Yusuf S, Pericak D, *et al.*: Comparison of candesartan, enalapril, and their combination in congestive heart failure: randomized evaluation of strategies for left ventricular dysfunction (RESOLVD) pilot study. The RESOLVD pilot study investigators. *Circulation* 1999, 100:1056–1064.

40. Granger CB, Ertl G, Kuch J, *et al.*: Randomized trial of candesartan cilexetil in the treatment of patients with congestive heart failure and a history of intolerance to angiotensin-converting enzyme inhibitors. *Am Heart J* 2000, 139:609–617.

41. Al-Khadra A, Salem D, Rand W, *et al.*: Antiplatelet agents and survival: a cohort analysis from the Studies of Left Ventricular Dysfunction (SOLVD) trial. *J Am Coll Cardiol* 1998, 31:419–425.

42. Spaulding C, Charbonnier B, Cohen-Solal A, *et al.*: Acute hemodynamic interaction of aspirin and ticlopidine with enalapril: results of a double-blind, randomized comparative trial. *Circulation* 1998, 98:757–765.

43. Exner DV, Dries DL, Domanski MJ, *et al.*: Lesser response to angiotensin-converting-enzyme inhibitor therapy in black as compared with white patients with left ventricular dysfunction. *N Engl J Med* 2001, 344:1351–1357.

44. Pitt B, Zannad F, Remme WJ, *et al.*: The effect of spironolactone on morbidity and mortality in patients with severe heart failure: randomized aldactone evaluation study investigators. *N Engl J Med* 1999, 341:709–717.

β-BLOCKERS

12
CHAPTER

Michael M. Givertz
and Wilson S. Colucci

The overall goals in the management of heart failure are to prevent or eliminate symptoms, improve quality of life, and prolong survival. Paradoxically, as has been demonstrated with positive inotropic agents such as vesnarinone and flosequinan, chronic heart failure therapy may improve quality of life and reduce symptoms while increasing mortality. As discussed in Chapter 11, several large randomized controlled trials have demonstrated the beneficial effects of angiotensin-converting enzyme (ACE) inhibitors on exercise tolerance, clinical signs and symptoms, neurohormonal stimulation, quality of life, and survival in patients with chronic heart failure.

β-Adrenergic antagonists were traditionally contraindicated in the treatment of heart failure because of concern for negative inotropic effects leading to clinical deterioration. In the 1980s, studies demonstrated that chronic overactivity of the sympathetic nervous system could contribute to disease progression and mortality in patients with chronic systolic heart failure. Small, uncontrolled trials suggested a beneficial effect of β-adrenergic antagonists in heart failure. Subsequent randomized controlled trials (US Carvedilol, MERIT-HF, CIBIS II) have demonstrated that β-blockers improve symptoms and left ventricular function, and reduce morbidity and mortality in patients with chronic heart failure. These drugs may have variable actions related in part to their non β-blocking effects, and must be titrated with caution in symptomatic patients. Consensus guidelines recommend β-blockers, in addition to ACE inhibitors and diuretics, for the long-term management of patients with mild to moderate heart failure. The recently completed COPERNICUS study demonstrated the safety and efficacy of β-blockers in patients with severe heart failure. The role of β-blockers in patients with asymptomatic left ventricular dysfunction has not been tested.

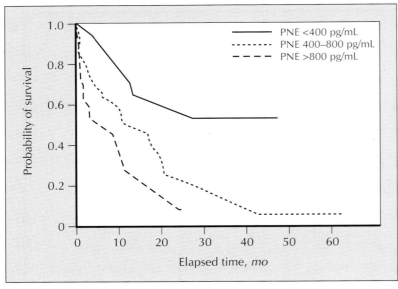

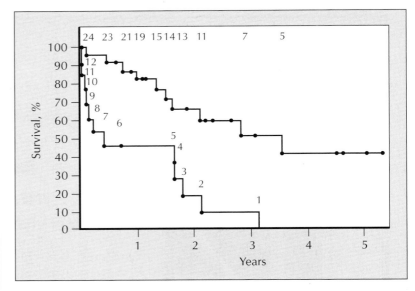

FIGURE 12-1. The level of activation of the sympathetic nervous system predicts survival in patients with chronic systolic heart failure. Cohn *et al.* [1] measured plasma norepinephrine (PNE) levels in 106 patients with functional class III to IV heart failure and followed them prospectively for a mean of 27 months. As shown by the survival curves, patients in the highest tercile (*dashed line*; PNE > 800 pg/mL) had significantly decreased long-term survival when compared with patients in either the middle (*dotted line*) or lowest terciles (*solid line*). Neurohormonal data from the Studies of Left Ventricular Dysfunction (SOLVD) [2] further demonstrated that norepinephrine levels are also increased in patients with asymptomatic left ventricular dysfunction. These and other studies have raised the possibility that chronic over-activity of the sympathetic nervous system could contribute to mortality in patients with heart failure, and might contribute to disease progression even in patients with early, asymptomatic disease. (*Adapted from* Cohn *et al.* [1].)

FIGURE 12-2. β-Adrenergic antagonists for treatment of dilated cardiomyopathy. In the 1970s, Swedberg *et al.* [3] in Goteberg, Sweden published a series of pioneering studies that suggested that β-adrenergic antagonists could be of clinical value in the treatment of patients with dilated cardiomyopathy. In these open-label studies, the addition of a β-adrenergic antagonist to standard treatment with digitalis and diuretics was associated with improvements in symptoms and ventricular function, and, as shown here, improved survival. In 24 patients treated with β-adrenergic antagonists (*upper curve*), the 3-year survival was improved when compared with a group of 12 historical controls (*lower curve*). (*Adapted from* Swedberg *et al.* [3].)

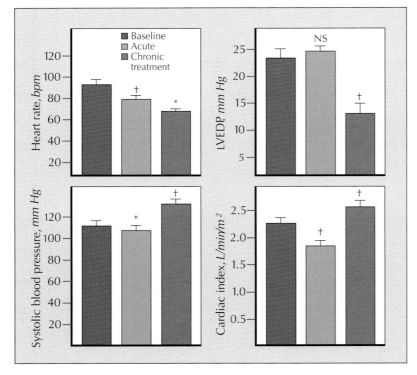

FIGURE 12-3. Acute and chronic hemodynamic effects of β-blockers in patients with heart failure: the role of the sympathetic nervous system. The sympathetic nervous system, acting via stimulation of myocardial β-adrenergic receptors, plays an important role in supporting cardiac pump function in patients with myocardial failure. Not surprisingly, in such patients the immediate effect of a β-blocker is a deterioration in hemodynamic performance. Intravenous administration of a low dose of the β-adrenergic antagonist metoprolol to patients with heart failure decreased heart rate and cardiac index, and caused a small increase in left ventricular end-diastolic pressure (LVEDP). Although the acute vascular effect of β-blockade is to increase systemic vascular resistance, systolic blood pressure decreased reflecting a decrease in cardiac output. In striking contrast, long-term administration of oral metoprolol to the same patients was associated with a decrease in LVEDP and an increase in cardiac index, despite a further decrease in heart rate indicative of more complete β-blockade (*Asterisk* indicates *P* < 0.01 vs baseline; *dagger* indicates *P* < 0.001 vs baseline). These data indicate that although the acute hemodynamic effect of β-adrenergic blockade is to worsen hemodynamics, long-term treatment is associated with improvement in ventricular function. (*Adapted from* Hjalmarson and Waagstein [4].)

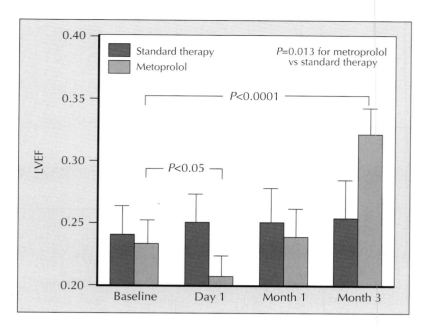

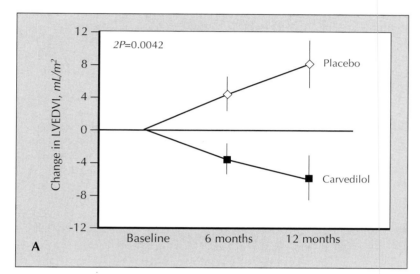

A

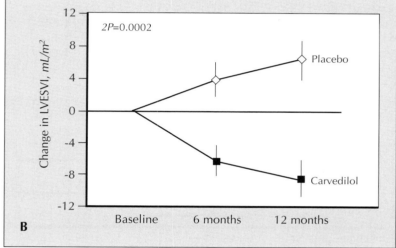

B

FIGURE 12-4. Time course of the increase in left ventricular ejection fraction (LVEF) with chronic β-blocker therapy in patients with heart failure. One of the most consistent findings in controlled trials of chronic β-blocker therapy in patients with heart failure has been an increase in LVEF. The increase in ejection fraction is time-dependent. Hall *et al.* [5] demonstrated that after 1 day of therapy with metoprolol, patients demonstrated a significant reduction in LVEF that was associated with an increase in end-systolic volume. However, with continued therapy, and despite uptitration to higher doses of metoprolol, LVEF returned to baseline by 1 month and was significantly increased over baseline by 3 months. Overall, LVEF increased from 23% to 32% ($P = 0.001$). In the placebo group, there were no significant changes in ejection fraction or left ventricular volumes. Data from this and other studies (*eg, see* Fig. 12-8) demonstrate that long-term improvements in LVEF are associated with improved outcomes. (*Adapted from* Hall *et al.* [5].)

FIGURE 12-5. Effect of chronic treatment with carvedilol on left ventricular volumes. The Australia-New Zealand (ANZ) Heart Failure Research Collaborative Group randomly assigned patients with ischemic heart failure and a left ventricular ejection fraction (LVEF) of less than 45% to carvedilol or placebo. An echocardiographic substudy was performed on 123 patients to determine the effects of treatment on left ventricular (LV) size and function at 6 and 12 months. After 6 months of therapy, LVEF had increased by 4.9% in the carvedilol group compared with a decrease of 0.9% in the placebo group ($2P < 0.001$). As shown, the LV end-diastolic (**A**) and end-systolic (**B**) volume indices (LVEDVI and LVESVI, respectively) increased in the placebo group at 12 months but were reduced in the carvedilol-treated patients. These data suggest that carvedilol exerted a beneficial reverse remodeling effect. (*Adapted from* Doughty *et al.* [6].)

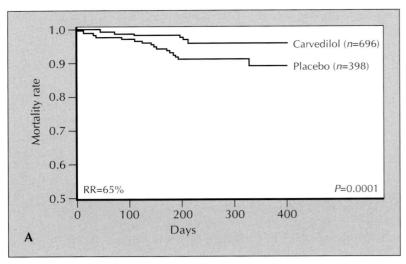

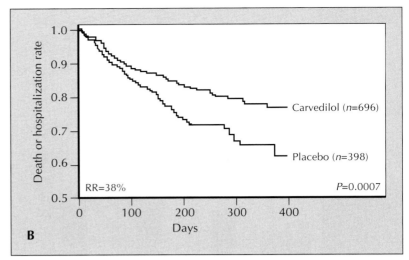

A　　　　　　　　　　　　　　　　　　　　**B**

FIGURE 12-6. US Carvedilol Heart Failure Trials Program: effect on major clinical events. In 1997, the US Food and Drug Administration approved carvedilol, a nonselective β-adrenergic antagonist with α_1-adrenergic receptor blocking and antioxidant properties, as adjunctive therapy for patients with mild to moderate heart failure. This decision was based in large part on the results of the US Carvedilol Heart Failure Trials Program, which randomly assigned 1094 patients with chronic heart failure and a left ventricular ejection fraction of 35% or less to placebo or carvedilol in addition to conventional therapy with an angiotensin-converting enzyme inhibitor, diuretics, and digoxin. Patients were assigned to one of four treatment protocols based on exercise capacity as assessed by a 6-minute walk test. After a mean follow-up of 7 months, the overall mortality rate was 7.8% in the placebo group versus 3.2% in the carvedilol group (risk reduction [RR], 65%; 95% CI, 39% to 80%; $P<0.001$) (**A**). In addition, carvedilol resulted in a 27% reduction in the risk of cardio-vascular hospitalization ($P = 0.036$) and a 38% reduction in the combined endpoint of death or cardiovascular hospitalization (**B**); ($P = 0.007$). (*Adapted from* Packer *et al* [7].)

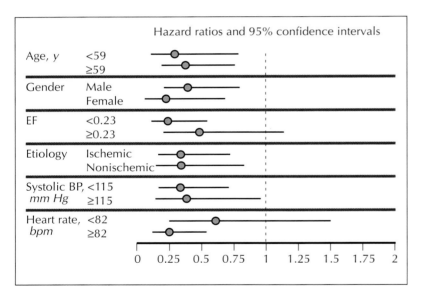

FIGURE 12-7. In the US Carvedilol Heart Failure Trials Program, the reduction in mortality with carvedilol was similar regardless of age, gender, left ventricular ejection fraction (EF), the etiology of heart failure, resting systolic blood pressure (BP), or heart rate. A meta-analysis of randomized clinical trials of β-adrenergic antagonists in heart failure [8] observed similar reductions in mortality for patients with ischemic (OR, 0.69; 95% CI, 0.45 to 0.98) and nonischemic cardiomyopathy (OR, 0.69; 95% CI, 0.47 to 0.99). (*Adapted from* Packer *et al*. [7].)

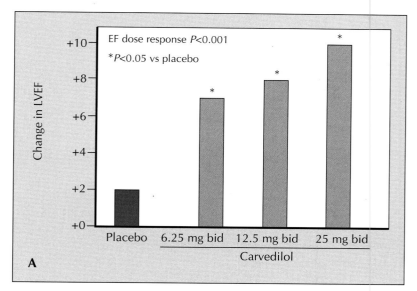

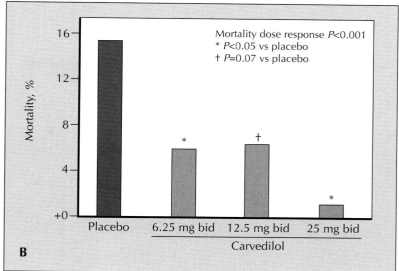

FIGURE 12-8. Dose-dependent effects of carvedilol on ejection fraction and mortality in the Multicenter Oral Carvedilol Heart Failure Assessment (MOCHA) trial. This trial, a component of the US Carvedilol Heart Failure Trials Program, tested whether the effects of carvedilol were dose-related. Patients ($n = 345$) with mild to moderate heart failure were randomly assigned to treatment with placebo or carvedilol in one of three target doses: 6.25 mg twice a day (low-dose group), 12.5 mg twice a day (medium-dose group), or 25 mg twice a day (high-dose group). Although carvedilol had no effect on the primary end-point of submaximal exercise, there was a significant dose-related improvement in left ventricular ejection fraction (LVEF) (**A**) and reduction in all-cause mortality (**B**). In this study, carvedilol also lowered the hospitalization rate by approximately 60%. bid—twice a day. (*Adapted from* Bristow *et al.* [9].)

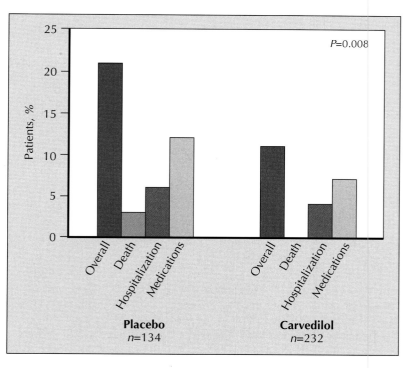

FIGURE 12-9. Effect of carvedilol on the clinical progression of heart failure. Another stratified trial within the US Carvedilol Heart Failure Trials Program examined the effect of carvedilol on the clinical progression of heart failure in 366 patients with only mild functional impairment. The primary endpoint of clinical progression was defined as death due to heart failure, hospitalization for heart failure or a sustained increase in heart failure medications for more than 30 days. As shown, heart failure progression occurred in 21% of placebo patients compared with 11% of carvedilol patients (48% risk reduction, $P = 0.008$). The effect of carvedilol was not influenced by gender, age, or the etiology of heart failure. Carvedilol also improved both physician and patient global assessments and reduced all-cause mortality. (*Adapted from* Colucci *et al.* [10].)

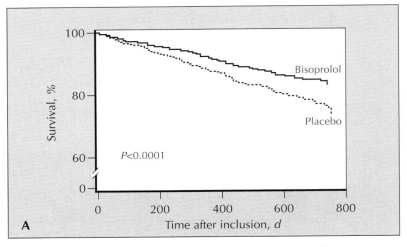

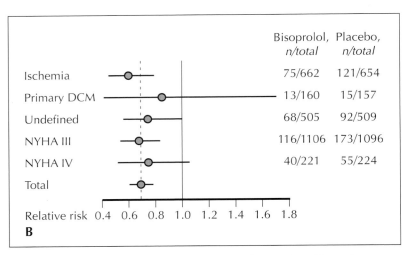

FIGURE 12-10. Survival results from the Cardiac Insufficiency Bisoprolol Study (CIBIS) II. This study randomly assigned 2647 patients with New York Heart Association (NYHA) functional class III and IV heart failure and a left ventricular ejection fraction of 35% or less to treatment with the β_1-selective antagonist bisoprolol (up to 10 mg daily) or placebo. The study was stopped early, after a mean follow-up of 1.3 years, when the second interim analysis demonstrated a 34% reduction in all-cause mortality with bisoprolol (**A**) ($P < 0.001$).

Bisoprolol also reduced sudden death by 42% and hospitalization for worsening heart failure by 32%. The number of permanent treatment withdrawals was similar in the two groups. Subgroup analyses (**B**) revealed that the treatment effects of bisoprolol were independent of heart failure etiology or NYHA class. Most patients (83%) were in NYHA class III and the annual mortality rate was only 13% in the placebo group, leading the investigators to caution against extrapolating the results to patients with severe heart failure. DCM—dilated cardiomyopathy. (*Adapted from* the CIBIS II Investigators [11].)

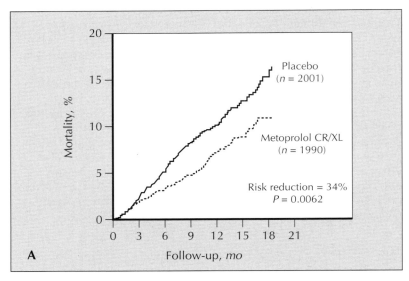

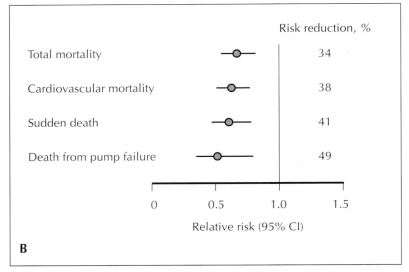

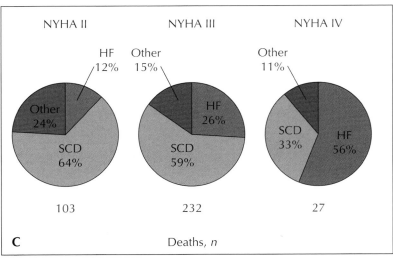

FIGURE 12-11. Results from the Metoprolol CR/XL Randomised Intervention Trial in Congestive Heart Failure (MERIT-HF). This trial randomly assigned 3991 patients with NYHA class II to IV heart failure and a left ventricular ejection fraction of 40% or less to metoprolol CR/XL (up to 200 mg daily) or placebo. After a mean follow-up of 1 year, an independent safety committee recommended stopping the study early because of a 34% reduction in all-cause mortality in the metoprolol CR/XL group (**A**) ($P = 0.0062$). Metoprolol CR/XL also reduced cardiovascular mortality by 38%, sudden death by 41%, and death due to worsening heart failure by 49% (**B**). In a post-hoc analysis, mode of death was analyzed in relation to NYHA class (**C**). The proportion of sudden deaths (SCD) decreased, and the proportion of deaths due to heart failure (HF) increased, with increasing severity of HF. (*Adapted from* the MERIT-HF Study Group [12].)

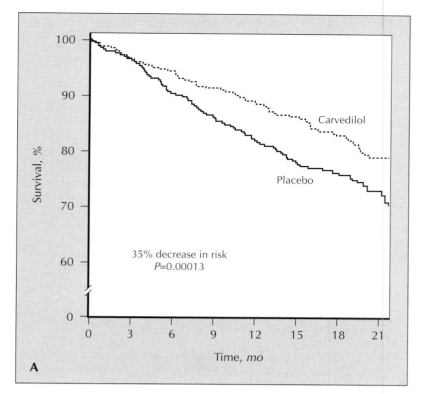

A

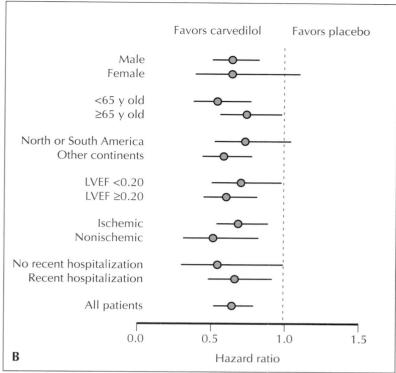

B

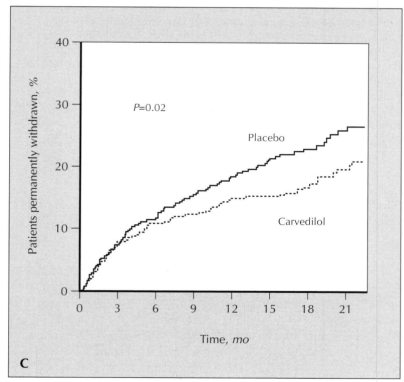

C

FIGURE 12-12. β-Adrenergic antagonists in severe heart failure. The US Carvedilol Program and CIBIS II and MERIT-HF studies confirmed that β-blockers reduce morbidity and mortality in patients with mild to moderate heart failure. To test the efficacy of β-blockers in patients with severe heart failure, the Carvedilol Prospective Randomized Cumulative Survival (COPERNICUS) Study randomly assigned 2289 patients with symptoms of heart failure at rest or on minimal exertion and an ejection fraction of less than 25% to carvedilol or placebo for a mean of 10.4 months. Patients were receiving standard therapy, including diuretics optimized to achieve euvolemia; they were excluded if they required intensive care or intravenous vasodilators or positive inotropes. The study was stopped early by the Data and Safety Monitoring Board due to the finding of a 35% decrease in the risk of death with carvedilol (95% CI, 19% to 48%; $P = 0.00013$ unadjusted) (**A**). The reduction in mortality was consistent across a range of subgroups defined according to sex, age, location of study center, left ventricular ejection fraction (LVEF), cause of heart failure, and history of recent heart failure hospitalization (**B**). Carvedilol was well tolerated in patients with severe heart failure as demonstrated by the fact that fewer patients in the carvedilol group were permanently withdrawn from study medication due to adverse effects (1 year withdrawal rate 18.5% in the placebo group vs 14.8% in the carvedilol group [$P = 0.02$]) (**C**). (*Adapted from* Packer *et al.* [13].)

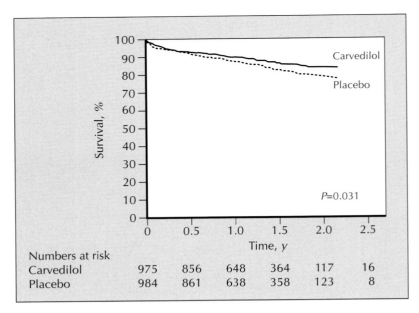

Numbers at risk

Carvedilol	975	856	648	364	117	16
Placebo	984	861	638	358	123	8

FIGURE 12-13. β-Blockers following acute myocardial infarction. The beneficial effects of β-blockers following acute myocardial infarction were demonstrated prior to the introduction of angiotensin-converting enzyme (ACE) inhibitors, thrombolytic therapy, and primary angioplasty, and prior studies tended to exclude patients with heart failure and did not measure left ventricular (LV) function. The Carvedilol Post-Infarct Survival Control in LV Dysfunction (CAPRICORN) study randomly assigned 1959 patients 3 to 21 days following acute myocardial infarction with an ejection fraction of 40% or less to carvedilol or placebo for a mean of 1.3 years. Reperfusion therapy, mainly thrombolysis, was used in 46% of patients, and 98% were receiving ACE inhibitors at the time of randomization. Although there was no difference between the treatment groups in the primary endpoint of death or cardiovascular hospitalization, carvedilol reduced all-cause mortality by 23%. There were 116 deaths in the carvedilol group compared with 151 deaths in the placebo group (hazard ratio, 0.77; 95% CI, 0.60 to 0.98; P = 0.031). Carvedilol had no significant effect on sudden death, but reduced the risk of nonfatal myocardial infarction by 41%. (*Adapted from* the CAPRICORN Investigators [14].)

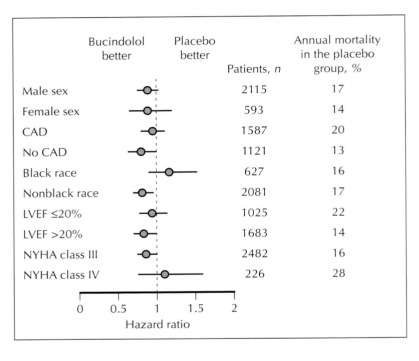

FIGURE 12-14. Race and the response to β-blockers in heart failure. The Beta-Blocker Evaluation of Survival Trial (BEST) randomly assigned 2708 patients with moderate to severe heart failure to double-blind therapy with placebo or bucindolol, a nonselective β-blocker and mild vasodilator. After an average follow-up of 2 years, there was a nonsignificant reduction in mortality with bucindolol (hazard ratio, 0.90; 95% CI, 0.78 to 1.02; adjusted P = 0.13). A prespecified subgroup analysis suggested a lack of benefit with bucindolol in black patients, whereas nonblack patients had a significant survival benefit (hazard ratio, 0.82; 95% CI, 0.70 to 0.96; P = 0.01). (*Adapted from* the BEST Investigators [15].)

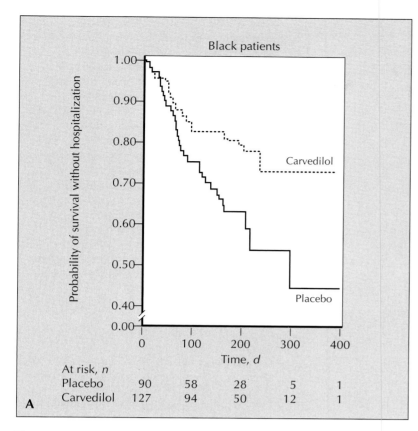

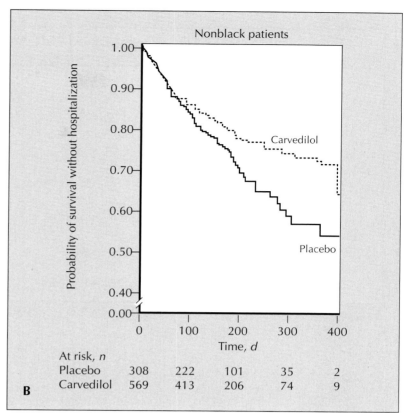

FIGURE 12-15. Race and the response to β-blockers in heart failure. A retrospective analysis of the US Carvedilol Heart Failure Trials Program was performed to determine whether race influences the response to carvedilol in patients with chronic heart failure. On average, black patients ($n = 217$) were younger, more likely to have hypertension, and less likely to have ischemic heart disease than nonblacks ($n = 877$). As compared with placebo, carvedilol lowered the risk of death or hospitalization by 48% in black patients (**A**) ($P = 0.01$) and 30% in nonblack patients (**B**) ($P = 0.01$). Carvedilol improved NYHA class and ejection fraction in both blacks and nonblacks with no significant interaction between treatment effect and race ($P > 0.05$). (*Adapted from* Yancy *et al.* [16].)

COMBINED ORAL POSITIVE INOTROPIC AND β-BLOCKER THERAPY IN REFRACTORY HEART FAILURE

	BASELINE	DURING THERAPY	P VALUE
LVEF, %	18 ± 2	28 ± 3	0.01
HR, *bpm*	101 ± 4	80 ± 4	0.0001
NYHA class	4 ± 0	2.8 ± 0.1	0.0001
Admissions per y	2.3 ± 0.3	1.0 ± 0.6	0.06

FIGURE 12-16. Combined oral positive inotropic and β-blocker therapy in refractory heart failure. Patients with refractory New York Heart Association (NYHA) class IV heart failure have a high 1-year mortality rate, and generally do not tolerate β-blocker therapy. Positive inotropic agents may be used acutely to treat severe decompensated heart failure, but prolonged oral use is associated with excess mortality. Combined therapy with an oral positive inotrope and β-blocker has the theoretical advantage of attenuating the adverse effects of the positive inotrope while allowing titration of the β-blocker. Twenty-three patients with severe heart failure (left ventricular ejection fraction [LVEF], 17 ± 1%; cardiac index, 1.6 ± 0.1 L/min/m^2; 60% inotrope-dependent) were treated with oral enoximone, a phosphodiesterase inhibitor, and metoprolol for a mean of 9 months. During combined therapy, LVEF increased from 18% to 28%, and this was associated with a decrease in heart rate (HR), improvement in NYHA functional class, and a trend toward decreased hospital admissions. Over the long-term, 48% of patients were weaned off enoximone and 30% underwent successful heart transplantation. These data suggest that combined oral inotropic and β-blocker therapy may play a role in palliation or as a bridge to transplantation in patients with end-stage heart failure. (*Adapted from* Shakar *et al.* [17].)

CLINICAL PHARMACOLOGY OF β-ADRENERGIC ANTAGONISTS

	β₁/β₂ ADRENERGIC RECEPTORS, *RELATIVE SELECTIVITY*	VASODILATOR MECHANISMS	INTRINSIC SYMPATHOMIMETIC ACTIVITY
Nebivolol	300	Direct	0
Bisoprolol	120	0	0
Metoprolol	75	0	0
Celiprolol	70	β₂ Agonist	+
Atenolol	40	0	0
Carvedilol	10	α₁ Antagonist	0
Propranolol	1	0	0
Pindolol	1	β₂ Agonist	+
Bucindolol	1	Direct	0
Labetalol	1	α₁ Antagonist	0

FIGURE 12-17. Clinical pharmacology of β-adrenergic antagonists. The pharmacology of β-adrenergic antagonists differs substantially with regard to properties such as the relative selectivity for $β_1$-versus $β_2$-adrenergic receptors and the presence or absence of various vasodilator mechanisms and intrinsic sympathomimetic activity. Shown are the major pharmacologic properties of several β-blockers. *Zero* indicates no activity; *plus signs* indicate activity; *direct* indicates a direct vasodilator action. In addition to these properties, carvedilol and its metabolite have been shown to exert antioxidant effects in vitro. Whether the non–β-blocking properties of these agents contribute to their clinical efficacy remains to be determined.

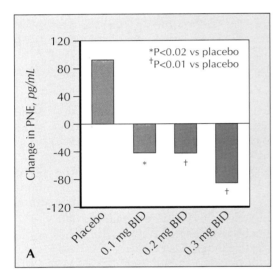

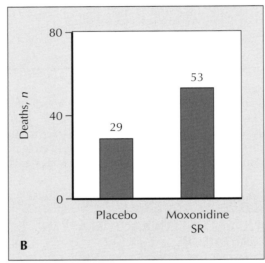

FIGURE 12-18. Central-acting sympathetic inhibitors as treatment for heart failure. Chronic overactivity of the sympathetic nervous system appears to contribute to the progression of myocardial failure (*see* Fig. 12-1). Agents acting via the central nervous system to inhibit sympathetic outflow might therefore provide another means of therapy in patients. In short-term studies, the central $α_2$-adrenergic agonist clonidine has been shown to reduce preload, heart rate, and mean arterial pressure in heart failure patients. However, chronic clonidine use may be limited by side effects (*eg*, dry mouth and fatigue). Moxonidine is a central sympatholytic agent whose actions are mediated primarily by brainstem imidazoline receptors. Moxonidine is currently approved in Europe for the treatment of hypertension, and preliminary data suggest that moxonidine causes dose-related reductions in plasma norepinephrine (PNE), blood pressure, and heart rate in patients with heart failure. **A,** Changes in PNE in patients with NYHA class II to III heart failure after 12 weeks of oral therapy with placebo or one of three doses of moxonidine.

B, The Moxonidine for Congestive Heart Failure (MOXCON) trial. This trial was designed to test the effect of sustained-release (SR) moxonidine on mortality in approximately 4500 patients with symptomatic left ventricular dysfunction. The study was stopped early by the Data and Safety Monitoring Board after a total of 1793 patients had been randomly assigned to moxonidine SR (0.25 to 1.5 mg bid) or placebo because early data suggested a higher mortality rate in the active treatment group. As shown, there were 53 deaths in the moxonidine group versus 29 deaths in the placebo group. Sudden death appeared to be the main cause of the moxonidine-related mortality. Moxonidine was also associated with a higher rate of heart failure hospital-izations and acute myocardial infarction. A potential explanation for these results is that moxonidine caused excessive blockade of the sympathetic nervous system. bid—twice a day. (*Panel A adapted from* Swedberg *et al.* [18]; *panel B adapted from* Jones and Cleland [19].)

REFERENCES

1. Cohn JN, Levine TB, Olivari MT, *et al.*: Plasma norepinephrine as a guide to prognosis in patients with chronic congestive heart failure. *N Engl J Med* 1984, 311:819–823.

2. Francis GS, Benedict C, Johnstone DE, *et al.*: Comparison of neuroendocrine activation in patients with left ventricular dysfunction with and without congestive heart failure: a substudy of the Studies of Left Ventricular Dysfunction (SOLVD). *Circulation* 1990, 82:1724–1729.

3. Swedberg K, Hjalmarson A, Waagstein F, Wallentin I: Prolongation of survival in congestive cardiomyopathy by beta-receptor blockade. *Lancet* 1979, 1(8131):1374–1376.

4. Hjalmarson A, Waagstein F: Use of beta-blockers in the treatment of dilated cardiomyopathy. In *Heart Failure: Basic Science and Clinical Aspects*. Edited by Gwathmey JK, Briggs GM, Allen PD. New York: Marcel Dekker; 1993:223–251.

5. Hall SA, Cigarroa CG, Marcoux L, *et al.*: Time course of improvement in left ventricular function, mass and geometry in patients with congestive heart failure treated with beta-adrenergic blockade. *J Am Coll Cardiol* 1995, 25:1154–1161.

6. Doughty RN, Whalley GA, Gamble G, *et al.*: Left ventricular remodeling with carvedilol in patients with congestive heart failure due to ischemic heart disease: Australia-New Zealand Heart Failure Research Collaborative Group. *J Am Coll Cardiol* 1997, 29:1060–1066.

7. Packer M, Bristow MR, Cohn JN, *et al.*: The effect of carvedilol on morbidity and mortality in patients with chronic heart failure: U.S. Carvedilol Heart Failure Study Group. *N Engl J Med* 1996, 334:1349–1355.

8. Heidenreich PA, Lee TT, Massie BM: Effect of beta-blockade on mortality in patients with heart failure: a meta-analysis of randomized clinical trials. *J Am Coll Cardiol* 1997, 30:27–34.

9. Bristow MR, Gilbert EM, Abraham WT, *et al.*: Carvedilol produces dose-related improvements in left ventricular function and survival in subjects with chronic heart failure. *Circulation* 1996, 94:2807–2816.

10. Colucci WS, Packer M, Bristow MR, *et al.*: Carvedilol inhibits clinical progression in patients with mild symptoms of heart failure: US Carvedilol Heart Failure Study Group. *Circulation* 1996, 94:2800–2806.

11. CIBIS II Investigators and Committees: The Cardiac Insufficiency Bisoprolol Study II (CIBIS-II): a randomised trial. *Lancet* 1999, 353:9–13.

12. MERIT-HF Study Group: Effect of metoprolol CR/XL in chronic heart failure: Metoprolol CR/XL Randomised Intervention Trial in Congestive Heart Failure (MERIT-HF). *Lancet* 1999, 353:2001–2007.

13. Packer M, Coats AJ, Fowler MB, *et al.*: Effect of carvedilol on survival in severe chronic heart failure. *N Engl J Med* 2001, 344:1651–1658.

14. The CAPRICORN Investigators: Effect of carvedilol on outcome after myocardial infarction in patients with left-ventricular dysfunction: the CAPRICORN randomised trial. *Lancet* 2001, 357:1385–1390.

15. The Beta-Blocker Evaluation of Survival Trial Investigators: A trial of the beta-blocker bucindolol in patients with advanced chronic heart failure. *N Engl J Med* 2001, 344:1659–1667.

16. Yancy CW, Fowler MB, Colucci WS, *et al.*: Race and the response to adrenergic blockade with carvedilol in patients with chronic heart failure. *N Engl J Med* 2001, 344:1358–1365.

17. Shakar SF, Abraham WT, Gilbert EM, *et al.*: Combined oral positive inotropic and beta-blocker therapy for treatment of refractory class IV heart failure. *J Am Coll Cardiol* 1998, 31:1336–1340.

18. Swedberg K, Bergh CH, Dickstein K, *et al.*: The effects of moxonidine, a novel imidazoline, on plasma norepinephrine in patients with congestive heart failure: Moxonidine Investigators. *J Am Coll Cardiol* 2000, 35:398–404.

19. Jones LG, Cleland JG: Meeting report: the LIDO, HOPE, MOXCON, and WASH studies. *Eur J Heart Fail* 1999, 1: 425–431.

New Approaches to the Treatment of Heart Failure

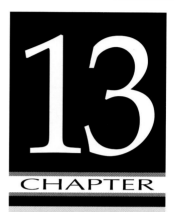

13

CHAPTER

Michael M. Givertz and Wilson S. Colucci

The major goals in the therapy of chronic heart failure include the amelioration of symptoms and the reduction of morbidity and mortality. There is overwhelming evidence that angiotensin-converting enzyme (ACE) inhibitors and β-blockers achieve both of these goals and therefore are first-line therapy. For patients who remain symptomatic, the clinical utility of digitalis and spironolactone has also been established. Despite the appropriate use of standard therapy, many patients will experience progressive symptoms and reduced survival. Fortunately, an unprecedented number of promising new therapeutic approaches to heart failure have been developed over the past few years.

The demonstration that β-blockers can slow disease progression has highlighted the importance of this goal of therapy. As discussed in Chapter 5, the progressive nature of myocardial dysfunction is due primarily to the process of ventricular remodeling. Remodeling is the result of a composite of molecular and cellular events, including myocyte hypertrophy and apoptosis, alteration in calcium handling proteins, and changes in the extracellular matrix, which taken together adversely affect cardiac structure and function. It is increasingly apparent that agents that alleviate myocardial wall stress or block the actions of angiotensin or norepinephrine (*eg*, ACE inhibitors and β-blockers) can slow the progression of myocardial dysfunction. It now appears likely that other neuro-hormones and biological mediators contribute to myocardial remodeling, including endothelin, arginine vasopressin, inflammatory cytokines, and reactive oxygen species. This appreciation has led to the development of novel agents and strategies that are now being subjected to clinical testing. Other biological therapies for myocardial rescue that are undergoing preclinical investigation include matrix metalloproteinase inhibition, gene therapy, and transplantation of myoblasts or stem cells. Finally, biventricular pacing and new pharmacologic approaches to inotropic support show promise in patients with advanced heart failure.

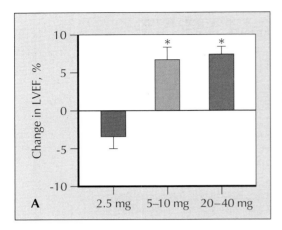

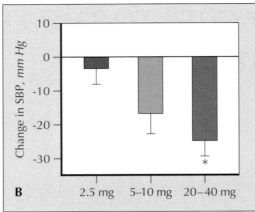

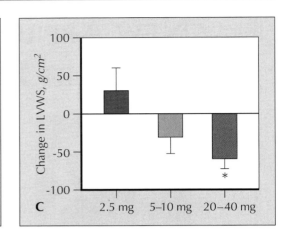

FIGURE 13-1. Vasopeptidase inhibition in heart failure. Vasopeptidase inhibitors are a novel class of neurohormonal antagonists that simultaneously inhibit neutral endopeptidase (NEP) and angiotensin-converting enzyme. The inhibition of NEP, an enzyme involved in the degradation of natriuretic peptides, results in increased circulating levels of atrial and brain (or B-type) natriuretic peptide. As discussed in Chapter 9, these neuro-hormones, which cause vasodilation, natriuresis, diuresis, and aldosterone antagonism, play a counterregulatory role in heart failure. In a dose-ranging pilot study of the vasopeptidase inhibitor omapatrilat, 48 patients with symptomatic left ventricular (LV) dysfunction were randomized to receive low dose (2.5 mg), moderate dose (5 to 10 mg), or high dose (20 to 40 mg) omapatrilat for 12 weeks. Omapatrilat improved the patients' score for functional status and resulted in a dose-dependent increase in left ventricular ejection fraction (LVEF) (**A**) and decreases in systolic blood pressure (SBP) (**B**) and LV end-systolic wall stress (LVWS) (**C**). (*Asterisk* indicates $P<0.05$ mg vs. 2.5 mg). Omapatrilat also increased ANP levels and induced natriuresis at high doses. (*Adapted from* McClean *et al* [1].)

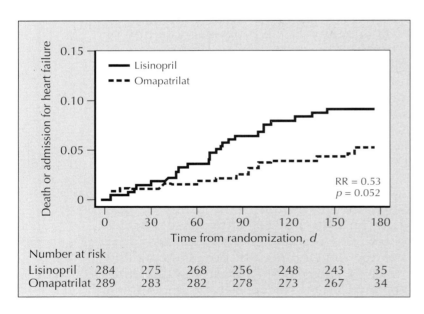

FIGURE 13-2. The effect of vasopeptidase inhibition on clinical outcomes in heart failure. The IMPRESS trial was designed to compare the effects of combined neutral endopeptidase (NEP) and angiotensin-converting enzyme (ACE) inhibition versus ACE inhibition alone on functional capacity and clinical outcomes in heart failure. IMPRESS randomized 573 patients with New York Heart Association (NYHA) functional class II–IV heart failure and an ejection fraction of 40% or less to receive omapatrilat (target dose 40 mg daily) or lisinopril (target dose 20 mg daily) for 24 weeks. At week 12, there were similar small increases in exercise duration in the omapatrilat and lisinopril groups (24 vs 31 seconds, $P=0.45$). Both treatments were fairly well tolerated, although there were more cardiovascular adverse events with lisinopril and more dizziness with omapatrilat. As shown in this Kaplan-Meier analysis, omapatrilat tended to reduce the risk of death or admission for worsening heart failure when compared to lisinopril (hazard ratio, 0.53; 95% CI, 0.27–1.02; $P=0.052$). In patients with NYHA functional class III–IV heart failure, omapatrilat improved NYHA class more than lisinopril. The OVERTURE study is currently testing the effect of omapatrilat on survival in patients with chronic heart failure. (*Adapted from* Rouleau *et al*. [2].)

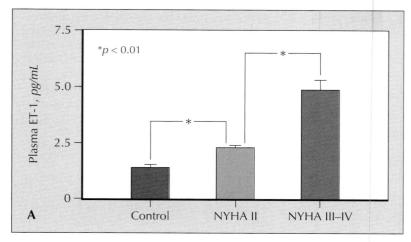

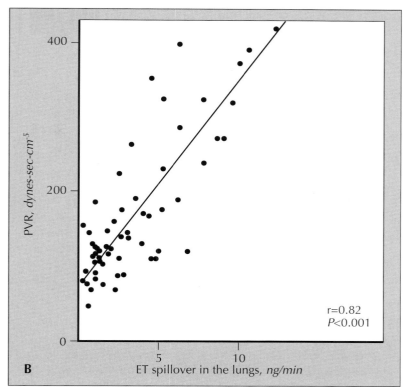

FIGURE 13-3. The relationship between plasma endothelin (ET) levels and the severity of heart failure. Endothelin is a potent vasoconstrictor peptide which can exert long-term effects on myocardial growth and phenotype. Plasma ET levels are elevated in patients with chronic heart failure and correlate with symptoms and hemodynamic compromise. **A,** Plasma ET-1 levels and severity of disease. Control subjects consisted of 20 age-matched normal subjects. Plasma ET-1 levels were elevated in patients with New York Heart Association (NYHA) functional class II ($n = 33$) and NYHA functional class III or IV ($n = 29$) heart failure and increased in relation to disease severity (*Asterisk* indicates $P<0.01$ by ANOVA). **B,** The correlation between resting pulmonary vascular resistance (PVR) and ET spillover in the lungs in the 62 patients in A. ET-1

spillover correlated strongly with PVR, suggesting that the pulmonary vascular bed is an important source of ET-1, which appears to be a key mediator of secondary pulmonary hypertension. (*Adapted from* Tsutamoto *et al.* [3].)

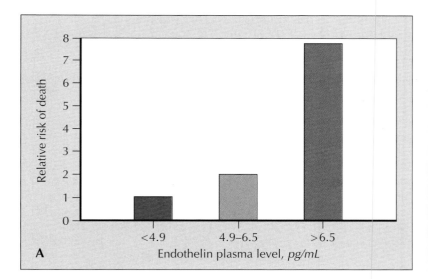

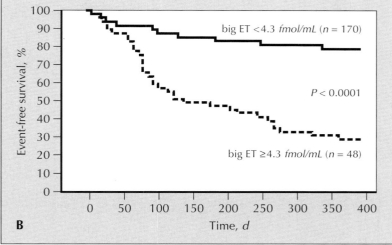

FIGURE 13-4. Endothelin (ET) and prognosis in heart failure. Since plasma ET levels correlate with disease severity, the degree of activation of the endothelin system may provide independent prognostic information. **A,** The relative risk of one-year mortality after acute myocardial infarction (MI) in 142 patients was related to plasma ET levels measured on day 3 post-MI, with the highest risk occurring in patients with plasma ET levels greater than 6.5 ($P=0.0116$). **B,** A Kaplan-Meier

analysis showed that the event-free survival, defined as freedom from death or need for urgent heart transplant, in 226 heart failure patients was significantly lower in patients with big ET-1 (Big ET) levels greater than or equal to 4.3 fmol/mL. By multivariate analysis, plasma big ET levels, New York Heart Association functional class, and exercise capacity provided independent prognostic information. (Part A *adapted from* Spieker *et al.* [4]; part B *adapted from* Hulsmann *et al.* [5].)

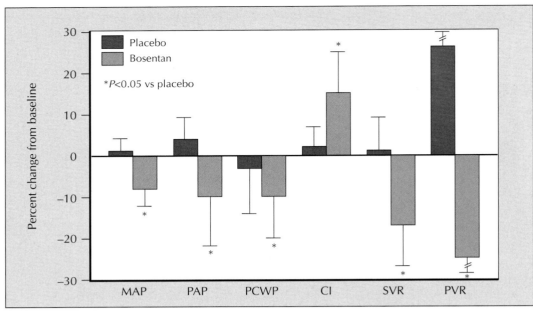

FIGURE 13-5. Acute hemodynamic effects of nonselective endothelin (ET) blockade. Understanding the actions of ET has been aided greatly by the development of several nonpeptide molecules that block ET receptors [6]. Whereas some of these antagonists are subtype selective (*eg*, BQ-123, ET_A selective), others are relatively nonselective (*eg*, bosentan, tezosentan). Encouraged by results in animal models of heart failure showing

beneficial effects of endothelin receptor antagonists on left ventricular remodeling and survival (see Fig. 13-7), clinical investigators have addressed the role of these agents in patients with heart failure. Kiowski *et al.* [7] randomly assigned 24 patients with New York Heart Association (NYHA) functional class III heart failure to intravenous bosentan or placebo. Shown here is the change in hemodynamics 60 minutes after drug administration, expressed as the percent change from baseline. Bosentan-decreased mean arterial pressure (MAP), mean pulmonary artery pressure (PAP), and mean pulmonary capillary wedge pressure (PCWP) and increased cardiac index (CI). Consistent with the strong relationship between plasma ET-1 and pulmonary hypertension, bosentan caused a greater decrease in pulmonary vascular resistance (PVR) than systemic vascular resistance (SVR). Additional decreases in PVR and SVR have been demonstrated after 2 weeks of oral bosentan therapy [8]. (*Adapted from* Kiowski *et al.* [7])

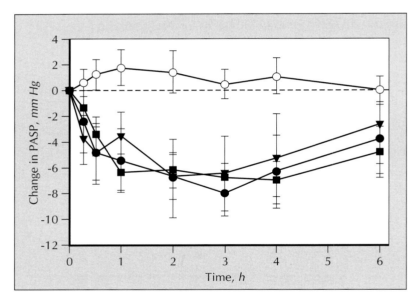

FIGURE 13-6. Acute hemodynamic effects of selective ET_A receptor blockade. This multicenter, double-blind study enrolled 48 patients with New York Heart Association functional class III or IV heart failure treated with angiotensin-converting enzyme (ACE) inhibitors and diuretics who had a pulmonary capillary wedge pressure (PCWP) ≥15 mm Hg and cardiac index (CI) ≤ 2.5 L/min/m². Patients were randomly assigned to receive the ET_A-selective receptor antagonist sitaxsentan in one of three doses (1.5 [*closed circles*], 3.0 [*closed squares*], 6.0 mg/kg [*closed triangles*], or placebo [*open circles*] over 15 minutes, and hemodynamics were measured for 6 hours. Compared to placebo, sitaxsentan decreased pulmonary artery systolic pressure (PASP) (*P*=0.001), pulmonary vascular resistance, and right atrial pressure, but had no effect on heart rate, mean arterial pressure, PCWP, CI, or systemic vascular resistance. These data suggest that in patients with moderate to severe heart failure, acute ET_A receptor blockade causes relatively selective pulmonary vasodilation and may be useful in the treatment of patients with heart failure who also have secondary pulmonary hypertension. (*Adapted from* Givertz *et al.* [9].)

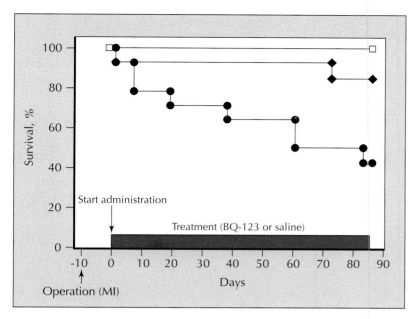

FIGURE 13-7. The pathophysiologic role of endothelin (ET) in the progression of heart failure. The observation that ET levels are elevated in patients with heart failure, taken together with the known actions of ET on cardiovascular tissues, has raised the possibility that ET plays a pathophysiologic role in the progression of myocardial failure. Support for this thesis comes from studies in animal models of heart failure in which beneficial long-term effects of ET receptor blockade have been demonstrated. Sakai *et al.* [10] studied the effects of the ET_A receptor antagonist BQ-123 on survival in rats after experimental myocardial infarction. Addition of BQ-123 to the drinking water beginning 10 days after coronary artery ligation (*closed diamonds*) resulted in a significant improvement in survival over animals treated with saline (*closed circles*). The *open squares* represent sham-operated animals treated with saline. The effects of chronic ET receptor blockade with bosentan on disease progression and survival in humans with heart failure is currently being tested in the Endothelin Antagonist Bosentan for Lowering Cardiac Events (ENABLE) trial. (*Adapted from* Sakai *et al.* [10].)

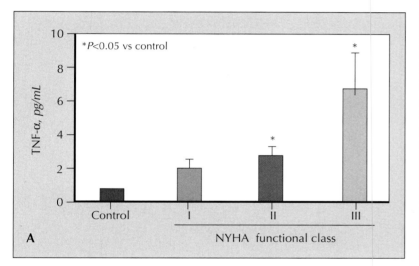

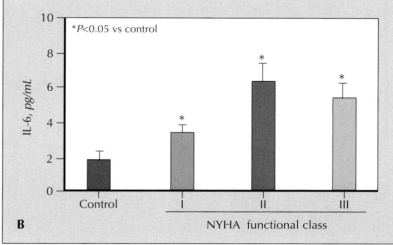

FIGURE 13-8. The role of proinflammatory cytokines in myocardial failure. Proinflammatory cytokines such as tumor necrosis factor-α (TNF-α), interleukin-1β (IL-1β), and interleukin-6 (IL-6) may play an important pathophysiologic role in the progression of myocardial failure. The circulating levels of TNF-α and IL-6 were analyzed in randomly selected plasma samples from 63 patients in New York Heart Association (NYHA) functional classes I to III enrolled in the neurohormonal substudies of the Studies of Left Ventricular Dysfunction (SOLVD) trial. Compared with age-matched controls, patients with left ventricular dysfunction had TNF-α levels (**A**) that were elevated in direct proportion to functional class. IL-6 levels (**B**) were also elevated in patients, although the levels did not appear to correlate with functional class. (*Adapted from* Torre-Amione *et al.* [11].)

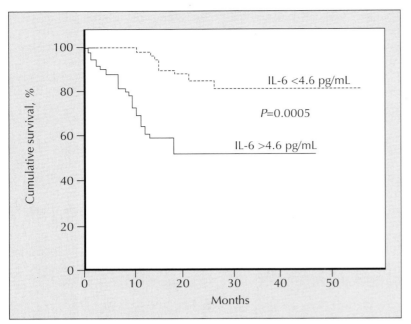

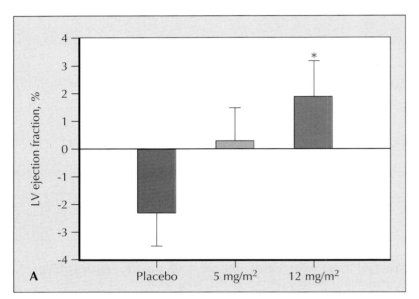

A

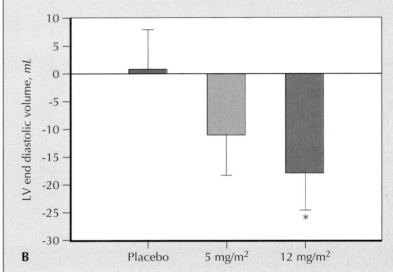

B

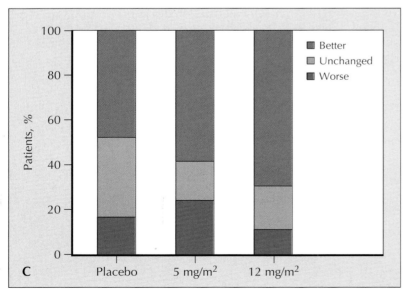

C

FIGURE 13-9. The effect of cytokines on mortality. To examine the prognostic role of circulating cytokines in patients, plasma interleukin-6 (IL-6) levels were measured in 100 patients with chronic heart failure who were followed for a mean of 28 months (range, 3 to 54). During the follow-up period, 31 patients had a cardiovascular death. When patients were stratified based on median plasma concentration (4.6 pg/mL) of IL-6, Kaplan-Meier analysis demonstrated reduced survival in patients with higher IL-6 levels (*solid line*). In a multivariate analysis, plasma levels of IL-6 ($P<0.0001$) and norepinephrine ($P=0.0004$) and left ventricular ejection fraction ($P=0.015$) were independent predictors of mortality. Although norepinephrine has been directly associated with the pathophysiology of myocardial failure, it is not yet clear whether IL-6 plays a role in the pathophysiology of heart failure, and if so, whether it is detrimental or beneficial. (*Adapted from* Tsutamoto *et al.* [12].)

disease progression in heart failure and other inflammatory disease states has led to the development of anti–TNF-α therapies. Etanercept is a recombinant fusion protein consisting of a soluble TNF receptor linked to the Fc portion of human immunoglobulin 1. Soluble TNF-α receptors bind to and inactivate TNF-α and have been shown to reduce disease activity in patients with rheumatoid arthritis. A phase I pilot study in patients with New York Heart Association functional class III heart failure demonstrated that etanercept was well tolerated, and that it reduced circulating levels of biologically active TNF-α [13]. Bozkurt *et al.* [14] randomly assigned 47 patients with moderate to severe heart failure to biweekly subcutaneous injections of etanercept (5mg/m^2 or 12 mg/m^2) or placebo for 3 months. Etanercept caused a dose-dependent improvement in left ventricular (LV) ejection fraction (**A**) and a reduction in LV end-diastolic volume (**B**).(*Asterisk* indicates $P<0.05$ vs control), which was associated with a trend toward improvement in functional status ($P=0.20$) (**C**). A clinical composite score was used to determine whether a patient was improved, unchanged, or worse at the end of the study. Despite these early positive results, two large phase III studies of etanercept in chronic heart failure (RENAISSANCE and RECOVER) were recently stopped due to lack of efficacy. (*Adapted from* Bozkurt *et al.* [14].)

FIGURE 13-10. Anticytokine therapy in chronic heart failure. The recognition that tumor necrosis factor-α (TNF-α) may contribute to

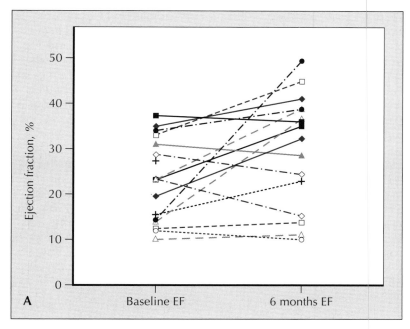

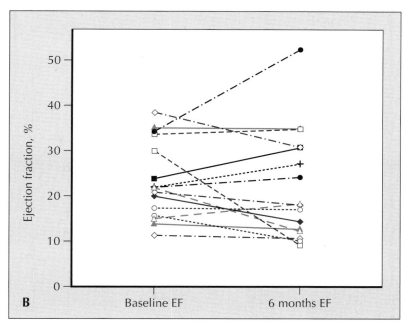

FIGURE 13-11. The effect of pentoxifylline on ejection fraction. Pentoxifylline, a xanthine derivative used for the treatment of claudication, suppresses tumor necrosis factor-α (TNF-α) production *in vitro* and *in vivo*. Improved outcomes have been reported in patients with rheumatoid arthritis and graft-versus-host disease. This single-center, controlled study tested the hypothesis that pentoxifylline would improve left ventricular function in patients with idiopathic dilated cardiomyopathy treated with angiotensin-converting enzyme (ACE) inhibitors and carvedilol. Thirty-nine patients with New York Heart Association functional class II or III heart failure with an ejection fraction (EF) less than 40% were randomized to receive pentoxifylline (400 mg three times daily) or placebo for 6 months. Pentoxifylline improved functional class and increased EF from 24% to 31% (vs 24% to 25% with placebo; *P*=0.03), but had no effect on TNF-α levels. Individual changes in EF are shown in the pentoxifylline (**A**) and placebo (**B**) groups. (*Adapted from* Skudicky *et al.* [15].)

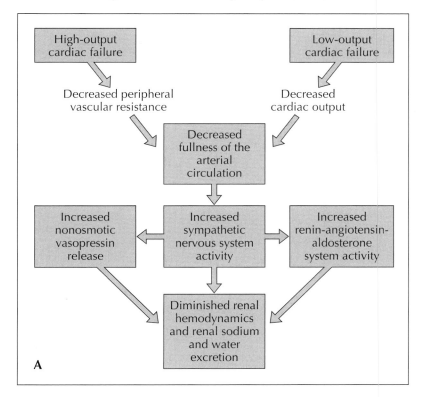

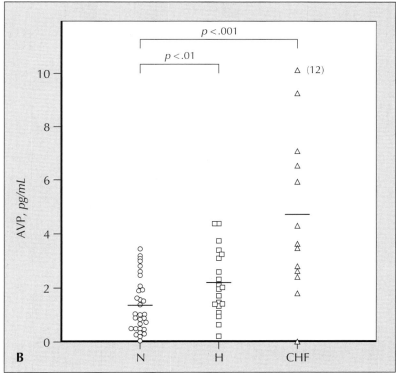

FIGURE 13-12. Arginine vasopressin (AVP) and heart failure. In patients with chronic heart failure, a decrease in effective circulating volume causes the nonosmotic release of AVP by the posterior pituitary gland. Other mediators of AVP secretion in heart failure include angiotensin II, adrenergic stimulation, and thirst. AVP may contribute to disease progression in heart failure by binding to both vascular (V_1) and renal (V_2) receptors that mediate vasoconstriction and free water retention, respectively. **A**, Proposed mechanisms by which high-output or low-output heart failure leads to neurohormonal activation and renal sodium and water retention. **B**, Plasma AVP levels in normal subjects (*N*), patients with hypertension (*H*) and patients with heart failure (*CHF*). Patients with hypertension demonstrate a small increase in the range and mean AVP levels compared with normal subjects. Patients with heart failure demonstrate a striking range of AVP levels, from very high to barely detectable. (Part A *adapted from* Shrier and Abraham [16]; part B *adapted from* Preibisz *et al.* [17].)

N EW APPROACHES TO THE TREATMENT OF HEART FAILURE

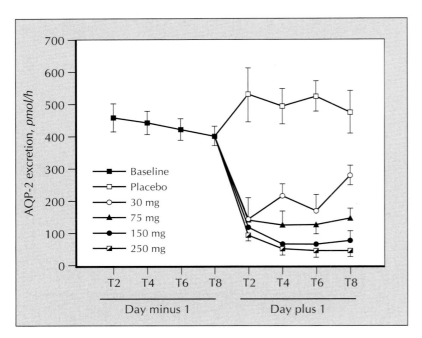

FIGURE 13-13. Selective V_2 receptor antagonism in heart failure. Vasopressin antagonists are a novel class of cardiovascular agents that are being developed to attenuate disease progression and improve survival in heart failure. Selective V_2 receptor antagonists cause free water diuresis (also termed *aquaresis*) and may reduce LV wall stress, prevent myocardial fibrosis, and improve ventricular compliance. In this preliminary dose-escalating study, heart failure patients received either placebo or one of four doses of an oral nonpeptide V_2 receptor antagonist (VPA-985) and urine was collected every 2 hours. The excretion of aquaporin-2 (AQP-2), a water channel located on the apical membrane of collecting duct cells that mediates water reabsorption under the influence of arginine vasopressin, was assessed by Western blot analysis. As shown, VPA-985 caused dose-dependent decreases in AQP-2 excretion over 8 hours (T2–T8), and this was associated with increases in free water clearance and urine output. These data suggest that selective V_2 receptor antagonists may prevent fluid retention and correct hyponatremia in patients with chronic heart failure. (*Adapted from* Martin *et al* [18].)

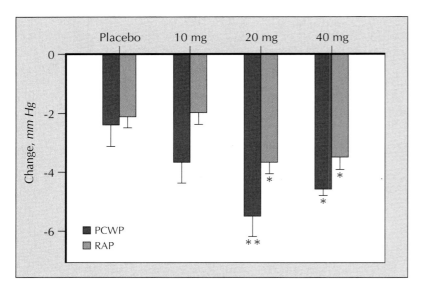

FIGURE 13-14. Combined V_{1a}/ V_2 receptor antagonism in heart failure. The safety and acute hemodynamic effects of conivaptan, a combined V_{1a}/ V_2 receptor antagonist, were studied in 142 patients with New York Heart Association functional class III or IV heart failure who had a pulmonary capillary wedge pressure (PCWP) ≥16 mm Hg and cardiac index (CI) ≤ 2.8 L/min/m². Patients were randomized in a double-blind fashion to receive one of three doses of conivaptan (10 mg, 20 mg, or 40 mg) or placebo given as an intravenous bolus, and central hemodynamics were measured for 12 hours. Mean baseline PCWP and CI were 24 mm Hg and 2.1 L/min/m², respectively. Between 3 to 6 hours postinfusion, conivaptan reduced PCWP and right atrial pressure (RAP) (*asterisk* indicates $P<0.05$ vs placebo; *double asterisk* indicates $P<0.005$ vs placebo) without a change in systolic blood pressure or heart rate, and was well tolerated. Compared to placebo, conivaptan caused a dose-dependent increase in urine output. (*Adapted from* Udelson *et al.* [19].)

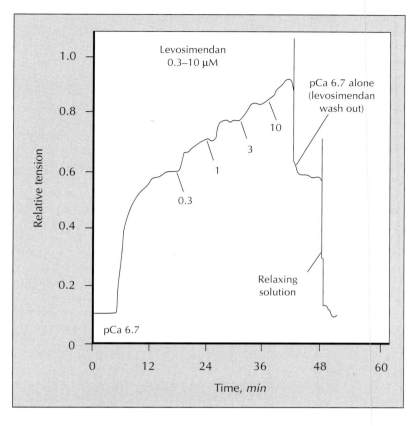

FIGURE 13-15. Calcium-sensitizing agents. A limitation of most positive inotropic agents (*eg*, β-adrenergic agonists, phosphodi-esterase [PDE] inhibitors) is that they act by increasing intra-cellular calcium in the myocyte and may thus increase heart rate and arrhythmias. Calcium-sensitizing agents act by directly increasing the sensitivity of the myofilament to calcium so that greater contractile force develops without an increase in calcium level. Levosimendan is a pyridazinone-dinitrile derivative that enhances calcium sensitivity of myofilaments via calcium-dependent binding to troponin C. Other pharmacologic actions observed include mild PDE III inhibition and activation of adenosine triphosphate–dependent potassium channels. Shown is the effect of several concentrations of levosimendan (0.3 to 10 μM) when applied to skinned fibers from guinea pig papillary muscle. Under these conditions, the calcium available to the myofilaments is fixed by the concentration in the bath, and the increase in contractile force therefore must reflect an increase in myofilament sensitivity to calcium. (*Adapted from* Haikala *et al.* [20].)

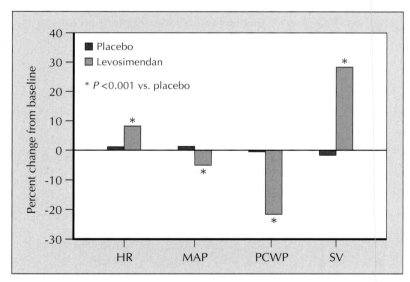

FIGURE 13-16. Levosimendan and the short-term treatment of patients with decompensated heart failure. The acute hemodynamic effects of intravenous levosimendan were studied in 146 patients with New York Heart Association functional class III or IV heart failure in a multicenter, double-blind, placebo-controlled trial. At baseline, the mean left ventricular ejection fraction was 21%, the cardiac index was 1.9 L/min/m^2, and the mean pulmonary capillary wedge pressure (PCWP) was 27 mm Hg. Shown is the percent change from baseline at 6 hours for heart rate (HR), mean arterial pressure (MAP), mean PCWP, and stroke volume (SV) for placebo and levosimendan. The increase in stroke volume resulted in a 39% increase in cardiac index (data not shown). Levosimendan also reduced systemic and pulmonary vascular resistance. Hemodynamic effects were maintained for a total of 24 hours and were associated with improved dyspnea and fatigue. This salutary hemodynamic profile suggests that levosimendan may be of value in the short-term treatment of patients with decompensated heart failure. A phase III study (REVIVE) will test the effect of a short-term infusion of levosimendan on clinical outcomes in patients with decom-pensated heart failure. (*Adapted from* Slawsky *et al.* [21].)

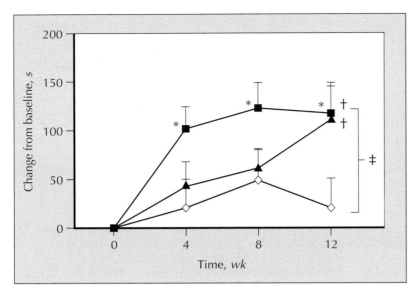

FIGURE 13-17. Low-dose phosphodiesterase inhibition in chronic heart failure. Enoximone is an oral positive inotropic agent intended for the treatment of patients with advanced chronic heart failure. Enoximone, which inhibits a high-affinity cyclic adenosine-monophosphate phosphodiesterase (PDE III), exerts both positive inotropic and vasodilator effects in patients with heart failure. As has been demonstrated with other oral positive inotropic agents (*eg*, milrinone, vesnarinone), enoximone when administered at higher doses (≥100 mg three times daily) to patients with stable chronic heart failure is associated with proarrhythmia and excess mortality [22]. However, low-dose enoximone (25 to 50 mg three times daily) given to patients with advanced heart failure appears to be well tolerated, allows weaning from intravenous inotropic agents, and may be used to bridge patients to cardiac transplantation or through the initiation of β-blocker therapy (*see* Fig. 12-16). To determine the effects of low-dose enoximone on exercise capacity and adverse events, 105 patients with New York Heart Association functional class II or III heart failure were randomized to placebo (*open diamonds*) or enoximone at 25 mg (*closed triangles*) or 50 mg (*closed squares*) three times daily for 12 weeks. Shown are the changes from baseline in exercise duration in the three treatment groups (*asterisk* indicates *P*<0.05 vs placebo; *dagger* indicates *P*<0.05 time-response vs placebo; *double dagger* indicates *P*=0.019 dose-time-response). Enoximone improved exercise capacity and was not associated with an increase in ventricular arrhythmias or death. A phase III study (ESSENTIAL) is planned that will test the safety and efficacy of low-dose enoximone in approximately 700 patients with advanced chronic heart failure. (*Adapted from* Lowes *et al*. [23].)

RESYNCHRONIZATION THERAPY

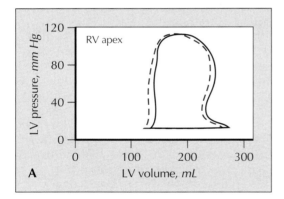

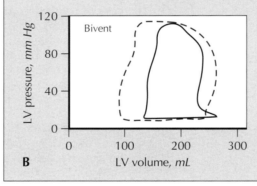

FIGURE 13-18. Acute biventricular pacing in patients with dilated cardiomyopathy and ventricular conduction delay. Interventricular conduction delay (IVCD) is common in patients with chronic heart failure, with a prevalence of 30% to 50%. The resulting impairment in the coordination of ventricular contraction and relaxation contributes to hemodynamic compromise and is associated with increased mortality. Simultaneous pacing from the right ventricular apex and left ventricular (LV) free wall (accessed via the coronary sinus) has been proposed as a novel means to "resynchronize" ventricular contraction. Acute biventricular pacing studies in patients with chronic heart failure and IVCD have demonstrated improved contractile function without an increase in myocardial oxygen consumption. In this study, patients with dilated cardiomyopathy (mean LV ejection fraction, 19%) and IVCD (mean QRS, 157 msec) underwent acute pacing from the right ventricular (RV) apex or combined RV apex and LV free wall. This figure displays pressure-volume loops from a patient with left bundle branch block during normal sinus rhythm (*solid lines*) and VDD pacing (*dashed lines*). **A**, RV apical pacing had a negligible effect on cardiac performance. **B**, Biventricular pacing (Bivent) produced loops with greater area (stroke work) and width (stroke volume) and increased LV dP/dt$_{max}$ by 13%. (*Adapted from* Kass *et al*. [24].)

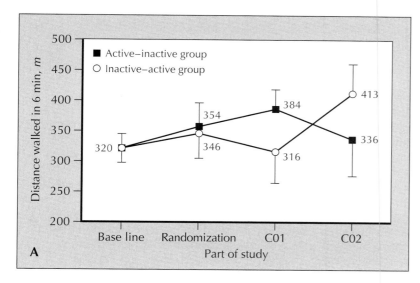

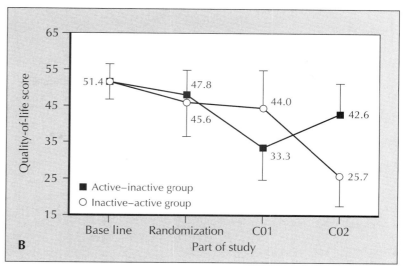

FIGURE 13-19. Chronic biventricular pacing in heart failure. The Multisite Stimulation in Cardiomyopathies (MUSTIC) Study enrolled 67 patients with New York Heart Association functional class III heart failure, an ejection fraction less than 35%, and a QRS duration of greater than 150 ms into a single-blind, randomized crossover study of biventricular pacing. Exercise capacity was measured by the distance walked in 6 minutes and the quality of life was assessed by a questionnaire during two periods—a 3-month period of inactive pacing (ventricular inhibited pacing at a back-up rate of 40 bpm) and a 3-month period of active (atriobiventricular) pacing. Implantation of a left ventricular lead was successful in 92% of patients, and 48 of 67 patients completed both phases of the study. During active pacing, the mean distance walked in 6 minutes (**A**) was 23% longer (*P*<0.001) and the quality-of-life score (**B**) decreased by a mean of 32% (*P*<0.001). The figures show the mean (±SD) values for each phase of the study in patients randomized to active-inactive and inactive-active groups. CO1—end of crossover period 1; CO2—end of crossover period 2. (*Adapted from* Cazeau *et al.* [25].)

OUTCOMES OF THE MULTICENTER INSYNC RANDOMIZED CLINICAL EVALUATION (MIRACLE) TRIAL

OUTCOME	CRT, *N* = 119	NO CRT, *N* = 125
Improvement in NYHA status by ≥ 1 class	69%	34%
Increase in 6-min walk by ≥ 50 m	50%	30%
LVEF	Increased 6%	No change
LVEDD	Decreased 5 mm	No change
HF hospitalization, *d*	56	296

FIGURE 13-20. Cardiac resynchronization therapy (CRT) in patients with advanced heart failure. The Multicenter InSync Randomized Clinical Evaluation (MIRACLE) trial [26] randomly assigned 244 patients with predominantly New York Heart Association (NYHA) class III heart failure (HF) and interventricular conduction delay to CRT or no CRT for 6 months. At baseline the mean left ventricular ejection fraction (LVEF) was 22% ± 6 %, the mean left ventricular end-diastolic diameter (LVEDD) was 70 mm ± 9 mm, and the mean QRS duration was 165 ms ± 19 ms. Biventricular pacing improved functional status and exercise capacity and had favorable effects on cardiac structure and function by promoting reverse remodeling of the failing left ventricle. Preliminary results also suggest that CRT reduced healthcare utilization. These data were instrumental in the decision by the US Food and Drug Administration's Circulatory Systems Device Panel to recommend approval of biventricular pacing as adjunctive therapy for patients with symptomatic heart failure.

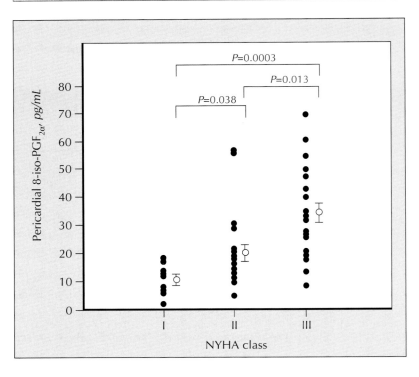

FIGURE 13-21. Oxidant stress and progression to heart failure. Reduced myocardial antioxidant activity and increased oxidant damage have been demonstrated in animal models of heart failure, and markers of oxidative stress are increased in patients with chronic heart failure, leading to the thesis that reactive oxygen species may contribute to the progression of myocardial dysfunction in patients. A specific technique for assessing oxidant stress *in vivo* involves measuring stable endproducts of lipid peroxidation, called F_2-*isoprostanes* [27]. 8-iso-prostaglandin $F_{2\alpha}$ (8-iso-PGF$_{2\alpha}$) levels were measured in the pericardial fluid of 51 consecutive patients with ischemic or valvular heart disease referred for cardiac surgery. Pericardial levels of 8-iso-PGF$_{2\alpha}$ increased with the severity of heart failure. In a subgroup of patients who underwent preoperative echocardiography, pericardial fluid levels of 8-iso-PGF$_{2\alpha}$ correlated with left ventricular end-diastolic dimension. (*Adapted from* Mallat *et al.* [28].)

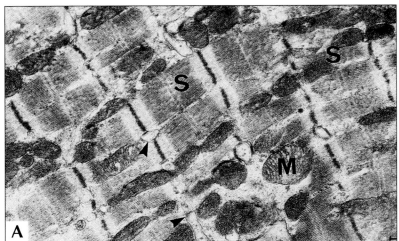

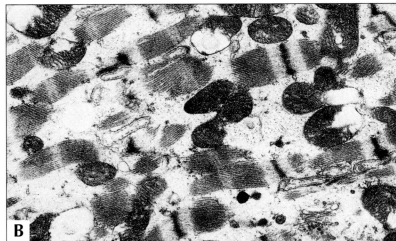

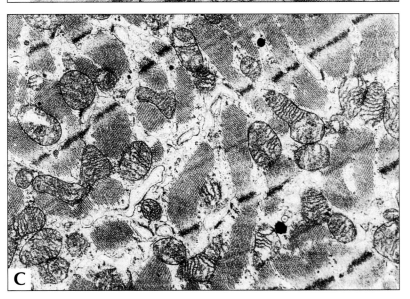

FIGURE 13-22. Role of antioxidants in heart failure. In animal models of ischemia-reperfusion, antioxidants have been shown to reduce free radical generation, prevent myocyte damage, and improve ventricular function. In this study, Dhalla *et al.* [29] examined the effects of vitamin E therapy in aortic-banded guinea pigs, a model of pressure overload–induced failure. **A,** An electron micrograph of a sham-operated guinea pig heart demonstrating normal ultrastructure, including myofibrils, sarcomeres (S), mitochondria (M), and T tubules (*arrowheads*). **B,** A micrograph from a guinea pig that was banded for 20 weeks and did not receive subcutaneous vitamin E implants. There is ultrastructural damage characterized by increased vacuolization, loss of contractile elements, and mitochondrial injury with dropout of christae membranes. **C,** A micrograph from a guinea pig with banding for 20 weeks and chronic treatment with vitamin E. There is less vacuolization, mitochondrial injury, and interstitial edema. This improvement in structure was associated with improved hemo-dynamics, decreased signs of heart failure, and reduced mortality. Despite these experimental findings, the role of antioxidant therapy in patients with chronic heart failure remains unproven. (*From* Dhalla *et al* [29]; with permission.)

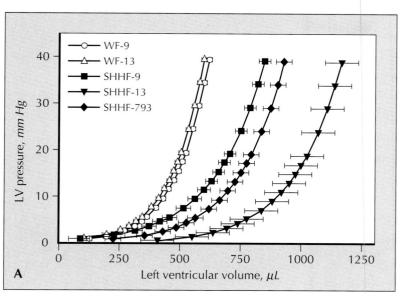

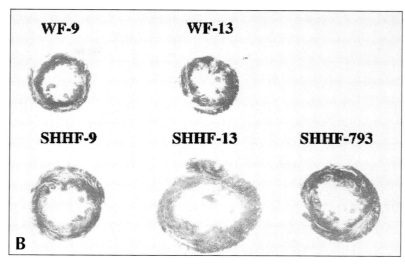

FIGURE 13-23. Role of matrix metalloproteinases in heart failure. The matrix metalloproteinases (MMPs) are a family of zinc-dependent enzymes that contribute to ventricular remodeling in heart failure by promoting collagen synthesis and degradation [30]. The activity of MMPs may be increased in failing human myocardium by the local action of neurohormones and proin-flammatory cytokines, or by the downregulation of tissue inhibitors of metalloproteinases (TIMPs). Upregulation of MMPs and downregulation of TIMPs have been demonstrated in venticular myocardium from patients with severe dilated cardiomyopathy of ischemic or idiopathic etiology [31]. Peterson *et al.* [32] tested the hypothesis that MMP inhibition would influence left ventricular (LV) remodeling during the development of heart failure in the spontaneously hypertensive heart failure (SHHF) rat. **A,** Shown are *ex vivo* LV pressure volume curves generated in 5 groups of rats: SHHF rats at 9

months (SHHF-9), SHHF rats at 13 months (SHHF-13), SHHF rats treated with an MMP inhibitor (PD166793) during months 9 to 13 (SHHF-793), and normotensive Wistar-Furth (WF) rats at 9 months (WF-9) and 13 months (WF-13). LV chamber size remained constant in both groups of normotensive WF rats. Significant chamber dilation was present in SHHF-9 rats compared with normotensive controls. Treatment with PD166793 reduced progressive chamber dilation at 13 months. **B,** Representative LV cross sections taken at the level of the papillary muscles and prepared with a Masson's trichrome stain. LV circumference is increased in the SHHF-9 rat and increased further in the SHHF-13 rat compared with the WF-9 and WF-13 normotensive controls. Treatment with PD166793 reduced LV chamber dilation at 13 months. These data suggest that MMP inhibition can attenuate disease progression in heart failure. (*Adapted from* Peterson *et al.* [32].)

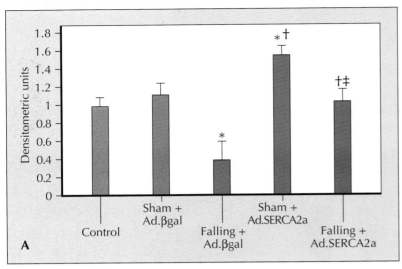

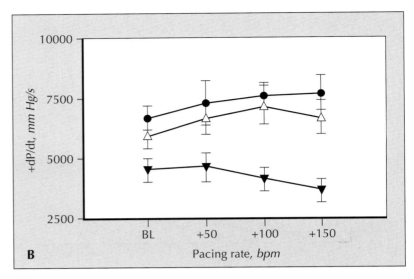

FIGURE 13-24. Gene therapy for heart failure. With increased understanding of the molecular pathogenesis of heart failure and improved techniques for cardiac gene delivery, investigators have begun to explore the potential of gene therapy to rescue failing myocardium [33]. Abnormal calcium handling in failing hearts, which results in impaired contraction and relaxation, is due in part due to decreased activity of sarcoplasmic reticulum Ca^{2+} ATPase (SERCA2a). To test whether increasing SERCA2a expression would improve ventricular function during the transition to heart failure, Miyamoto *et al.* [34] overexpressed cardiac SERCA2a in aortic-banded rats by using a catheter-based, adenoviral gene transfer technique. After 4 months of banding, rats were randomized to receive an adenovirus carrying the SERCA2a gene (Ad.SERCA2a) or β-galatosidase (Ad.βgal) as a control, and were compared with sham-operated controls. **A,** Bar graph shows the protein levels of SERCA2a from sham rats infected with Ad.βgal (*n*=7) or Ad.SERCA2a (*n*=8), and from rats with heart failure infected with Ad.βgal (*n*= 8) or

Ad.SERCA2a (*n*=9). The protein expression of SERCA2a was significantly decreased in failing rat hearts compared with sham-operated controls. Adenoviral gene transfer of SERCA2a in failing hearts restored SERCA2a levels to that of nonfailing controls. (*Asterisk* indicates *P*<0.05 vs. Sham + Ad.βgal; *dagger* indicates *P*<0.05 vs. failing + Ad.βgal; *double dagger* indicates *P*<0.05 vs. Sham + Ad.SERCA2a.) **B,** Correction of the force-frequency relationship with adenoviral gene transfer of SERCA2a. Seven days following gene transfer, rats underwent hemodynamic studies with a high-fidelity micromanometer catheter in the left ventricle (LV) to measure the maximal rate of pressure rise (+dP/dt) and an epicardial pacing lead on an atrial appendage to increase heart rate above baseline. LV +dP/dt decreased with higher heart rates in the failing hearts infected with Ad.βgal (*closed triangles*) consistent with a negative force-frequency relationship. Overexpression of SERCA2a in the failing hearts (*open triangles*) restored the force-frequency response to values near sham-operated controls (*closed circles*). (*Adapted from* Miyamoto *et al.* [34].)

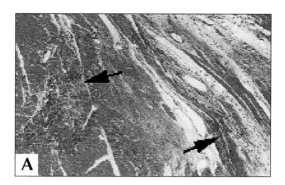

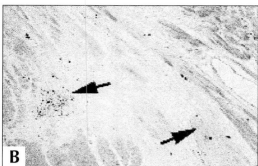

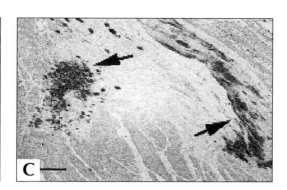

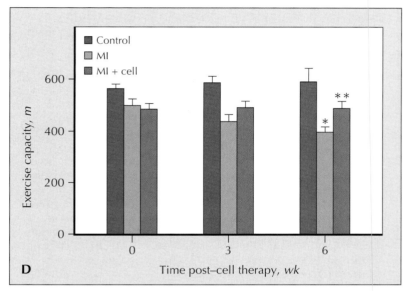

FIGURE 13-25. Cell therapy to attenuate ventricular remodeling after myocardial infarction. Cardiomyocyte loss following myocardial infarction is believed to be irreversible, and the degree of left ventricular dysfunction is an independent predictor of mortality. Recently, cell therapy with skeletal myoblasts or stem cells has been suggested as a novel treatment for ischemic cardiomyopathy. When implanted into myocardium, myoblasts and stem cells may retain the ability to proliferate and differentiate into myotubes with the capability of forming functional muscle fibers. Jain *et al.* [35] injected syngeneic skeletal myoblasts directly into the infarct region of rats one week following experimental myocardial infarction. Twelve weeks after implantation, myoblast survival is demonstrated in infarcted left ventricular free wall with trichrome staining (**A**), and immunohistochemical staining for myogenin (**B**) or skeletal-specific myosin heavy chain (**C**). Maximum exercise capacity, as assessed by the distance run on a rodent treadmill until exhaustion, was used as a measure of *in vivo* ventricular function and overall cardiac performance (**D**). Exercise capacity was measured before cell implantation, and at 3 and 6 weeks post-implantation in three groups of animals (noninfarcted control rats, infarcted rats without cell therapy [MI], and infarcted rats receiving myoblast cell therapy [MI + cell]). Both MI and MI + cell animals demonstrated a comparable reduction (~10%) in exercise capacity at baseline compared with controls. Control animals maintained a stable exercise capacity over time, while MI animals demonstrated a progressive decrease in exercise capacity. Cell therapy prevented the continued decline in exercise capacity suggesting a protective effect on cardiac function. (*Asterisk* indicates *P*<0.05 vs 0 weeks; *double asterisk* indicates *P*<0.05 vs MI.) (*Adapted from* Jain *et al.* [35].)

REFERENCES

1. McClean DR, Ikram H, Garlick AH, *et al.*: The clinical, cardiac, renal, arterial and neurohormonal effects of omapatrilat, a vasopeptidase inhibitor, in patients with chronic heart failure. *J Am Coll Cardiol* 2000, 36:479–486.

2. Rouleau JL, Pfeffer MA, Stewart DJ, *et al.*: Comparison of vasopeptidase inhibitor, omapatrilat, and lisinopril on exercise tolerance and morbidity in patients with heart failure: IMPRESS randomised trial. *Lancet* 2000, 356:615–620.

3. Tsutamoto T, Wada A, Maeda Y, *et al.*: Relation between endothelin-1 spillover in the lungs and pulmonary vascular resistance in patients with chronic heart failure. *J Am Coll Cardiol* 1994, 23:1427–1433.

4. Spieker LE, Noll G, Ruschitzka FT, *et al.*: Endothelin receptor antagonists in congestive heart failure: a new therapeutic principle for the future? *J Am Coll Cardiol* 2001, 37:1493–1505.

5. Hulsmann M, Stanek B, Frey B, *et al.*: Value of cardiopulmonary exercise testing and big endothelin plasma levels to predict short-term prognosis of patients with chronic heart failure. *J Am Coll Cardiol* 1998, 32:1695–1700.

6. Luscher TF, Barton M: Endothelins and endothelin receptor antagonists: therapeutic considerations for a novel class of cardio-vascular drugs. *Circulation* 2000, 102:2434–2440.

7. Kiowski W, Sutsch G, Hunziker P, *et al.*: Evidence for endothelin-1–mediated vasoconstriction in severe chronic heart failure. *Lancet* 1995, 346:732–736.

8. Sutsch G, Kiowski W, Yan XW, *et al.*: Short-term oral endothelin-receptor antagonist therapy in conventionally treated patients with symptomatic severe chronic heart failure. *Circulation* 1998, 98:2262–2268.

9. Givertz MM, Colucci WS, LeJemtel TH, *et al.*: Acute endothelin A receptor blockade causes selective pulmonary vasodilation in patients with chronic heart failure. *Circulation* 2000, 101:2922–2927.

10. Sakai S, Miyauchi T, Kobayashi M, *et al.*: Inhibition of myocardial endothelin pathway improves long-term survival in heart failure. *Nature* 1996, 384:353–355.

11. Torre-Amione G, Kapadia S, Benedict C, *et al.*: Proinflammatory cytokine levels in patients with depressed left ventricular ejection fraction: a report from the Studies of Left Ventricular Dysfunction (SOLVD). *J Am Coll Cardiol* 1996, 27:1201–1206.

12. Tsutamoto T, Hisanaga T, Wada A, *et al.*: Interleukin-6 spillover in the peripheral circulation increases with the severity of heart failure, and the high plasma level of interleukin-6 is an important prognostic predictor in patients with congestive heart failure. *J Am Coll Cardiol* 1998, 31:391–398.

13. Deswal A, Bozkurt B, Seta Y, *et al.*: Safety and efficacy of a soluble P75 tumor necrosis factor receptor (Enbrel, etanercept) in patients with advanced heart failure. *Circulation* 1999, 99:3224–3226.

14. Bozkurt B, Torre-Amione G, Warren MS, *et al.*: Results of targeted anti-tumor necrosis factor therapy with etanercept (ENBREL) in patients with advanced heart failure. *Circulation* 2001, 103:1044–1047.

15. Skudicky D, Bergemann A, Sliwa K, *et al.*: Beneficial effects of pentoxifylline in patients with idiopathic dilated cardiomyopathy treated with angiotensin-converting enzyme inhibitors and carvedilol: results of a randomized study. *Circulation* 2001, 103:1083–1088.

16. Schrier RW, Abraham WT: Hormones and hemodynamics in heart failure. *N Engl J Med* 1999, 341:577–585.

17. Preibisz JJ, Sealey JE, Laragh JH, *et al.*: Plasma and platelet vasopressin in essential hypertension and congestive heart failure. *Hypertension* 1983, 5:I129–I138.

18. Martin PY, Abraham WT, Lieming X, *et al.*: Selective V_2-receptor vasopressin antagonism decreases urinary aquaporin-2 excretion in patients with chronic heart failure. *J Am Soc Nephrol* 1999, 10:2165–2170.

19. Udelson JE, Smith WB, Hendrix GH, *et al.*: Hemodynamic effects of conivaptan hydrochloride (YM087, CI-1025) a combined vasopressin V_{1a} and V_2 receptor antagonist in patients with advanced heart failure. *Circulation* 2000, 102:II–593.

20. Haikala H, Nissinen E, Etemadzadeh E, *et al.*: Troponin C-mediated calcium sensitization induced by levosimendan does not impair relaxation. *J Cardiovasc Pharmacol* 1995, 25:794–801.

21. Slawsky MT, Colucci WS, Gottlieb SS, *et al.*: Acute hemodynamic and clinical effects of levosimendan in patients with severe heart failure. *Circulation* 2000, 102:2222–2227.

22. Uretsky BF, Jessup M, Konstam MA, *et al.*: Multicenter trial of oral enoximone in patients with moderate to moderately severe congestive heart failure. Lack of benefit compared with placebo. Enoximone Multicenter Trial Group. *Circulation* 1990, 82:774–780.

23. Lowes BD, Higginbotham M, Petrovich L, *et al.*: Low-dose enoximone improves exercise capacity in chronic heart failure. Enoximone Study Group. *J Am Coll Cardiol* 2000, 36:501–508.

24. Kass DA, Chen CH, Curry C, *et al.*: Improved left ventricular mechanics from acute VDD pacing in patients with dilated cardiomyopathy and ventricular conduction delay. *Circulation* 1999, 99:1567–1573.

25. Cazeau S, Leclercq C, Lavergne T, *et al.*: Effects of multisite biventricular pacing in patients with heart failure and intraventricular conduction delay. *N Engl J Med* 2001, 344:873–880.

26. Abraham WT: Rationale and design of a randomized clinical trial to assess the safety and efficacy of cardiac resynchronization therapy in patients with advanced heart failure: the Multicenter InSync Randomized Clinical Evaluation (MIRACLE). *J Card Fail* 2000, 6:369–380.

27. Morrow JD, Hill KE, Burk RF, *et al.*: A series of prostaglandin F2-like compounds are produced in vivo in humans by a non-cyclooxygenase, free radical-catalyzed mechanism. *Proc Natl Acad Sci U S A* 1990, 87:9383–9387.

28. Mallat Z, Philip I, Lebret M, *et al.*: Elevated levels of 8-iso-prostaglandin F2alpha in pericardial fluid of patients with heart failure: a potential role for in vivo oxidant stress in ventricular dilatation and progression to heart failure. *Circulation* 1998, 97:1536–1539.

29. Dhalla AK, Hill MF, Singal PK: Role of oxidative stress in transition of hypertrophy to heart failure. *J Am Coll Cardiol* 1996, 28:506–514.

30. Mann DL, Spinale FG: Activation of matrix metalloproteinases in the failing human heart: breaking the tie that binds. *Circulation* 1998, 98:1699–1702.

31. Li YY, Feldman AM, Sun Y, *et al.*: Differential expression of tissue inhibitors of metalloproteinases in the failing human heart. *Circulation* 1998, 98:1728–1734.

32. Peterson JT, Hallak H, Johnson L, *et al.*: Matrix metalloproteinase inhibition attenuates left ventricular remodeling and dysfunction in a rat model of progressive heart failure. *Circulation* 2001, 103:2303–2309.

33. Hajjar RJ, del Monte F, Matsui T, *et al.*: Prospects for gene therapy for heart failure. *Circ Res* 2000, 86:616–621.

34. Miyamoto MI, del Monte F, Schmidt U, *et al.*: Adenoviral gene transfer of SERCA2a improves left-ventricular function in aortic-banded rats in transition to heart failure. *Proc Natl Acad Sci U S A* 2000, 97:793–798.

35. Jain M, DerSimonian H, Brenner DA, *et al.*: Cell therapy attenuates deleterious ventricular remodeling and improves cardiac performance after myocardial infarction. *Circulation* 2001, 103:1920–1927.

CARDIAC TRANSPLANTATION

Donna Mancini and Mat Williams

Since the first human heart transplantation in 1967 [1], cardiac transplantation has evolved from a medical curiosity to an accepted therapy for end-stage cardiomyopathy. Initial 1-year survival was only about 20%. With the general availability of cyclosporine in 1986, 1-year survival improved to more than 80%. This highly effective immunosuppressive agent stimulated the growth of cardiac transplantation, and the number of transplantations increased worldwide from 90 in 1981 to 2000 in 1988 [2].

Immunosuppressive agents have become more selective in targeting allograft rejection; nevertheless, significant morbidity still exists following transplantation primarily due to the consequences of immunosuppression or the side effects of the immunosuppressive drugs [3]. Current immunosuppression includes triple therapy with cyclosporine, prednisone, and azathioprine or mycophenolate mofetil. Early transplantation-related problems include allograft rejection and infection. Chronic clinical problems of hypertension, nephrotoxicity, steroid-induced diabetes, obesity, and osteoporosis are frequently observed. Transplantation-related coronary artery disease as a manifestation of chronic rejection is the major long-term morbidity. It currently represents the major limitation to long-term survival after transplantation [4]. Efforts have been directed at prevention of this complication by the identification of risk factors responsible for its development. Once established, this vasculopathy becomes so diffuse and extensive that the only possible treatment is retransplantation.

Despite the comorbidities related to transplantation, the quality of life of these patients is frequently dramatically improved. Exercise performance is greatly enhanced, although it remains submaximal compared with normal age-matched subjects. Diastolic dysfunction, chronotropic incompetence, and recipient-donor size mismatch are some potential limitations to exercise performance in transplantation patients [5].

The sustained improvement in survival following heart transplantation has lead to a broadening of recipient selection criteria and an increase in the number of potential transplantation candidates. Current estimates indicate that between 14,000 and 15,000 people per year could benefit from heart transplantation. The continued expansion of heart transplantation is limited by the availability of donor organs, which has remained stagnant at approximately 2000 per year [6]. Public awareness campaigns have minimally increased the donor pool. Improved medical therapy for heart failure and refined risk stratification has helped to defer transplantation in large numbers of patients. Despite these efforts, the waiting lists for transplantation candidates continue to lengthen. Alternatives to transplantation with mechanical-assist devices are actively being investigated. Several new mechanical assist devices have been developed for single or biventricular support [7]. The use of these devices is presently limited to bridge therapy to transplant but future applications of these devices will include destination therapy. Additionally, other surgical options aimed at left ventricular remodeling and unloading are being investigated. Several of these approaches are illustrated in this chapter.

POSTTRANSPLANTATION SURVIVAL

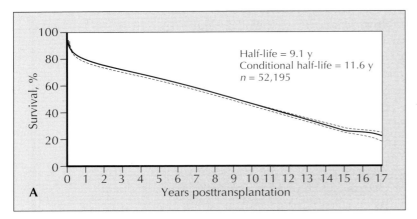
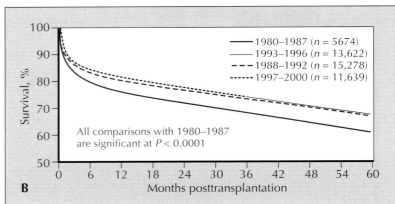

FIGURE 14-1. Heart transplantation actuarial survival. Survival following cardiac transplantation has significantly improved following the addition of cyclosporine to the immunosuppressive regimen. **A,** Actuarial heart transplantation survival for 57,818 heart transplantations performed between 1982 and 2000. **B,** Survival by era with improved survival demonstrated after 1987 following the clinical availability of cyclosporine A. (*Adapted from* Hosenpud *et al.* [8].)

CANDIDATE SELECTION

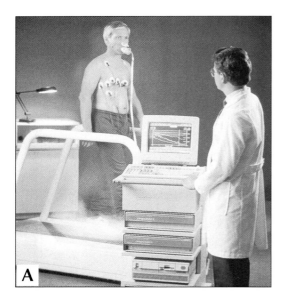

FIGURE 14-2. Cardiopulmonary stress testing. Application of cardiopulmonary stress testing has been an extremely valuable tool for guiding the transplantation selection process in ambulatory patients. **A,** The equipment used to conduct this form of testing. The patient breathes through a disposable pneumotach into a metabolic cart (Medical Graphics 2001, Minneapolis, MN) while exercising on a treadmill or bicycle. The metabolic cart is equipped with rapidly responding CO_2 and O_2 analyzers enabling online measurement of oxygen consumption (VO_2) and CO_2 production.

Because VO_2 equals the cardiac output times the arterial-venous oxygen difference, peak VO_2 provides an indirect noninvasive assessment of cardiac output response to exercise. Cardiopulmonary stress testing was first used in candidate selection in 1986.

(continued)

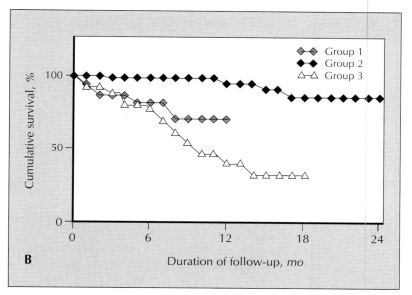

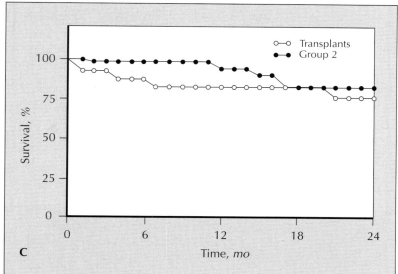

FIGURE 14-2. (*continued*) **B,** In a study by Mancini *et al.* [9], 114 transplantation candidates were divided into three groups on the basis of exercise capacity. In patients with a VO_2 level greater than 14 mL/kg/min, cardiac transplantation was deferred (group 2). Patients with a VO_2 of 14 mL/kg/min or less were accepted for transplantation in the absence of any other contraindications (group 1). Patients with a significant comorbidity that excluded transplantation and with VO_2 less than 14 mL/kg/min constituted a medical control group (group 3). Cumulative survival curves for the three groups are shown here. For group 1, transplant was

considered a censored observation. The 52 patients with a preserved exercise capacity (*ie*, peak $VO_2 > 14$ mL/kg/min) had a 1-year survival rate of 94%.

This was significantly better than the survival of patients with reduced exercise capacity (*ie*, VO_2 of 14 mL/kg/min or less). **C,** The survival of the heart failure patients with VO_2 greater than 14 mL/kg/min (group 2) was similar to the survival of patients in group 1 who underwent cardiac transplantation. (Parts B and C *adapted from* Mancini *et al.* [9].)

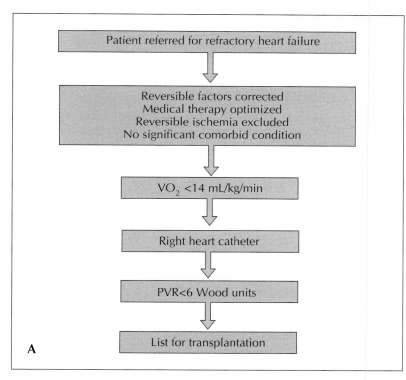

B. EXCLUSION CRITERIA FOR CARDIAC TRANSPLANTATION

Age >65 years
Fixed PVR >6 Wood units
Peptic ulcer disease or pulmonary infarct within 3 months
Brittle diabetes mellitus or diabetes with end-organ damage
Major debilitating comorbid disease
Symptomatic severe peripheral vascular or carotid disease
Symptomatic hypertension requiring multidrug therapy
Active infection
Renal insufficiency (creatinine level >2.5 mg/dL or creatine clearance <50 mL/min)
Severe liver dysfunction (bilirubin level >2.5 mg/dL or transaminase level >two times normal)
Significant obstructive pulmonary disease (FEV_1 <1 L/min)
Significant intrinsic coagulation abnormalities
Active or recent malignancy (within 2 years)
HIV seroconversion
Amyloidosis
Excessive obesity (>33% above ideal body weight)
Evidence of active tobacco, alcohol, or drug abuse
History of severe mental illness or psychosocial instability

FIGURE 14-3. Proposed algorithm for cardiac transplantation recipient selection (**A**). All referred candidates should be New York Heart Association class III or IV after optimization of medical therapy. A list of clinical contraindications to transplantation is included here (**B**) [10]. FEV_1—1-sec forced expiratory volume; PVR—pulmonary vascular resistance.

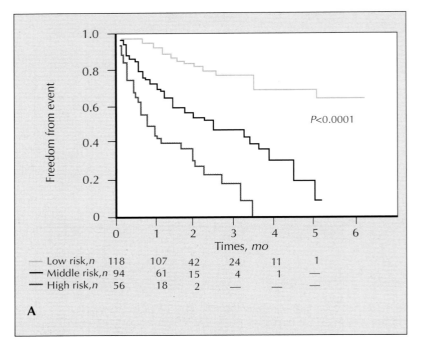

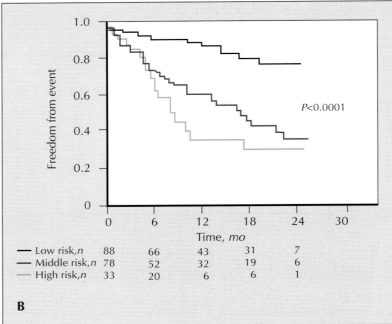

C. CALCULATION OF PROGNOSTIC SCORE

CLINICAL CHARACTERISTIC	VALUE (χ)	COEFFICIENT (β)	PRODUCT
Ischemic cardiomyopathy	1	+0.06931	+0.6931
Resting heart rate	90	+0.0216	+1.9440
LVEF	17	-0.0464	-0.7888
Mean BP	80	-0.0255	-2.0400
IVCD	0	+0.6083	0
Peak VO_2	16.2	-0.0546	-0.8845
Serum sodium	132	-0.0470	-6.2040
PROGNOSTIC SCORE	$=\Sigma\beta_1\chi_1+\beta_2\chi_2+...+\beta n\chi n$		
	=SUM OF THE PRODUCTS		=7.2802

absence of intraventricular conduction defect, peak VO_2 in mL/kg/min, and serum sodium. The heart failure survival score is calculated as the absolute value of the sum of the products of the identified prognostic variables and their computed coefficients.

Noncontinuous variables were graded as 1 if present or 0 if absent. Low-risk patients are identified as those with a score of more than 8.10; medium- and high-risk patients have scores below 8.1. Medium- and high-risk candidates are appropriate for listing for transplantation. **A,** Survival curve for the derivation sample. **B,** Survival curve for the validation group. **C,** An example of the calculation of the heart failure survival score for a 55-year-old man with an ischemic cardiomyopathy; resting heart rate of 90 bpm; left ventricular ejection fraction (LVEF) of 17%; mean arterial blood pressure (BP) of 80 mm Hg; absence of an intraventricular conduction defect (IVCD); peak VO_2 level of 16.2 mL/kg/min; and a serum sodium level of 132. The prognostic score below 8.1 places the patient in the medium-to high-risk group. In the absence of any major contraindications, the patient should be activated on the transplantation list. (*Adapted from* Aaronson *et al.* [11].)

FIGURE 14-4. In an attempt to further refine the use of oxygen consumption (VO_2) in the selection of ambulatory transplantation candidates, a clinical index was developed and prospectively validated to predict survival [11].

Multivariable proportional hazards modeling was used to develop the model from 80 clinical characteristics in 268 ambulatory patients with severe heart failure. The statistical model was subsequently validated in 199 patients. The smallest number of prognostic variables that accurately predicted 1-year survival was used to develop the heart failure survival score. The most significant prognostic factors were etiology of heart failure, resting heart rate and mean arterial blood pressure, left ventricular ejection fraction, presence or

FIGURE 14-5. Reevaluation of the need for transplantation. Heart failure is a dynamic state and therefore requires periodic reevaluation of the continued need for transplantation. A protocol for reevaluation is listed here. Left ventricular ejection fraction (LVEF) and exercise capacity are reassessed within 3 months of the initial evaluation in patients with major alterations in therapy or with symptomatic improvement. In the majority of patients, reevaluation is performed every 6 months. Patients selected using criteria emphasizing reduced oxygen consumption (VO_2) generally continue to have a high mortality, with few patients being deactivated from the transplantation list. Thus, accumulated time on the list remains a good parameter by which to allocate organs. PRA—panel of reactive antibodies; PVR—pulmonary vascular resistance.

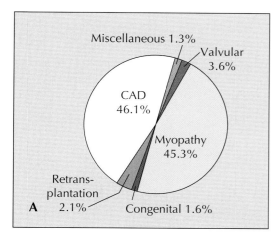

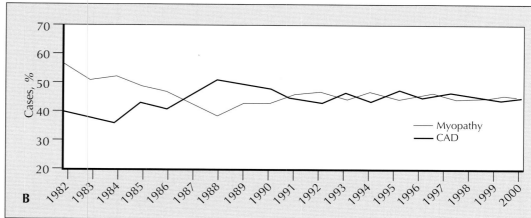

FIGURE 14-6. Indications for adult heart transplantation. In 2000, the most common indications for cardiac transplantation were coronary artery disease (CAD) (46.1%), followed closely by dilated cardiomyopathy (45.3%). (*Adapted from* Hosenpud *et al.* [8].)

DONOR SELECTION CRITERIA

FIGURE 14-7. Donor criteria. The major limitation to the growth of cardiac transplantation has been the scarcity of donor organs. Attempts have been made to expand the donor pool by accepting hearts from older candidates, serologic-positive organs (*ie*, hepatitis C positive), and even marginal hearts with high inotropic requirements and small segmental wall abnormalities pretransplant. Guidelines for selecting suitable heart donors at Columbia-Presbyterian Medical Center (New York, NY) are shown here. Bs Ag—hepatitis B surface antigen; ECG—electrocardiogram; ECHO—echocardiogram.

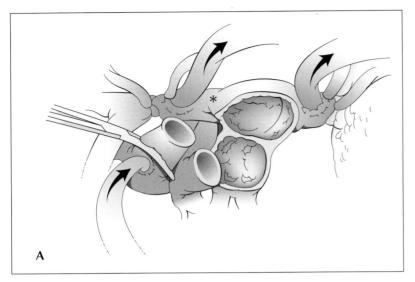

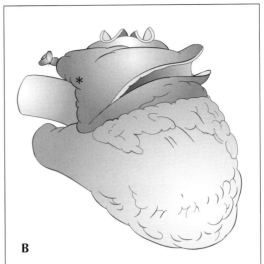

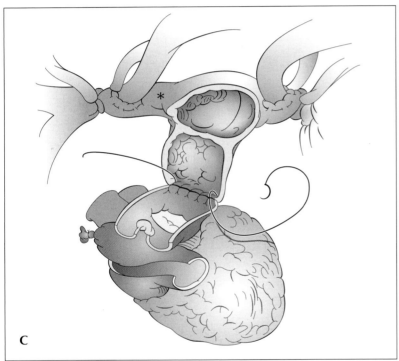

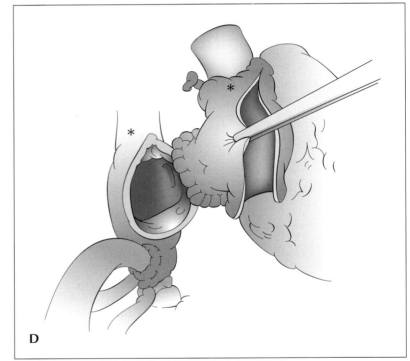

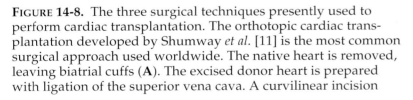

FIGURE 14-8. The three surgical techniques presently used to perform cardiac transplantation. The orthotopic cardiac transplantation developed by Shumway *et al.* [11] is the most common surgical approach used worldwide. The native heart is removed, leaving biatrial cuffs (**A**). The excised donor heart is prepared with ligation of the superior vena cava. A curvilinear incision into the right atrium is made to protect the donor sinus node (*asterisk*) (**B**). Biatrial anastomoses are performed, beginning with the left-to-left atrial anastomoses. This is followed by right atrial anastomoses (**C** and **D**) and finally by the pulmonary (**E**) and aortic (**F**) anastomoses.

(continued)

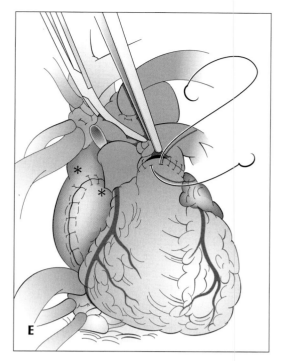

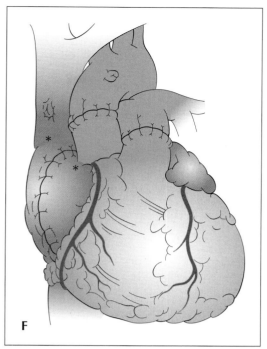

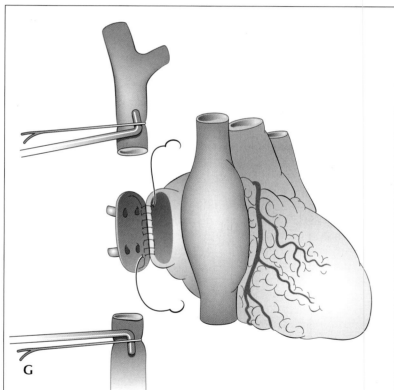

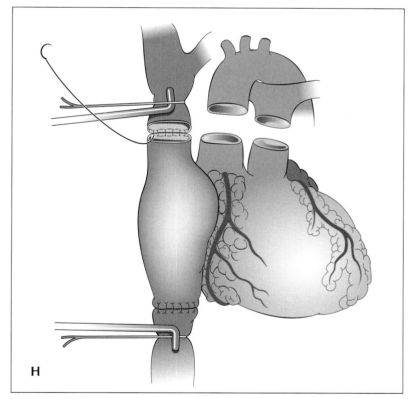

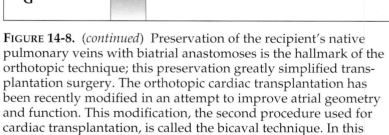

FIGURE 14-8. (*continued*) Preservation of the recipient's native pulmonary veins with biatrial anastomoses is the hallmark of the orthotopic technique; this preservation greatly simplified transplantation surgery. The orthotopic cardiac transplantation has been recently modified in an attempt to improve atrial geometry and function. This modification, the second procedure used for cardiac transplantation, is called the bicaval technique. In this modification, the recipient's atria are completely excised, with the exception of one or two small left-atrial cuffs containing the pulmonary veins. Direct anastomoses are then performed between the donor and recipient inferior and superior venae cavae, and then the left atrial cuff on the donor heart is anastomosed to the pulmonary venous cuff on the recipient side (**G**). The aorta and pulmonary artery are then anastomosed (**H**). (*continued*)

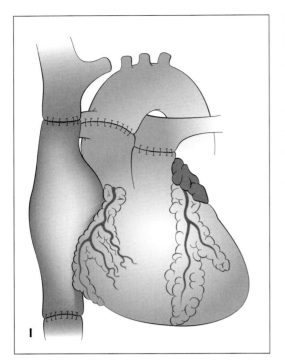

FIGURE 14-8. (*continued*) The completed bicaval transplant (**I**) thus preserves atrial geometry. The third technique for transplantation currently utilized is the heterotopic technique (not shown), which was the original transplantation performed by Dr. Christian Barnard in 1967. In this technique, the donor organ is "piggybacked" to the recipient heart. The two aortas are anastomosed, and a Dacron graft is interposed between the donor and recipient pulmonary artery. The right and left ventricular circulations are connected parallel. In a recent modification of this technique, the donor pulmonary artery is anastomosed to the recipient right atrium. This modification places the right ventricles in series; the left ventricles remain in parallel circuits. Heterotopic transplantation permits transplantation of patients with fixed elevated pulmonary vascular resistances who are not eligible for orthotopic transplantation. However, this approach is limited by a lower long-term survival, need for chronic anticoagulation, development of arrhythmias, and potential for refractory angina in some patients [13]. (Parts A to G *adapted from* Cooley [14]; parts H to J *adapted from* El Gamel *et al.* [15].)

ALLOGRAFT REJECTION

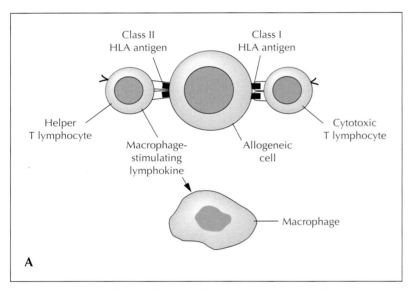

A

FIGURE 14-9. (*See* Color Plate.) Allograft rejection. **A,** The rejection of an allograft is primarily determined by the recognition of foreign antigens on the surface of engrafted cells. The major surface histocompatibility antigens are determined by a single complex genetic region called the HLA region in humans. The loci are divided into two classes, I and II, based on structure, function, and tissue distribution of their cell surface protein products. Cell-mediated rejection is the primary cause of rejection. T lymphocytes are crucial to the initiation and execution of cellular rejection. Donor antigens are presented either directly (*ie*, on the surface of a donor cell) or indirectly. The subsequent recognition of foreign or donor HLA antigens by highly specific T-cell receptors remains the critical control element for the immune response. However, the recognition of foreign HLA protein by a T-cell receptor is not sufficient to provoke the rejection response. The interaction between the antigen-presenting cell and the T-cell receptor must be aligned with integrins and adhesion molecules such that a conformational change can occur in the T-cell receptor. T-cell surface molecules that promote adhesion include lymphocyte-associated antigen (LFA-1). LFA-1 binds to intra-cellular adhesion molecule (ICAM-I), which is a glycoprotein expressed on endothelial cells, fibroblasts, lymphocytes, and monocytes. Interleukin-2 is the main cytotrophic factor to T lymphocytes that causes allospecific clonal expansion activation of cytotoxic and helper T cells, as well as activation of B lymphocytes. The complexity of the cellular interaction provides many potential targets for immunosuppression. Development of monoclonal antibodies against these cellular molecules has been an active area of research. Humoral rejection can occur early after transplantation. It is characterized histologically by immunoglobulin and complement deposition in the absence of cellular rejection. It is frequently associated with hemodynamic compromise and occurs in about 10% of cases. (*continued*)

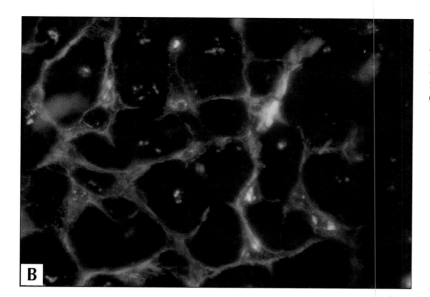

B

FIGURE 14-9. (*continued*) **B,** Immunofluorescent staining of a myocardial biopsy with fluorescein-conjugated anti-human IgG. The green fluorescent stain demonstrates the linear deposition of IgG on the endothelial capillaries; the yellow stain represents auto-fluorescent lipofusion within the myocytes. (Part A *adapted from* Cerilli [16].)

A. IMMUNOSUPPRESSIVE DRUGS

DRUG	MECHANISM OF ACTION	DOSE	SIDE EFFECTS
ANTIMETABOLITES			
Azathioprine	Inhibition of purine metabolism	2 mg/kg/d (titrated to WBC count of 5000/cc)	Leukopenia, bone marrow suppression, hepatotoxicity, nausea
Mycophenolate mofetil	Inhibition of purine metabolism	1500 mg bid	Nausea, diarrhea, leukopenia
Brequinar sodium*	Inhibition of pyrimidine metabolism	—	Leukopenia, thrombo-cytopenia, diarrhea
Cytoxan	Inhibition of pyrimidine metabolism	1 g/m^2 every 3–4 wk	Leukopenia, mucositis, thrombocytopenia, hemorrhagic cystitis
ANTIPROLIFERATIVES			
Prednisone	Inhibits macrophage migration factor; inhibits processing and display of antigen; inhibits IL1 release & synthesis of IL1 & 2	0–10 mg/d	Diabetes, osteoporosis, obesity, dyslipidemia, myopathy, cataracts, mood swings
Cyclosporine	Interferes with transcription of IL2 by binding cyclophilin on T cells	4–6 mg/kg/d bid (titrated to trough blood levels)	Nephrotoxicity, headache, tremors, hyperkalemia, photosensitivity, gingival hyperplasia
Tacrolimus	Binds cyclophilin on T cells and interferes with IL2 transcription	0.15–0.3 mg/kg/d bid	Nephrotoxicity, hyperkalemia, seizures, headache, tremor
Rapamycin*	Binds to cyclophin causing IL2 receptor blockade	—	Thrombocytopenia, nausea
ANTIBODY THERAPY			
OKT3	Monoclonal antibody to the CD3 receptor that prevents IL2 release	5 mg/d	Pulmonary edema with cytokine release, fever, myalgias, aseptic meningitis
Daclizumab*	Monoclonal antibody to the IL2 receptor	1 mg/kg on day 1, then every 2 wk for 2 mo	Gastrointestinal disorders
ATGAM	Polyclonal antibody	15–20mg/kg for 14 d	Fever, serum sickness, thrombocytopenia

FIGURE 14-10. Immunosuppressive drugs. The immunosuppressive drugs can be grouped into three categories: antimetabolites, antiproliferatives, and antibodies. **A,** Doses and side effects for the most commonly used drugs. Antimetabolites block purine or pyrimidine synthesis clonal lymphocyte expansion; antiproliferatives inhibit clonal expansion of cell lines that modulate rejection; and antibody therapy includes targeted and specific inhibition of cell lines that modulate rejection. (*continued*)

B. MAINTENANCE IMMUNOSUPPRESSIVE THERAPY

WEEK POSTTRANSPLANT	PREDNISONE, MG/D	CYCLOSPORINE TROUGH LEVEL	MYCOPHENOLATE MOFETIL	OR	AZATHIOPRINE
2	30	300–500			
3	25	300–500			
4	20	300–500			
6	15	300–500			
8	10	300–500			
12	7.5	200–300			
16	5	200–300	1500 mg bid orally		2 mg/kg titrated to a WBC count of 5
20	5	200–300			
24	4	200–300			
28	3	100–200			
36	2	100–200			
44	1	100–200			
52	0	100–200			

FIGURE 14-10. (*continued*) **B,** The maintenance immunosuppressive regimen used after cardiac transplantation at Columbia-Presbyterian Medical Center (New York, NY). Rapid withdrawal of corticosteroids is attempted to minimize steroid associated side effects. bid—twice a day; IL—interleukin; WBC—white blood cell.

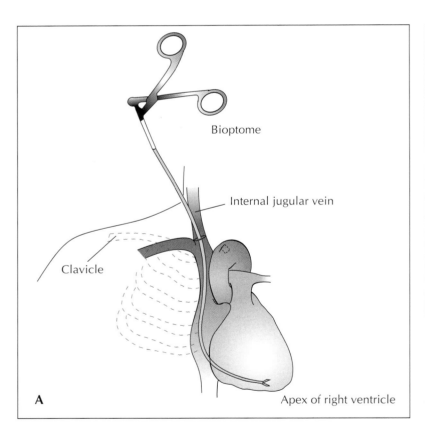

A

Bioptome

Internal jugular vein

Clavicle

Apex of right ventricle

B. ISHLT ENDOMYOCARDIAL GRADING SYSTEM

GRADE	HISTOLOGIC DESCRIPTION
0	No rejection
1A	Focal perivascular or interstitial infiltrate without necrosis
1B	Diffuse but sparse infiltrate without necrosis
2	One focus of aggressive infiltration or focal myocyte damage
3A	Multifocal aggressive infiltrates or myocyte damage
3B	Diffuse inflammatory process with necrosis
4	Diffuse aggressive polymorphous infiltrate with necrosis ±edema, ±hemorrhage, ±vasculitis

FIGURE 14-11. Histologic grading of allograft rejection. In order to monitor rejection, periodic endomyocardial biopsies are performed. **A,** The percutaneous technique of endomyocardial biopsy using the Caves bioptome. The bioptome is inserted through the internal jugular vein to the right ventricular portion of the interventricular septum under fluoroscopy. Four to six specimens containing at least 50% myocytes are required for 90% to 95% confidence in the interpretation. **B,** The standardization of histologic biopsy grading according to the International Society for Heart Transplantation (ISHLT). (Part A *adapted from* Unverferth [17].)

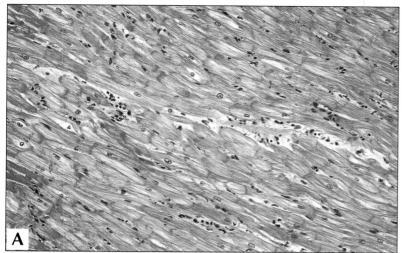

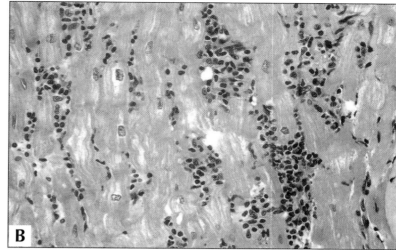

FIGURE 14-12. Hematoxylin and eosin staining of representative endomyocardial biopsies at a magnification of 100 × showing grade 1B rejection with focal lymphocytic infiltrate without evidence of myocardial necrosis (**A**), grade 3A rejection demonstrating more intensive lymphocytic infiltration and myocyte necrosis (**B**), and grade 4 allograft rejection with extensive lymphocyte infiltration, myocyte necrosis, and hemorrhage (**C**).

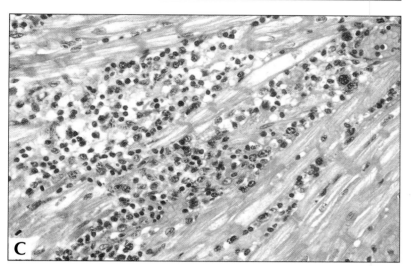

FIGURE 14-13. Infections associated with posttransplant immunosuppression. Because of reduced cellular immunity, the cardiac transplantation recipient is subject to development of typical bacterial as well as atypical viral, protozoal, and fungal infections. **A,** The typical posttransplant infections and the times at which they occur.

(continued)

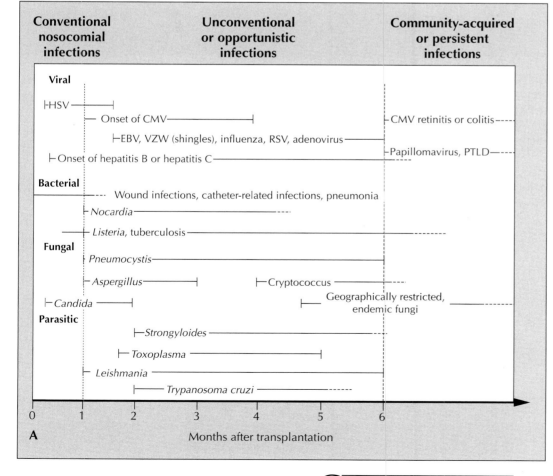

B. ANTIMICROBIAL PROPHYLAXIS

BACTERIAL PROPHYLAXIS

Cefazolin 1.5 g IV preoperatively and 1 g IV every 6 hours for 24 hours

Isoniazid 300 mg and pyridoxine 50 mg orally daily for 1 year for PPD-positive
candidates and recipients

Pneumococcal vaccine IM pretransplant

VIRAL PROPHYLAXIS (CMV, HSV, INFLUENZA)

Acyclovir 800 mg orally qid for 3 months in all patients; CytoGam 150 mg/kg IV within
72 hs of transplant, then 100 mg/kg on weeks 2, 4, 6, 8, then 50 mg/kg on weeks 12
and 16 in all CMV-positive recipients or in all recipients of CMV-positive donor hearts

CMV-positive recipients who receive CMV-negative hearts receive HSV prophylaxis with
acyclovir 400 mg orally tid

CMV-negative blood products to all transplant recipients

Influenza A and B vaccine every November to all recipients after year 1

PROTOZOAL PROPHYLAXIS (PCP, TOXOPLASMOSIS)

Trimethaprin-sulfamethoxazole single-strength tablet daily for 1 year or monthly 300 mg
of aerosolized pentamidine isethionate in patients with sulfa allergy

Pyrimethamine 50 mg daily and folinic acid 5 mg orally bid for 6 weeks for all recipients
with negative titers for toxoplasmosis who receive a heart that is positive for toxoplasmosis

FUNGAL PROPHYLAXIS

Mycostatin swish and swallow 5 cc orally qid for 2 months or clotrimazole troches orally
5 times per day for 2 months

FIGURE 14-13. (*continued*) **B,** In an attempt to prevent the various infections, the antimicrobial prophylactic regimen is implemented. bid—twice a day; CMV—cytomegalovirus; CNS—central nervous system; EBV—Epstein Barr virus; HSV—herpes simplex virus; IM—intramuscular; IV—intravenous; PCP—*Pneumocystis carinii* pneumonia; qid—four times a day; TB—tuberculosis; tid—three times a day; UTI—urinary tract infection; VZV—varicella zoster virus. (Part A *adapted from* Fishman and Rubin [18].)

QUALITY OF LIFE AFTER TRANSPLANTATION

A. DETERMINANTS OF DECREASED EXERCISE CAPACITY AFTER CARDIAC TRANSPLANTATION

DONOR

Abnormal LV relaxation or diastolic dysfunction

Reduced systolic performance due to rejection or
accelerated atherosclerosis

Chronotropic incompetence

RECIPIENT

Effects of immunosuppressive drugs: steroid-induced
myopathy

Persistent pulmonary abnormalities

Persistent skeletal muscle abnormalities

FIGURE 14-14. Exercise capacity after transplantation. Quality of life after transplantation is generally excellent. Many recipients are able to return to work and an active lifestyle [19]. However, multiple studies have demonstrated that cardiac transplantation recipients exhibit a 30% to 40% reduction in exercise capacity compared with normal individuals [5]. **A,** Determinants of decreased exercise capacity after cardiac transplantation. There are many theories to explain this reduced exercise capacity some that relate to the recipient and others to the donor characteristics. An important determinant of reduced exercise capacity is chronotropic incompetence due to graft denervation. As a consequence of denervation, the heart rate response is determined primarily by the transplanted heart response to circulating catecholamines.

(continued)

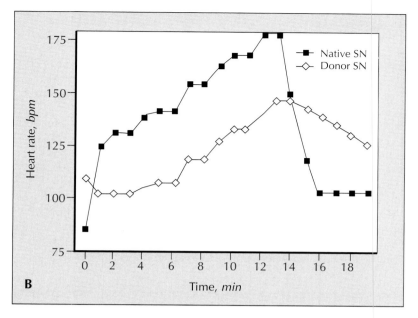

FIGURE 14-14. (*continued*) **B,** Simultaneous esophageal electrode recordings of the remnant native sinus node (SN) and the surface electrocardiogram recordings of donor heart rate from a patient 2 years after transplantation. The heart rate recorded from the native sinus node quickly increases at the onset of exercise and decreases precipitously with its termination. In contrast, the donor heart rate does not increase until minute 8 of exercise, consistent with its catecholamine-dependent response. Deceleration is also delayed as catecholamines are cleared from the circulation. LV—left ventricular. (*Adapted from* Beniaminovitz *et al.* [20].)

ACCELERATED TRANSPLANTATION ATHEROSCLEROSIS AND RETRANSPLANTATION

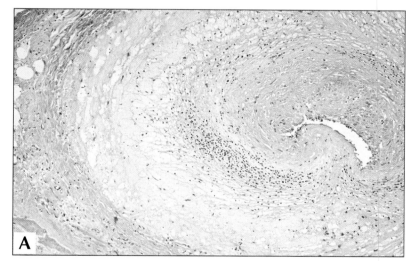

FIGURE 14-15. Transplantation coronary allograft disease (TCAD). The major cause of late death after cardiac transplantation is the development of TCAD, a unique accelerated form of coronary artery disease. By 1 year posttransplant, about 30% of patients demonstrate some TCAD, and the incidence and severity continue to increase with time [21]. The pathogenesis of TCAD is thought to begin with immunologic and nonimmunologic injury to the arterial endothelium, with resultant loss of endothelial integrity [22]. Microthrombi, cellular proliferation, and plasma lipids accumulate at the site of the injured intima. **A,** This leads to further cellular proliferation and finally profound myointimal hyperplasia leading to diffuse coronary artery lumen narrowing.

(*continued*)

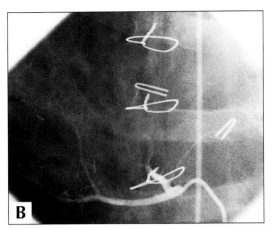

FIGURE 14-15. (*continued*) **B,** Selective left coronary angiography from a patient with severe TCAD, which shows diffuse tapering of the left anterior descending and circumflex arteries as well as pruning of all the secondary vessels. Immunologic mechanisms resulting in endothelial injury include both cellular and humoral factors [23]. Nonimmunologic risk factors also contribute to the development of cardiac allograft vasculopathy. Recipient age and gender, donor age and gender, obesity, hyperlipidemia, and donor ischemic time may impact on the development of vasculopathy [24]. An association has also been found between the presence of active cytomegalovirus infection and the development of vasculopathy [25]. Given the diffuse, concentric nature of this disease, percutaneous transluminal coronary angioplasty and coronary artery bypass grafting are not useful strategies for management. Unfortunately, patients with TCAD have a fivefold greater risk of cardiac events such as myocardial infarction, severe refractory heart failure, and sudden death. Presently, retransplantation is the only treatment for severe TCAD; however, survival after repeat transplantation is significantly reduced. Consequently, preventative strategies have assumed clinical importance. Hyperlipidemia management with HMG Co-A (3-hydroxy-3-methylglutaryl-coenzyme A) reductase inhibitors and routine aspirin use are two such approaches.

MECHANICAL-ASSIST DEVICES

PATIENT SELECTION CRITERIA FOR LEFT VENTRICULAR ASSIST DEVICES

Transplant candidate
Hemodynamic parameters
    Cardiac index <2 L/min/m^2
    Systolic blood pressure <80 mm Hg
    Pulmonary capillary wedge > 20 mm Hg
Technical considerations for exclusion
    Body surface area <1.5 m^2
    Aortic insufficiency
    Right to left shunt
    Abdominal aortic aneurysm
    Prosthetic valves
    Left ventricular thrombus
Severe right ventricular failure
Preoperative risk factors
    Right atrial pressure >16 mm Hg
    Prothrombin time >16 s
    Reoperation
    White blood cell count >15
    Urine output <30 cc/h
    Mechanically ventilated
    Temperature >101.5°F

FIGURE 14-16. Approximately 25% of the patients listed for cardiac transplantation die before a suitable donor heart becomes available. Consequently, several types of short-term and more permanent mechanical-assist devices have been developed to bridge patients to transplantation. Commonly used short- and long-term devices for support in patients with postcardiotomy failure, acute cardiogenic shock from extensive acute myocardial infarction or myocarditis or in patients with medically refractory heart failure are shown this table. Devices can be divided into extracorporeal and intracorporeal systems that can provide single or biventricular support.

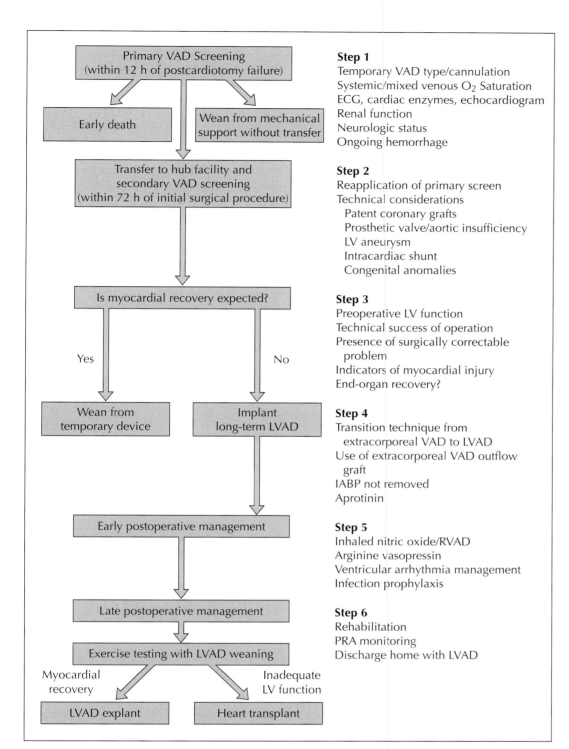

Step 1
Temporary VAD type/cannulation
Systemic/mixed venous O_2 Saturation
ECG, cardiac enzymes, echocardiogram
Renal function
Neurologic status
Ongoing hemorrhage

Step 2
Reapplication of primary screen
Technical considerations
  Patent coronary grafts
  Prosthetic valve/aortic insufficiency
  LV aneurysm
  Intracardiac shunt
  Congenital anomalies

Step 3
Preoperative LV function
Technical success of operation
Presence of surgically correctable
  problem
Indicators of myocardial injury
End-organ recovery?

Step 4
Transition technique from
  extracorporeal VAD to LVAD
Use of extracorporeal VAD outflow
  graft
IABP not removed
Aprotinin

Step 5
Inhaled nitric oxide/RVAD
Arginine vasopressin
Ventricular arrhythmia management
Infection prophylaxis

Step 6
Rehabilitation
PRA monitoring
Discharge home with LVAD

FIGURE 14-17. Proposed algorithm for insertion of mechanical-assist devices in patients with postcardiotomy failure occurring at outside institutions. VAD—ventricular assist device; LVAD—left ventricular assist device; LV—left ventricle; ECG—electrocardiogram; IABP— intra-aortic balloon pump; RVAD—right ventricular assist device; PRA— panel reactive antibody. (*Adapted from* Helman [26].)

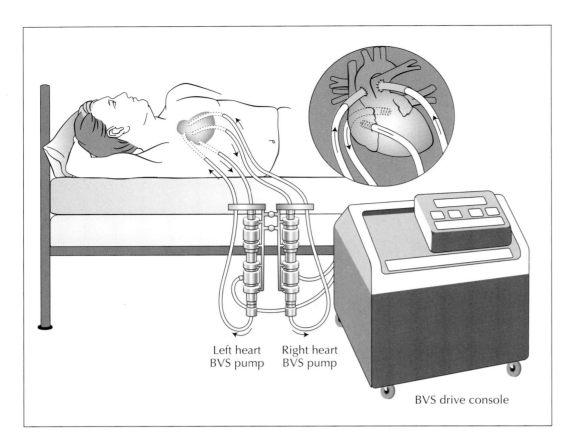

FIGURE 14-18. The Abiomed Bi-Ventricular Support (BVS) 5000 (Abiomed, Inc., Danvers, MA) is a pulsatile pneumatically driven extracorporeal assist device that can provide univentricular or biventricular support. Inflow cannulae are placed in either the right or left atrium. The device consists of two chambers with flow direction controlled by two polyurethane valves. Each chamber consists of a 100-mL, smooth-surfaced, polyurethane bladder. The device's top chamber (atrial) fills passively by gravity and the lower chamber (ventricular) has a bladder that fills and empties through pneumatic compression by an external console. The control console is self regulated based on preload filling of the atrial chamber and can achieve flows of up to 6 L/min. Outflow is generally achieved by direct anastamosis of a synthetic graft to either the aorta or pulmonary artery. The primary indication for this device is short-term support for postcardiotomy failure but it can also be used to facilitate transfer of patients in acute cardiogenic shock to a specialized center for either transplantation or long-term LVAD placement. The device is self-regulating and thus does not require special support staff to operate; however, the patient must be maintained on intravenous heparin throughout support. (*Adapted from* Higgins *et al.* [27].)

Left heart BVS pump   Right heart BVS pump

BVS drive console

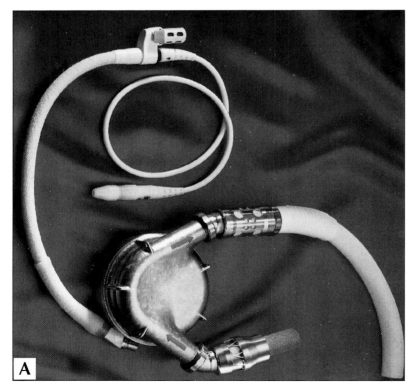

FIGURE 14-19. The HeartMate XVE (Thoratec Corp., Pleasanton, CA) uses pusher plate technology with a polyurethane diaphragm to propel the blood in a pulsatile fashion. This device can only be utilized for left-sided support [28]. It has a sintered titanium housing that promotes adherence of blood elements and development of a pseudointima. Because of this innovation and the use of xenograft valves, anticoagulation can be avoided with a very low thromboembolic rate (2.7%). The HeartMate device can achieve flow rates of 10 L/min and can be operated in a fixed rate mode or an automatic mode that self regulates rate based on the available preload. The device is implanted in the right upper abdomen. Inflow to the device is provided from the left ventricular apex and the outflow from a Dacron graft anastomosed to the ascending aorta. The driveline that connects to the power source is tunneled percutaneously exiting via the left abdomen. It can be connected to two external portable batteries providing patients with free mobility to engage in a variety of indoor and outdoor activities for up to 6 to 8 hours. Overnight, the patients are linked to a power base station. The driveline also allows for manual pneumatic activation in the event of an electrical or motor failure. Unfortunately, the driveline also serves as the major site of complications in this population with an infection rate near 50%. The device is shown in Figure 14-19A with a schematic of the positioning of the device in Figure 14-19B. (*continued*)

A

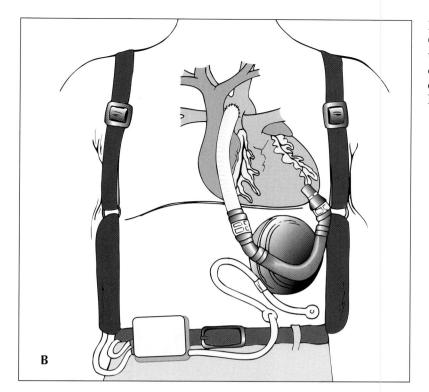

B

FIGURE 14-19. (*continued*) The Novacor system (Baxter Healthcare Corp., Deerfield, IL; not shown) is the other most commonly used left ventricular assist device (LVAD) bridge. The Novacor system does not contain a textured surface. Despite anticoagulation, the incidence of embolic cardiovascular accidents remain high with the present Novacor system.

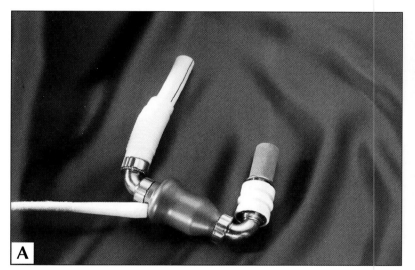

A

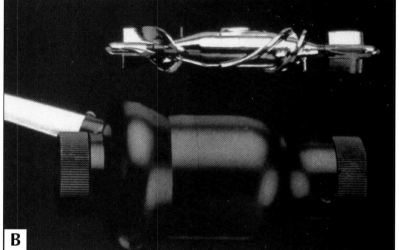

B

FIGURE 14-20. The newest generation of devices are axial flow pumps. The HeartMate II, Jarvik, and Debakey VADs are all axial flow pumps currently in clinical trial. The device illustrated in this figure is of the HeartMate II (Thoratec Corp., Pleasanton, CA) axial flow pump [29]. These small pumps utilize an impellar blade and circulate blood somewhat similar to a boat propellar. Flow is nonpulsatile. These devices have potential advantages in that they are small with minimal blood contact, simple mechanics, and lack of valves. They are extremely lightweight yet can generate flows in excess of 10 L/min without promoting hemolysis. No adverse end-organ function have been shown from the use of nonpulsatile devices in animal studies. These devices may very well represent the future of left sided support due to their simplicity and potential for better durability. **A,** The HeartMate 2 device. **B,** The propeller-like design of the pump is shown. (*Courtesy of* Thoratec Corp., Pleasanton, CA.)

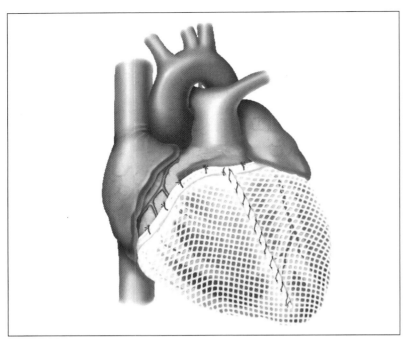

Figure 14-21. Passive cardiac restraint devices such as the CorCap (Acorn Cardiovascular, Inc., St. Paul, MN) are being investigated to prevent cardiac dilation and promote recovery. The development of this device originated from the passive benefit observed in patients undergoing cardiomyoplasty. The support device is made of a biocompatible mesh that is positioned around the epicardial surface of the heart like a sock. This specially weaved mesh is tightened to reduce the end-systolic volume of the heart by 10%. Animal and early clinical data have demonstrated slowing of the progression of heart failure and functional improvement [30]. Currently the device is placed with open chest techniques, but ultimately may be amenable to minimally invasive placement. (*Courtesy of* Acorn Cardiovascular, Inc.)

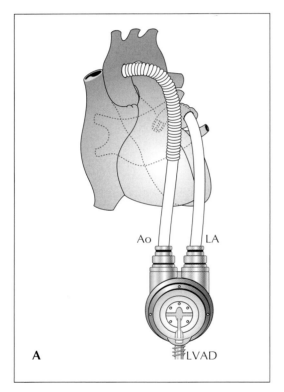
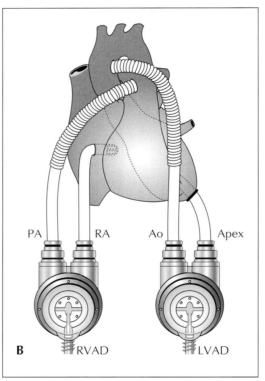
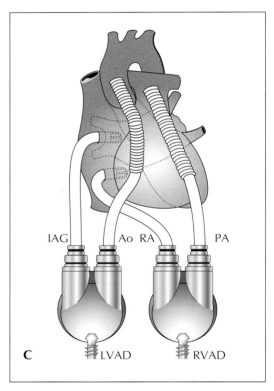

Figure 14-22. The Thoratec VAD (Thoratec Corp., Pleasanton, CA) is a polyurethane-lined pneumatically driven pusher plate device that can be used for both left- or right-sided support. The device has a stroke volume of 65 mL and can achieve flows up to 7 L/min. It is connected to the heart via special inflow cannulae that can be placed in the right atrium (**B,C**), left atrium (**A,C**) or left ventricle (**B**) depending on the type of support required. The outflow graft is sewn directly to the aorta or pulmonary artery, thereby providing stability. The extracorporeal pump is connected via cannulae that are tunneled from the chest subcutaneously, and exit in the upper abdominal wall. The main advantages to this device include its versatility for biventricular support and the ability to use it in small patients.

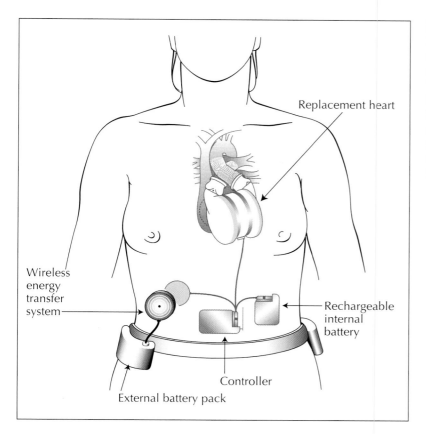

Replacement heart

Wireless energy transfer system

Rechargeable internal battery

Controller

External battery pack

FIGURE 14-23. The Abiocor total artificial heart (Abiomed Corp., Danvers, MA) is implanted in the orthotopic position. Driven by an internal motor, this device uses hydraulically coupled chambers that alternate left sided ejection with right-sided filling. The device is completely implantable with an internal battery. A transcutaneous energy transfer system permits recharging of the battery and device operation via an external coil. The valves of the device are made of polyurethane material thus patients will require chronic anticoagulation. This total artificial heart is undergoing clinical trials in patients who are not potential cardiac transplant recipients. (*Courtesy of* Abiomed Corp., Danvers, MA.)

REFERENCES

1. Barnard CN: A human cardiac transplant: an interim report of a successful operation performed at Groote Schuur Hospital, Cape Town. *S Afr Med J* 1967, 41:1271–1274.

2. Fragomeni LS, Kaye MP: The Registry of the International Society for Heart Transplantation: Fifth Official Report 1988. *J Heart Transplant* 1988, 7:249–253.

3. Gummert JF, Ikonen T, Morris RE: Newer immunosuppressive drugs: a review. *J Am Soc Nephrol* 1999, 10:1366–1380.

4. Kobashigawa JA: Postoperative management following heart transplantation. *Transplant Proc* 1999, 31:2038–2046.

5. Young JB, Winters WL, Bourge R, Uretsky BF: 24th Bethesda Conference: Cardiac Transplantation. Task Force 4: Function of the Heart Transplant Recipient. *J Am Coll Cardiol* 1993, 22:31–41.

6. Evans RW, Manninen DL, Garrison LP Jr, Maier AM: Donor availability as the primary determinant of the future of heart transplantation. *JAMA* 1986, 255:1892–1898.

7. Goldstein D, Oz M, Rose E: Implantable left ventricular assist devices *N Engl J Med* 1998, 339:1522–1533.

8. Hosenpud J, Bennett L, Keck B, *et al.*: The Registry of the International Society for Heart and Lung Transplantation: Fourteenth Official Report 2001. *J Heart Lung Transplant* 2001, 20:805–815.

9. Mancini DM, Eisen H, Kussmaul W, *et al.*: Value of peak exercise oxygen consumption for optimal timing of cardiac transplantation in ambulatory patients with heart failure. *Circulation* 1991, 83:778–786.

10. Costanzo MR: Selection and treatment of candidates for heart transplantation: a statement for health professionals from the Committee on Heart Failure and Cardiac Transplantation of the Council on Clinical Cardiology, American Heart Association. *Circulation* 1995, 92:3593–3612.

11. Aaronson KD, Schwartz JS, Chen TM, *et al.*: Development and prospective validation of a clinical index to predict survival in ambulatory patients referred for cardiac transplant evaluation. *Circulation* 1997, 95:2597–2599.

12. Shumway NE, Lower RR, Stofer RC: Transplantation of the heart. *Adv Surg* 1966, 2:265–284.

13. Kawaguchi A, Gandjbakhch I, Pavie A, *et al.*: Factors affecting survival after heterotopic heart transplantation. *J Thorac Cardiovasc Surg* 1989, 98:928–934.

14. Cooley DA: *Techniques in Cardiac Surgery*, edn 2. Philadelphia: WB Saunders; 1984:372.

15. El Gamel A, Yonan NA, Grant S, *et al.*: Orthotopic cardiac transplantation: a comparison of standard and bicaval Wythenshawe techniques. *J Thorac Cardiovasc Surg* 1995, 109:721–730.

16. Cerilli GJ: *Organ Transplantation and Replacement*. Philadelphia: JB Lippincott; 1988:120.

17. Unverferth DV: *Dilated Cardiomyopathy*. Mt. Kisco, NY: Futura Publishing Co; 1985.

18. Fishman J, Rubin R: Infection in organ transplant recipients. *N Engl J Med* 1998, 338:1741–1751.

19. Paris W, Woodbury A, Thompson S, *et al.*: Returning to work after heart transplantation. *J Heart Lung Transplant* 1993, 12:46–54.

20. Beniaminovitz A, Coromilas J, Oz M, *et al.*: Electrical connection of native and transplanted sinus nodes via atrial pacing improves exercise performance after cardiac transplantation. *Am J Cardiol* 1998, 81:1373–1377.

21. Michler RE, McLaughlin MJ, Chen JM, *et al.*: Clinical experience with cardiac retransplantation. *J Thorac Cardiovasc Surg* 1993, 106:622–629.

22. Ventura HO, Mehra MR, Smart FW, Stapleton DD: Cardiac allograft vasculopathy: current concepts. *Am Heart J* 1995, 129:791–798.

23. Costanzo-Nordin MR: Cardiac allograft vasculopathy: relationship with acute cellular rejection and histocompatibility. *J Heart Lung Transplant* 1992, 11(suppl):90–104.

24. Johnson MR: Transplant coronary artery disease: nonimmunologic risk factors. *J Heart Lung Transplant* 1992, 11(suppl):124–132.

25. McDonald K, Rector TS, Braunlin EA, *et al.*: Association of coronary artery disease in transplant recipients with cytomegalovirus infection. *Am J Cardiol* 1989, 64:359–362.

26. Helman D, Morales D, Edwards N, *et al.*: Left ventricular assist device bridge-to-transplant network improves survival after failed cardiotomy. *Ann Thorac Surg* 1999, 68:1187–1194.

27. Higgins RSD, Silverman NA: Status of permanent cardiac replacement for end-stage congestive heart failure. *Heart Failure Reviews* 1996, 1:39–52.

28. Rose EA, Goldstein DJ: Wearable long-term mechanical support for patients with end-stage heart disease: a tenable goal. *Ann Thorac Surg* 1996, 61:399–402.

29. Kaplon R, Oz M, Kwiatowski K, *et al*: Miniature axial flow pump for ventricular assistance in children and small adults. *J Thorac Cardiovasc Surg* 1996, 111:13–18.

30. Sabbah H, Chaudhry P, Paone G, *et al.*: Passive ventricular constraint with the ACORN prosthetic jacket prevents progressive left ventricular dilation and improves ejection fraction in dogs with moderate heart failure. *J Am Coll Cardiol* 1999, 33:207A.

DIASTOLIC DYSFUNCTION: PATHOPHYSIOLOGY, CLINICAL FEATURES, AND TREATMENT

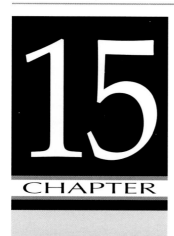

15

CHAPTER

Carl S. Apstein

Diastolic dysfunction occurs when the normal mechanisms that allow the left ventricle (LV) to fill under low pressure become deficient. Diastolic dysfunction may also affect the right ventricle (RV), but there is relatively little information about RV diastolic dysfunction. Therefore this chapter focuses exclusively on LV diastolic dysfunction with the understanding that the same principles undoubtedly apply to the RV.

The cardinal symptom of diastolic dysfunction is dyspnea with exertion, which reflects underlying pulmonary congestion. During exercise, diastolic function must be enhanced so that LV input remains precisely matched to LV output. The rate of diastolic filling must increase because the duration of diastole is shortened by the tachycardia of exercise, and the LV filling rate must increase without increasing pulmonary capillary pressure if pulmonary congestion is to be avoided.

Several elegant mechanisms combine to promote LV diastolic filling during exercise without increasing pulmonary capillary pressure. Myocyte relaxation is normally enhanced by exercise. A greater elastic recoil of the LV in early diastole enhances LV filling by means of a suction effect. The failure of these mechanisms, usually in combination with an increase in LV passive stiffness, results in the dyspnea with exertion that is characteristic of the patient with diastolic dysfunction.

This chapter first reviews normal diastolic physiology and the response to exercise at both the cell and organ level. The clinical settings of diastolic dysfunction are discussed in terms of their different etiologies and time courses. For example, acute ischemia can result in sudden diastolic dysfunction, which resolves rapidly with appropriate therapy; such acute diastolic dysfunction is responsible for the symptoms of chest tightness, wheezing, and dyspnea that often accompany an anginal episode. However, long-standing hypertension and LV hypertrophy (LVH) cause chronic diastolic dysfunction, which is difficult to treat satisfactorily. The effect of normal aging on diastolic function and the high prevalence in the elderly of CHF due to diastolic dysfunction is considered. Last, approaches to the treatment of diastolic dysfunction are outlined, including evidence that exercise training can improve diastolic dysfunction in the elderly.

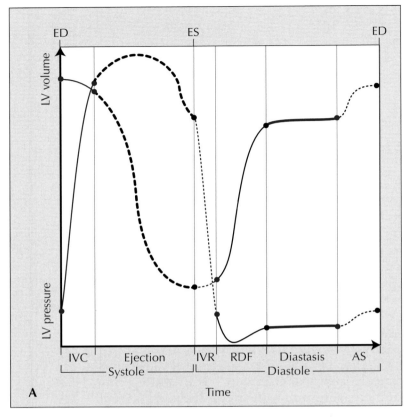

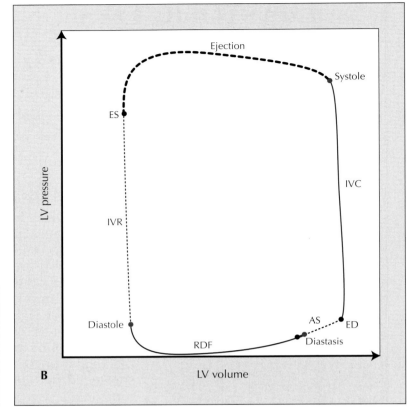

FIGURE 15-1. The place of diastole in the cardiac cycle. The heart is a phasic pump. The function of the diastolic phase is to fill the ventricle with an adequate volume for ejection during the subsequent systole. Classically, diastole has been defined as beginning at aortic valve closure and continuing until mitral valve opening. This figure shows the time-course of LV pressure, volume and the pressure-volume (PV) loop. **A,** The time-course of LV pressure and volume during a single cardiac cycle. **B,** The PV loop for the same cycle. The corresponding phases of systole and diastole are color coded. AS—atrial systole; ED—end diastole; ES—end systole; IVC—isovolumic contraction; IVR—isovolumic relaxation; RDF—rapid diastolic filling. (Courtesy of Dr. Robert Bonow.)

NORMAL LEFT VENTRICULAR DIASTOLIC FILLING AND RESPONSE TO EXERCISE

The Major Determinants of Normal LV Filling

Rate and extent of LV pressure decay

Elastic recoil or restoring force of myocardium

Small transmitral pressure gradients

Low resistance mitral valve orifice and inflow tract

High distensibility or low passive stiffness of LV chamber

Force of atrial contraction

Lack of external constraint from pericardium, pleura, lungs, intrathoracic pressure

Normal Diastolic Reponse to Exercise: Increased Flow Rate Across Mitral Valve

Increased LV elastic recoil and early diastolic LV suction

Increased rate of calcium reuptake

Deinhibition of SERCA by phosholamban

Accelerated titin expansion from greater end-systolic compression

Increased force of atrial contraction

FIGURE 15-2. The major determinants and features of left ventricular (LV) filling. Abnormalities of one or more of these factors can impair normal LV filling and result in diastolic dysfunction. Cardiac function during exercise is critically dependent on mechanisms to increase LV filling (cardiac input) in parallel with LV ejection (cardiac output). Further, pulmonary function and the work of breathing during exercise is also dependent on LV diastolic function because LV diastolic pressure directly affects pulmonary capillary pressure.

TIME COURSE OF DIASTOLE

Early diastole

Myocyte relaxation and relengthening

Cytosolic calcium removal

SR calcium reuptake (SERCA)

SL calcium extrusion (sodium/calcium exchange; Ca^{2+} ATPase)

Actin-myosin cross-bridge detachment

Expansion of compressed titin

LV elastic recoil

Transmitral pressure gradient from LV suction

Late diastole

LV passive stiffness

Left atrial function

FIGURE 15-3. Early and late diastolic physiology. Different factors regulate diastolic function in early and late diastole. Myocyte relaxation, the first step, results from the removal of cytosolic calcium and the expansion of the springlike molecule, titin, which is compressed during systolic cell shortening. Removal of cytosolic calcium reverses the

Both calcium removal and titin expansion are responsive to exercise. The rate of calcium uptake by the sarcoplasmic reticulum is regulated by phospholamban. Unphosphorylated phospholamban inhibits the SR calcium ATPase (SERCA). During exercise, phospholamban is phosphorylated by c-AMP dependent kinases that are activated by the increased sympathetic activity and adrenal catecholamine release that occurs during exercise. The increased SERCA activity accelerates calcium reuptake and relaxation.

During exercise, myocyte shortening and titin compression are greater than in the resting state due to the inotropic effects of the increased sympathetic activity and circulating catecholamines. As a result, titin expands at a greater velocity from its shorter end-systolic position, and myocyte lengthening is more rapid during exercise. The expansion of titin is responsible for the "restoring force" or "elastic recoil" that increases the LV suction effect in early diastole during exercise.

In late diastole during exercise the force of atrial contraction is increased due to the inotropic effect of increased sympathetic activity and circulating catecholamines.

process of excitation-contraction coupling and comprises repolarization-relaxation coupling. Calcium is removed from the cytosol by the sarcoplasmic reticulum (SR), and the sarcolemmal (SL) Na^+/Ca^{2+} exchanger and Ca^{2+} ATPase. As the cytosolic calcium is removed, the actin-myosin cross-bridges release, myofilament active tension in the shortening direction decreases, and the compressed titin expands and lengthens the cell. The movement of calcium through the calcium-handling subcellular organelles during excitation-contraction and repolarization-relaxation is illustrated earlier in this atlas. The rapid relengthening at the cellular level imparts an elastic recoil or restoring force to the left ventricular (LV) wall that creates an LV suction effect that draws blood across the mitral valve. In late diastole, LV passive stiffness and left atrial contraction are the major determinants of LV filling.

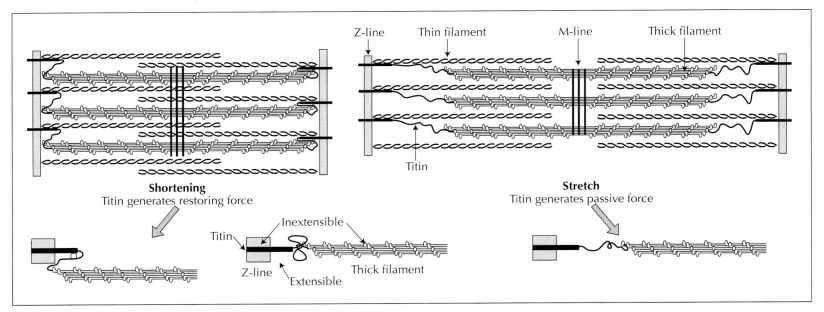

FIGURE 15-4. The role of titin in diastolic function. Titin is a protein that plays a critical role in diastolic function by functioning as a bidirectional spring located between the myosin thick filament and the Z-line. During systolic shortening, titin is compressed. At the start of cell relaxation, the compressed titin re-expands and generates an intracellular "restoring force," to restore sarcomere length to its diastolic position. This restoring force creates ventricular elastic recoil that is important in generating a negative LV pressure in early diastole to draw blood across the mitral valve and facilitate LV filling at low LV and left atrial diastolic (filling) pressures. Later in diastole, as the ventricle fills and the sarcomeres lengthen, titin is stretched and generates a passive force that contributes to LV passive stiffness. (*Courtesy of Dr. Michael Helms and Dr. Douglas Sawyer.*)

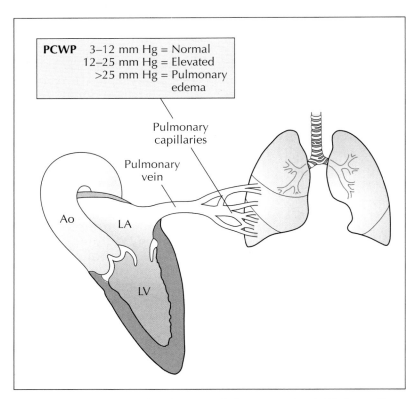

FIGURE 15-5. Relationship between left ventricular (LV) diastolic pressure and pulmonary capillary pressure. Shown here is the heart drawn in diastole with the mitral valve open to illustrate that the LV, left atrium, and pulmonary veins form a common chamber, continuous with the pulmonary capillary bed. Thus, LV diastolic pressure determines pulmonary capillary pressure and the presence or absence of pulmonary congestion and edema.

Left ventricular diastolic pressure is determined by the volume of blood in the LV during diastole and by LV diastolic distensibility or compliance. At the onset of diastole relaxation of the contracted myocardium occurs. This is a dynamic process that takes place during isovolumic relaxation (between aortic valve closure and mitral valve opening) and during early rapid filling of the ventricle. The rapid pressure decay, and the concomitant "untwisting" and elastic recoil of the left ventricle produce a ventricular suction that augments the left atrial–ventricular pressure gradient and thus enhances diastolic filling. During the later phases of diastole the normal LV is composed of completely relaxed myocytes and is very compliant and easily distensible, offering minimal resistance to LV filling over a normal volume range. Therefore, LV filling can normally be accomplished by very low "filling" pressures in the left atrium and pulmonary veins, preserving a low pulmonary capillary pressure (normal pulmonary capillary pressure is < 12 mm Hg), and high degree of lung distensibility. A loss of normal LV diastolic relaxation and distensibility, due to either structural or functional causes, impairs LV filling, resulting in increases in LV diastolic, left atrial, and pulmonary venous pressures, which directly increase pulmonary capillary pressure. The increase in pulmonary capillary pressure results in pulmonary congestion and edema, an increased work of breathing, hypoxemia, and the symptom of dyspnea. (*Adapted from* Apstein *et al.* [1].)

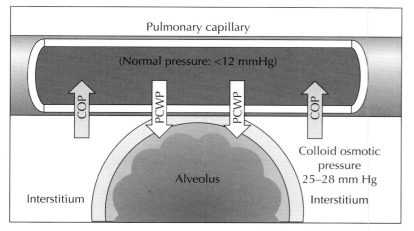

FIGURE 15-6. Mechanism of pulmonary edema in congestive heart failure (CHF). The development of cardiogenic pulmonary edema results from an abnormal imbalance of the pulmonary capillary "wedge" pressure (PCWP) and the colloid osmotic pressure (COP) at the alveolar-pulmonary capillary junction or membrane. The PCWP is normally less than 12 mm Hg and tends to move fluid into the pulmonary interstitium. Normally the PCWP is more than balanced by the COP, whose normal value of 25 to 28 mm Hg exceeds a normal PCWP; thus the net normal force balance tends to retain fluid in the pulmonary capillaries and the lung parenchyma remains dry. When the PCWP exceeds the COP, interstitial pulmonary edema occurs and is drained by pulmonary lymphatics. Alveolar edema occurs when lymphatic capacity is exceeded. With chronic elevation of PCWP, the lymphatic removal capacity is enhanced.

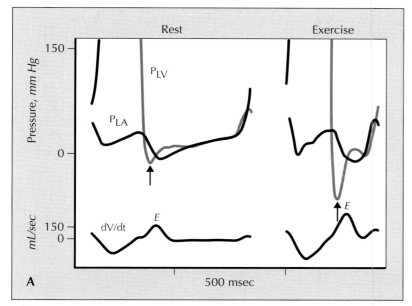

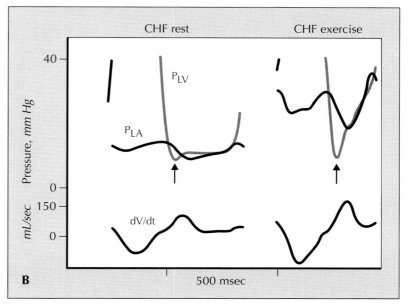

FIGURE 15-7. Effects of exercise and heart failure on early diastolic LV filling (LV suction effect). This figure illustrates the effects of exercise with and without heart failure on LV filling dynamics. **A,** Recording of left ventricular pressure (P_{LV} and left atrial pressure (P_{LA}) and the rate of change of left ventricular volume (dV/dt) at rest and during exercise in a normal dog. During exercise, minimal left ventricular pressure (*arrow*) decreases without any increase in left atrial pressure. This leads to an increase in the peak mitral valve gradient (area between P_{LA} and P_{LV} curves) and produces a larger peak filling rate (E).

B, Effect of heart failure. In a format similar to that of **A,** data are shown at rest and after exercise in a dog following the development of congestive heart failure (CHF). CHF was induced by several weeks of rapid pacing. During exercise after CHF, peak left ventricular filling rate (E wave) increases due to an increase in the early transmitral valve pressure gradient. However, the gradient is produced by an increase in left atrial pressure, instead

of a decrease in LV pressure as occurred during exercise prior to CHF, as shown in **A.**

Thus, the "LV suction effect" comprises these characteristics: the elastic recoil or restoring force contributes to LV pressure decay and drives LV pressure below LA pressure in early diastole to create a transmitral pressure gradient that provides the hydraulic force for early LV filling. In **A,** during exercise in the absence of congestive heart failure (CHF), the nadir of LV pressure decay (*arrow*) reaches a level of a *negative* 10 mm Hg. In **B,** during exercise after CHF, the nadir of LV pressure decay (*arrow*) does not fall below a *positive* 10 mm Hg. Thus, the occurrence of heart failure reduced the suction ability of the LV elastic recoil by approximately 20 mm Hg. This is an example of CHF due to systolic dysfunction (rapid pacing tachycardia model) causing secondary diastolic dysfunction with a loss of the force of early elastic LV recoil. (*Adapted from* Cheng et al. [2,3] and Little and Cheng [4].)

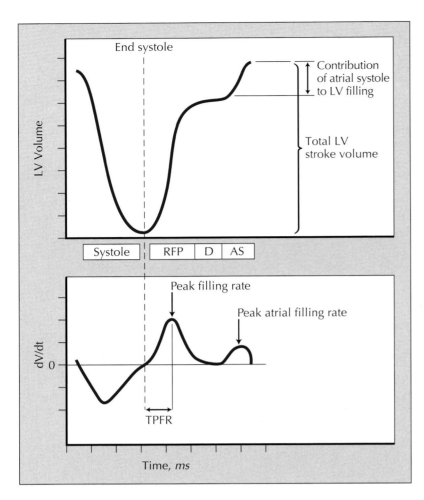

FIGURE 15-8. Left ventricular filling dynamics. The normal left ventricle (LV) has a characteristic pattern of inflow velocities that are altered with the development of diastolic dysfunction. This figure depicts an idealized change of LV volume versus time during systole and diastole. Normally, LV inflow velocity and the volume rate of LV filling is greatest early in diastole, immediately after mitral valve opening; relatively little LV filling occurs in late diastole because most atrial-to-ventricular transfer of blood has occurred in early and mid-diastole and the amount of blood transported by atrial contraction is relatively small.

This figure shows an idealized plot of left ventricular volume versus time (*top*) and the rate of change of volume (dV/dt) versus time (*bottom*) as might be obtained from radionuclide ventriculography. The representative cardiac cycle begins at end diastole. Subsequent events as depicted by the bars in the center of the figure include 1) systole, during which left ventricular volume decreases to a minimum; and 2) diastole, the beginning of which is signaled by the opening of the mitral valve and the onset of left ventricular filling. Diastole has three distinct phases in normal individuals: 1) the rapid filling phase (RFP) during which the LV fills rapidly, dV/dt reaches its maximum, the peak filling rate occurs; 2) diastasis (D) during which relatively little left ventricular volume change occurs; and 3) atrial systole (AS), in which active atrial contraction fills the LV to its end-diastolic volume. The diastolic parameters that have been derived from such analysis are the peak filling rate, the time to peak filling rate (TPFR), the percent contribution of atrial systole, and the first third filling fraction. (*Adapted from* Labovitz and Pearson [5].)

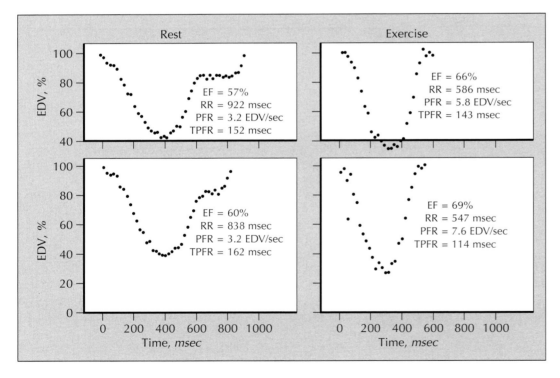

FIGURE 15-9. Effect of exercise on left ventricular (LV) filling dynamics in normal humans. These time-activity curves illustrate the effect of exercise tachycardia on indices of LV diastolic filling in a normal subject. Two time-activity curves obtained under resting conditions are shown (*left*) at two different resting cycle lengths (RR intervals). Differences in resting cycle length are buffered by changes in the diastasis interval, with little change in the characteristics of the rapid filling phase as assessed by peak filling rate (PFR) and time to peak filling rate (TPFR). During submaximal and then maximal exercise (*right*), with reduction of cycle length and disappearance of the diastasis period, diastolic indices become highly sensitive to heart rate fluctuations. Peak filling rate and time to peak filling rate change substantially between cycle lengths of 586 msec (heart rate, 102) and 547 msec (heart rate, 110). EDV—end-diastolic volume; EF—ejection fraction. (*Adapted from* Bonow [6].)

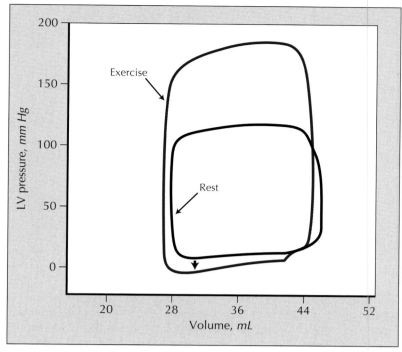

FIGURE 15-10. Pressure-volume (P-V) loops from a normal conscious dog during rest and exercise. The *arrow* denotes the decreased minimal left ventricular (LV) pressure and increased elastic recoil during exercise leading to a maintained filling volume at normal pressure despite a decreased filling time. Therefore, the higher flow velocities were achieved by a higher pressure gradient due to a lower LV pressure, thus maintaining the integrity of the lungs. (*Adapted from* Cheng *et al.* [7].)

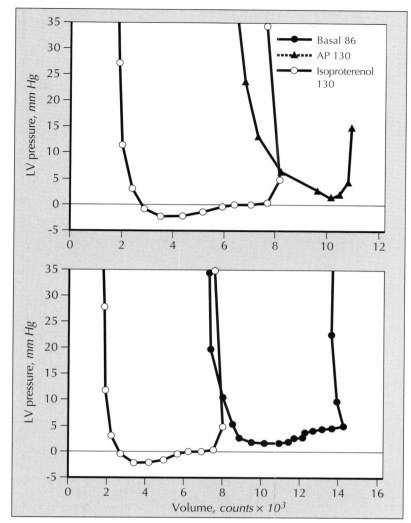

FIGURE 15-11. Left ventricular (LV) diastolic suction in normal humans. This figure shows the LV diastolic pressure-volume (P-V) relationship in a patient without significant cardiovascular disease. **A,** Diastolic P-V relations are shown during atrial pacing (AP) and during isoproterenol at similar heart rates (130 beats per minute). With pacing, LV pressure declines throughout most of the filling period. With isoproterenol, pressure fall is complete early in diastole with the subsequent development of negative diastolic pressure. **B,** baseline (basal) and isoproterenol data are compared. The contours of the filling portion of the curves are similar, but the extent of pressure fall during isoproterenol (from a smaller end-systolic volume) is greater, resulting in negative diastolic pressure. The P-V loops were obtained with simultaneous radionuclide angiography and a micro-manometer-tipped LV catheter. (*Adapted from* Udelson *et al.* [8].)

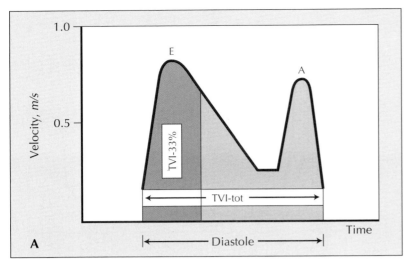

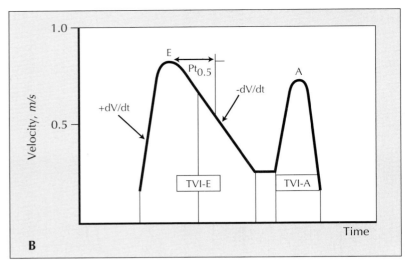

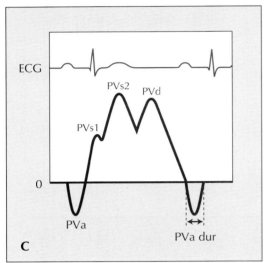

FIGURE 15-12. Assessment of LV diastolic function by Doppler echocardiography. Transmitral and pulmonary venous flow patterns. **A,** Early diastolic (*E*) and atrial filling velocity (*A*). **B,** Pressure half time ($PT_{0.5}$). **C,** The pulmonary vein flow pattern (PV): atrial flow reversal (Pva), early systolic (PVs1) and midsystolic (PVs2) flow

velocity as well as diastolic flow velocity (PVd). Pva*dur* represents the duration of atrial flow reversal.

Left ventricular (LV) diastolic function can be assessed by Doppler echocardiography and analysis of the transmitral and pulmonary venous flow patterns. The normal patterns are illustrated in this figure. Normally, LV inflow velocity and the volume rate of LV filling is greatest early in diastole, immediately after mitral valve opening, and is responsible for the normally tall E wave of the Doppler echocardiogram. Relatively little LV filling occurs in late diastole because most atrial-to-ventricular transfer of blood has occurred in early and mid-diastole. The amount of blood transported by atrial contraction is relatively small, the velocity imparted by the atrial contraction (the A wave of the Doppler echocardiogram) is relatively low, and the normal E/A wave ratio is greater than 1, and approaches a value of 2 in younger individuals.

With the diastolic dysfunction that accompanies ischemia and/or hypertrophy, myocardial relaxation is characteristically impaired and the rate and amount of early diastolic LV filling is reduced with a resultant shift of LV filling to the later part of diastole. The Doppler E wave is decreased. The hemodynamic load on the atrium is increased, and atrial contraction makes a more important contribution to ventricular filling than in normal subjects. This is reflected by an increase in the Doppler A wave, and decrease in the E/A ratio. The chronic atrial overload often eventually results in atrial fibrillation, and the loss of atrial contraction can dramatically reduce LV filling, left atrial emptying, and LV stroke-volume. The redistribution of filling from early to late diastole also means that LV filling and left atrial emptying are compromised more in patients with diastolic dysfunction than in normal subjects by the occurrence of tachycardia; an increased heart rate shortens the duration of diastole and truncates the important late phase of diastolic filling. TVI-tot—total time-velocity integral; TVI-33%—first third filling fraction; TVI-E, TVI-A—time-velocity integrals of E and A waves, respectively. (*Adapted from* Mandinov *et al.* [9].)

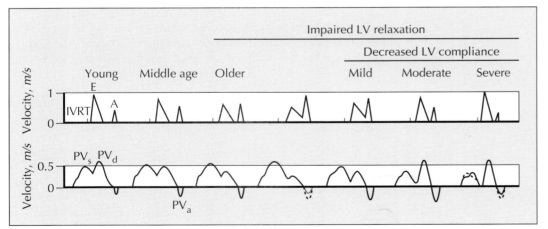

FIGURE 15-13. Doppler transmitral (*upper tracing*) and pulmonary (*lower tracing*) venous flow patterns with diastolic dysfunction. The transmitral velocity pattern provides valuable information regarding LV diastolic function. In healthy young individuals, most diastolic filling occurs early in diastole so that the E/A ratio is greater than 1. When relaxation is impaired, early diastolic filling decreases, and more blood is

transported late in diastole by atrial contraction; this is reflected by a reversed E/A ratio (E/A < 1, or "delayed relaxation pattern"), increased deceleration time, and increased isovolumic relaxation time (IVRT). With disease progression, LV compliance decreases, and filling pressure (LV and left atrial diastolic pressure) increases with the effect of increasing early LV filling ("pseudonormalization pattern" with E/A > 1). This pattern results from abnormalities of both relaxation and compliance, and is distinguished from a normal filling pattern by a shortened early deceleration time. With a severe decrease in LV compliance, left atrial pressure becomes markedly elevated, and this maintains diastolic filling that results in a "restrictive" pattern with E/A greater than 1. (*Adapted from* Mandinov *et al.* [9].)

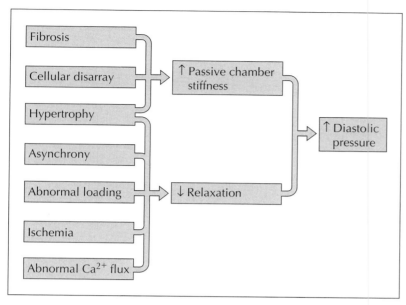

FIGURE 15-14. Factors that contribute to diastolic dysfunction. **Structural or compositional factors.** Fibrosis and myocyte hypertrophy are the two most common and important structural or compositional abnormalities that increase resistance to filling. Myocardial fibrosis commonly is present in coronary artery disease, LVH, and with dilated cardiomyopathy from almost any cause. The scarring that follows myocardial infarctions can be regional or diffuse

depending on the distributions, size, and numbers of the infarcts and whether they are transmural or subendocardial. Diffuse interstitial fibrosis is common when LVH occurs in response to a pressure overload such as hypertension or aortic stenosis. Several mechanisms may contribute to the interstitial fibrosis of LVH including a "compensatory response" to tether myocytes subjected to increased wall stress, a response to the recurrent ischemia and/or hypoxia that occurs in the hypertrophied myocardium, the replacement of necrotic myocytes, and hormonal factors (angiotensin; nitric oxide deficiency). Rarer causes of myocardial fibrosis include hemochromatosis and sarcoidosis. Cardiac amyloid deposition and myocardial edema are other compositional alterations that increase resistance to filling. Additional factors now shown in the figure include vascular turgidity, extrinsic factors, and ventricular interaction.

Vascular turgidity. The myocardium is a richly vascular tissue. Increased pressure and volume in the coronary arteries or veins increase vascular turgidity and LV chamber stiffness.

Extrinsic factors and ventricular interaction. Resistance to ventricular filling can also come from the pericardium, or from increased pleural or mediastinal pressure. The pericardium may be fibrotic or calcified and/or contain an effusion large enough to impair ventricular filling. Even a normal pericardium can impair LV diastolic filling by a mechanism of ventricular interaction in which right ventricular dilation results in pericardial constraint of the LV. An increase in right ventricular diastolic pressure and/or volume can also contribute to LV diastolic dysfunction by resisting interventricular septal movement during LV filling. (*Adapted from* Braunwald *et al.* [10].)

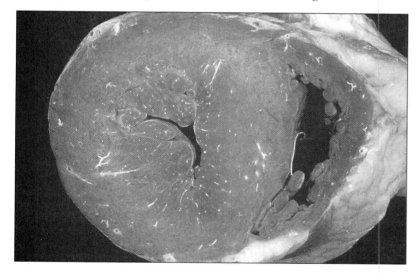

FIGURE 15-15. Marked LV hypertrophy (LVH). Shown is a cross-section through the LV of a case of marked concentric LVH. The marked increase in muscle mass and streaks of fibrosis make it easy to envision how such a ventricle would have an increased resistance to filling. (*From* Becker and Anderson [11]; with permission.)

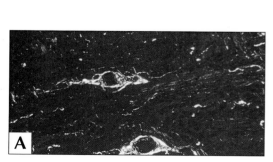

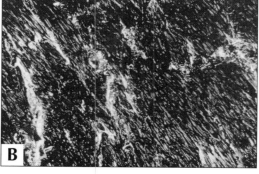

FIGURE 15-16. (SEE COLOR PLATE.) Pathologic hypertrophy and cardiac interstitium. These are photomicrographs of normal and hypertensive human left ventricles. The picrosirius

polarization technique is used to highlight fibrillar collagen in birefringent red, green, and yellow. **A,** The small amount of normal fibrillar collagen present in the interstitium and adventitia of intramyocardial vasculature is shown (magnification, × 40). **B,** The diffuse fibrous tissue response that occurs with hypertensive LV hypertrophy. This marked increase in fibrillar collagen contributes importantly to the increased resistance to filling and resultant diastolic dysfunction in patient with concentric LVH secondary to hypertension (magnification, × 10). (*From* Weber and Brilla [12]; with permission.)

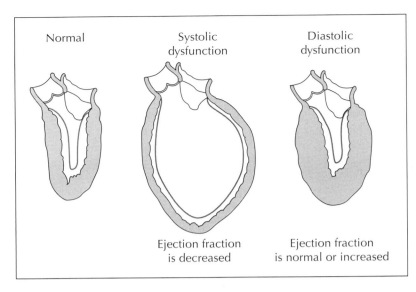

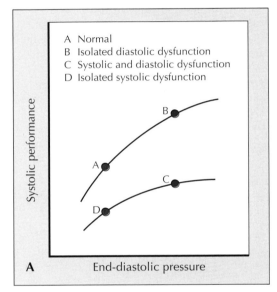

FIGURE 15-17. Typical LV geometry with systolic and diastolic dysfunction. This figures illustrates the LV long axis view in diastole (note open mitral valve and closed aortic valve) of

examples of a normal (*left*), a dilated cardiomyopathy with systolic dysfunction (*center*), and a concentric LVH with "pure" (strain-independent) diastolic dysfunction (*right*). The *thin lines* indicate the extent of wall motion during systolic contraction.

Systolic dysfunction (*center*) is characterized by a reduced extent of contraction, a decreased ejection fraction, and LV dilation. Strain-dependent diastolic dysfunction occurs when dilated ventricles with systolic dysfunction approach their limit of dilation and distensibility, and resistance to diastolic filling increases. Thus many patients have both systolic and diastolic dysfunction.

Pure diastolic dysfunction (*right*), without systolic dysfunction, commonly occurs with concentric LV hypertrophy (LVH), and is associated with a normal or supernormal extent of contraction and ejection fraction. An increased resistance to diastolic filling results from the increased mass itself, impaired relaxation of the hypertrophied myocytes, interstitial fibrosis, and subendocardial ischemia, which is often present with concentric LVH. Diastolic dysfunction can occur in the absence of LVH with myocardial infiltrative or fibrotic disease processes. The increased resistance to filling results in elevated LV diastolic (filling) pressures that are transmitted to the pulmonary capillaries and can cause pulmonary edema.

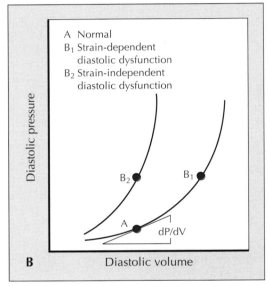

FIGURE 15-18. Hemodynamic differences between left ventricular systolic and diastolic dysfunction. A, Systolic performance is plotted against an index of end-diastolic fiber strain (*ie*, end-diastolic pressure). *Point A* defines the coordinate of a normal ventricle. If this heart were subjected to an excessive volume load, the coordinates of systolic performance and end-diastolic pressure would move up along the curve to *point B*;

thus the signs and symptoms of congestive failure would exist in the presence of normal systolic performance. The *lower curve* represents a typical patient with dilated cardiomyopathy; *point C* indicates the coordinate of an untreated patient with systolic and diastolic dysfunction. Diuretic therapy might cause a transition to *point D* (isolated systolic dysfunction), in which the patient would no longer exhibit venous congestion or diastolic dysfunction.

B, Diastolic pressure-volume relations. The slope of a tangent to this nonlinear relation represents chamber stiffness (dP/dV). *Point A* defines the coordinate of a normal heart. A volume load causes a strain-dependent increase in chamber stiffness (a shift from *point A* to *point B₁*). In the second example (B2), filling pressure is increased, but end-diastolic volume and muscle strain are normal; this is a typical example of increased chamber stiffness that is strain-independent. (*Adapted from* Levine and Gaasch [13].)

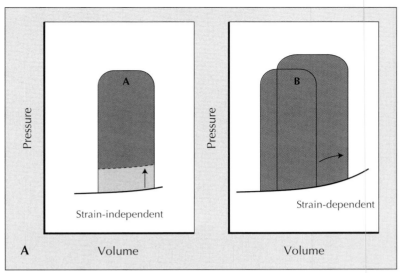

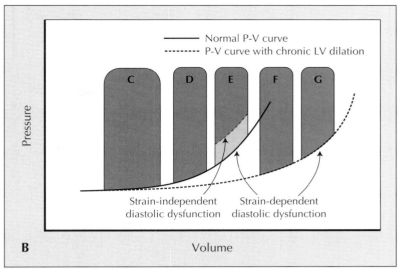

FIGURE 15-19. LV pressure-volume loops with systolic and diastolic function. **A,** Pure diastolic dysfunction. Different types of diastolic dysfunction are illustrated by schematic LV pressure-volume (PV) loops. Shown are two examples of the two types of diastolic dysfunction, *strain-independent* and *strain-dependent*, in the setting of normal systolic function. The terms "pure" or "isolated" diastolic dysfunction indicate the absence of systolic dysfunction. The *dashed line* in the left panel (PV loop A) shows *strain-independent* diastolic dysfunction: the diastolic portion of the PV loop is shifted upwards (*dashed line*) so that diastolic pressure is increased relative to a given volume. A common cause of strain-independent diastolic dysfunction is concentric LVH due to chronic hypertension or aortic stenosis. Chronic constrictive pericardial disease is a rarer cause. The right panel (PV loop B) shows *strain-dependent* diastolic dysfunction. The PV loop has shifted rightwards because of an increase in diastolic volume that imparts an increase in length or strain to the myofibrils during diastole. Diastolic filling pressures and LV diastolic chamber stiffness (*ie,* the slope of the PV curve) are increased because of this volume or strain increase. A typical example of pure strain-dependent diastolic dysfunction is a case of intravenous volume overload in a patient with normal systolic function. In such a case, restoration of a normal LV volume will restore the PV loop to its normal position and reverse the strain-dependent diastolic dysfunction. An acute, reversible rightward shift of the PV loop needs to be distinguished from a chronic volume overload that increases LV volume by a process of remodeling with resultant chronic LV dilation (see right panel).

B, Combined systolic and diastolic dysfunction. *Loop C* represents a normal PV loop. *Loop E,* with the diastolic portion inscribed by the *solid line* and lying on the extended normal PV curve, illustrates strain-dependent diastolic dysfunction in combination with systolic dysfunction, such as could occur in a case of acute myocarditis in a previously normal ventricle. The decreased loop area and rightward shift are characteristic of systolic dysfunction. The diastolic portion of the PV loop falls along an extended normal LV diastolic PV curve, *ie,* a diastolic PV curve that would be recorded from an acute increase in LV volume without chronic LV dilation. Movement of loop E rightwards from the normal loop C position indicates an increase in LV volume and diastolic filling pressures. Because the

diastolic pressure-volume relation is curvilinear, its slope increases as volume increases reflecting an increase in chamber stiffness and increased resistance to LV filling at larger LV volumes.

The *dashed line* diastolic portion drawn in loop E illustrates a case in which both strain-dependent and strain-independent diastolic dysfunction occur in the setting of acute systolic dysfunction. An example of this combination could be a large acute MI that resulted in acute systolic dysfunction and LV dilation, rightward loop movement, and strain-dependent diastolic dysfunction; in addition, myocardial ischemia could cause superimposed strain-independent diastolic dysfunction, which shifts the diastolic PV loop portion upward as indicated by the *arrow* and *dashed line.*

Loop D represents a case of pure systolic dysfunction in which LV diastolic volume is not increased enough to increase LVEDP significantly. Loop D could result from appropriate therapy to reduce LV volume and preload in the acute myocarditis example of loop E. Such treatment would alleviate the strain-dependent diastolic dysfunction, but the systolic dysfunction would persist as indicated by the rightward shift and the abnormally low area of loop D.

Loops F and G represent chronically remodeled ventricles with chronic volume overload from valvular insufficiency or chronic LV dilation from dilated cardiomyopathy. In loop F, LV volume is abnormally large, but because the ventricle is chronically dilated, the P-V curve is flatter than normal, and a normal or reduced LV diastolic chamber stiffness is present. Thus, in loop F, diastolic dysfunction is absent, and the chamber operates at a normal compliance, despite chronic LV dilation. Systolic dysfunction is indicated by the reduced PV loop area and rightward shift. Loop G represents a case in which acute strain-dependent diastolic dysfunction has been superimposed on a chronically dilated ventricle. Such a case could occur when a patient with dilated cardiomyopathy and "compensated" CHF discontinues diuretic and vasodilator therapy and LV volume increases acutely; clinical "decompensation" then follows as strain-dependent diastolic dysfunction occurs. Loop G is also characteristic of a patient with dilated cardiomyopathy and combined systolic and diastolic dysfunction prior to any therapy.

STRAIN-DEPENDENT AND -INDEPENDENT CAUSES OF LV DIASTOLIC DYSFUNCTION

Strain-dependent	Strain-independent
Iatrogenic volume overload	Acute myocardial ischemia or hypoxia
Nephrogenic congestive failure (*eg,* obstructive uropathy)	Chronic ischemic heart disease (*eg,* small fibrotic ventricle)
Anemia	Concentric LV hypertrophy (*eg,* aortic stenosis, hypertension)
Cirrhosis	Hypertrophic cardiomyopathy
Hyperplastic bone disease (*eg,* Paget's disease)	Endocardial fibroelastosis
Arteriovenous fistula	Infiltrative myocardial disease (*eg,* amyloid)
Heart rate mismatch	Constrictive pericardial disease
Thyrotoxicosis	
Thiamine deficiency	
Chronic volume overload (eg, valvular insufficiency)	
Dilated cardiomyopathy (eg, MI with post-MI remodeling and LV dilation	

FIGURE 15-20. Causes of LV diastolic dysfunction. The most common cause of "pure" (strain-independent) diastolic dysfunction is concentric LVH from hypertension. (*Adapted from* Levine and Gaasch [13].)

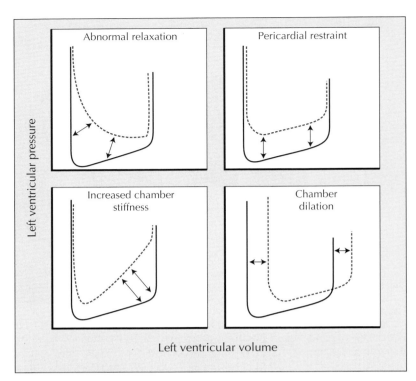

FIGURE 15-21. Diastolic dysfunction reflected in the pressure-volume relation. This figure illustrates the mechanisms that cause diastolic dysfunction. Only the bottom half of the pressure-volume loop in depicted. *Solid lines* represent normal subjects; *dashed lines* represent patients with diastolic dysfunction. (*Adapted from* Zile [14].)

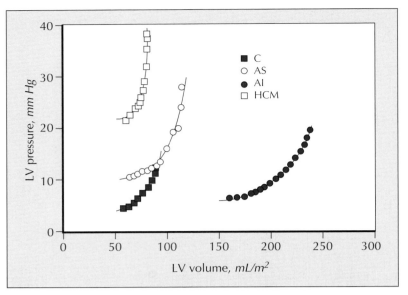

FIGURE 15-22. The diastolic pressure-volume (PV) relation with different types of heart disease. This figure shows the diastolic PV relationship in a control (C) subject and a patient with aortic stenosis (AS), aortic insufficiency (AI), and hypertrophic cardiomyopathy (HCM), respectively. Note that the PV relation is shifted upwards in the AS patient but even more in the patient with HCM, whereas the curve is shifted to the right in the volume overload hypertrophy (AI). The calculated slope of the P-V relation represents the constant of chamber stiffness. Chamber stiffness is increased in AS and HCM (decreased compliance), whereas stiffness is decreased in chronic volume overload (AI) due to LV remodeling with an increase in chamber size (increased compliance). (*Adapted from* Mandinov *et al.* [9].)

FIGURE 15-23. Parameters and causes of diastolic dysfunction. IVRT—isovolumic relaxation time; LV—left ventricular; LVH—left ventricular hypertrophy. (*Adapted from* Apstein [1].)

DIASTOLIC DYSFUNCTION: PARAMETERS AND ETIOLOGY

PHYSIOLOGIC ABNORMALITY	ALTERATION IN PARAMETER OF ASSESSMENT	COMMON ETIOLOGY
Delayed or incomplete relaxation	↑ Tau*	LV hypertrophy
	↑ IVRT	Myocardial ischemia
	↓ E/A ratio†	LV asynchrony
		Abnormal loading
Early diastolic filling abnormalities	↓ Peak filling rate ‡	Delayed relaxation
	↑ Time to peak filling §	LV asynchrony
	↓ E/A ratio	
Late diastolic filling abnormalities	↑ Diastolic P/V relationship	LV chamber dilation
	Normal or ↑ E/A ratio	Restrictive/constrictive filling pattern
Increased LV passive chamber stiffness	↑ Diastolic P/V relation ¶	↑ Collagen and fibrosis
	↑ Stiffness constant**	Myocardial infiltration (eg, amyloid)
		↑ Vascular turgor
		Concentric LVH
		Post-MI hypertrophy and fibrosis
		LV chamber dilation

*Time constant of isovolumic pressure decay.
†Ratio of early and late LV inflow as detected by Doppler echocardiography.
‡dV/dt max.
§Time to dV/dt max.
¶Upward shift of chamber stiffness.

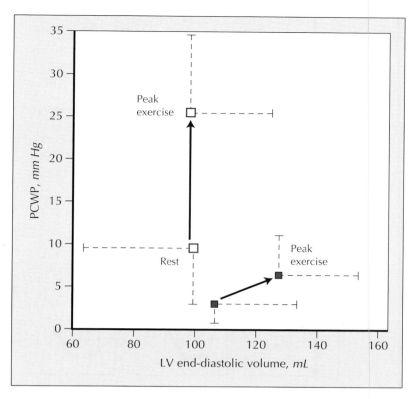

FIGURE 15-24. Effect of exercise on pulmonary capillary pressure in patients with diastolic dysfunction. This figure plots pulmonary capillary wedge pressure versus left ventricular (LV) end-diastolic volume. *Arrows* indicate the changes from rest to peak exercise in patients and control subjects during symptom-limited upright bicycle exercise.

The patients in this study had severe clinical heart failure (New York Heart Association class III or IV), but normal systolic function, *ie,* normal ejection fractions, and no significant valvular, pericardial, or coronary artery disease. Most had concentric LV hypertrophy secondary to hypertension, but four elderly patients had only chronic hypertension. These patients were compared to age and gender-matched controls during symptom-limited upright bicycle exercise.

The controls (*closed boxes*) had more distensible left ventricles at rest, as manifested by a lower pulmonary capillary wedge pressure (PCWP) at a larger LV end-diastolic volume (LVEDV). During exercise, the control subjects increased their LVEDV, consistent with utilization of the Frank-Starling mechanism, and the increase in LVEDV was associated with a modest and proportional increase in PCWP that stayed within normal range.

In contrast, during exercise the patients with diastolic dysfunction (*open boxes*) did not increase their LVEDV, *ie,* they were unable to utilize the Frank-Starling mechanism, presumably because their stiff, nondistensible ventricles resisted any increase in end-diastolic volume. Rather, during exercise in these patients, the PCWP increased markedly to pulmonary edema levels. This dramatic increase in PCWP, undoubtedly reflecting a comparable increase in LV diastolic pressures, suggests a very stiff ventricle that is unable to accommodate even a small increase in volume. Alternatively, the marked increase in PCWP suggests the occurrence of subendocardial ischemia and an "exaggerated" impairment of diastolic relaxation of the hypertrophied myocardium secondary to ischemia. (*Adapted from* Kitzman *et al.* [15].)

DIASTOLIC DYSFUNCTION WITH ISCHEMIA, HYPERTROPHY AND OTHER CAUSES

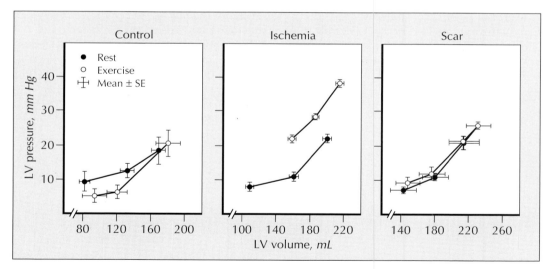

FIGURE 15-25. Effect of exercise, ischemia, and infarction on the diastolic pressure-volume (P-V) relationship. This figure reports LV diastolic P-V curves in the three patient groups at rest and during exercise. The simultaneous measures of LV diastolic pressure and volume define LV distensibility or compliance or chamber stiffness. In normal patients ("Control"), during the rest state LV pressure was approximately 9 mm Hg in early diastole, and increased to about 15 mm Hg at end-diastole. Exercise caused a marked downward shift of the LV diastolic P-V curve in early diastole, and a lesser decrease of mean LV diastolic pressure relative to the rest state. During exercise, these control patients increased their cardiac output three- to fourfold. Because of this physiologic increase in LV diastolic distensibility, the increase in cardiac output was accomplished without an increase of LV diastolic pressure and pulmonary capillary pressure. This increase in measured early diastolic distensibility results from the elegant mechanisms that ensure that cardiac input keeps pace with cardiac output during exercise with preservation of a low pulmonary capillary pressure. To increase systolic function during exercise, the β-adrenergic system increases cAMP levels to increase systolic calcium entry and SR calcium release, with a consequent increase in contractility, systolic fiber shortening, and compression of titin. But the rate of diastolic SR calcium reuptake is also accelerated by the cAMP increase, and the greater extent of systolic fiber shortening results in an increased early diastolic recoil mechanism, decreasing intra-LV pressure in early diastole, to "pull" blood into the LV and facilitate LV filling. These mechanisms result in an increase in measured LV distensibility during exercise in normal patients, manifested by a downward shift of the LV diastolic P-V curve during early diastole, in the control panel (*left*) of this figure.

Effects of ischemia. The *middle panel* reports the LV diastolic P-V curve in patients with coronary artery disease who developed angina and ischemia with exercise. (*continued*)

FIGURE 15-25. (*continued*) The P-V curve at rest was similar to that of the control patients, but with exercise a marked upward shift occurred, such that LV end-diastolic pressure was 40 mm Hg and mean diastolic pressure was approximately 30 mm Hg. Such an increase in LV diastolic pressure would cause significant pulmonary congestion.

This upward shift of the LV diastolic P-V curve, and the consequent pulmonary congestion during exercise-induced ischemia, explains why many patients with coronary disease have respiratory symptoms together with their anginal pain, often complaining of wheezing, chest tightness, inability to take a deep breath, or shortness of breath. Such respiratory symptoms may occur in the absence of anginal pain and are often referred to as "anginal equivalents." Often these "anginal" symptoms are quite similar to symptoms of heart failure, which is not surprising

because the responsible mechanism is an increase of pulmonary capillary pressure in both cases. Airway resistance and lung compliance decrease during an anginal episode concomitant with the increase in LV diastolic chamber stiffness and LV diastolic pressure. This upward shift of the LV diastolic P-V curve was completely reversible with recovery after exercise.

Effect of healed infarction (scar). The *right* panel reports the LV diastolic P-V curves in patients with a healed myocardial infarction but without exercise-induced ischemia. Such patients lost the early diastolic increase in distensibility during exercise that was seen in the control patients, so that LV diastolic filling was not facilitated by an increase in distensibility. Because exercise-induced ischemia did not occur, there was no upward shift of the LV diastolic P-V curve. (*Adapted from* Carroll *et al.* [16,17] and Pepine and Wiener [18].)

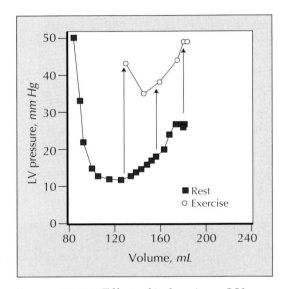

FIGURE 15-26. Effect of ischemia on LV pressure-volume (P-V) relation. The classic P-V shift of ischemia is shown by this patient with coronary disease who had ischemia during exercise. At all diastolic volumes, pressure is clearly elevated versus the resting coordinates. (*Adapted from* Carroll and Carroll [19].)

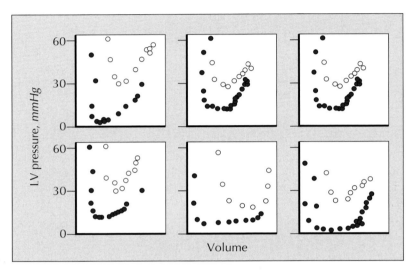

FIGURE 15-27. Six left ventricular diastolic-volume plots from different patients with coronary artery disease illustrate some of the heterogeneity seen with ischemia. By end-diastole, some patients, *eg*, those represented in the *middle panel lower row*, have no or little shift in their diastolic pressure-volume relation. The *open circles* are during exercise-induced ischemia. The *closed circles* are at rest. (*Adapted from* Carroll and Carroll [19].)

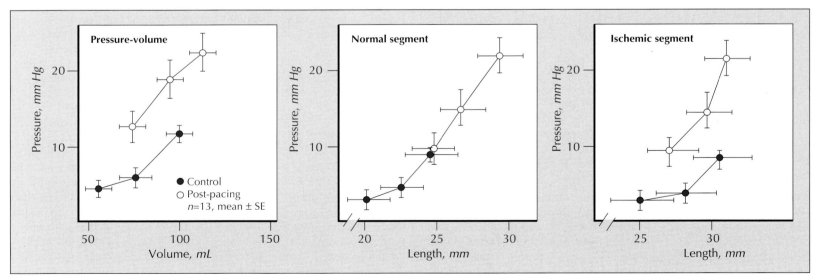

FIGURE 15-28. Left ventricular diastolic pressure-volume (P-V) and pressure-length relations before and after pacing-induced angina pectoris. In the postpacing state (*left panel*), diastolic P-V coordinates are shifted upwards. The pressure-length analysis

(*middle and right panels*) reveals that the nonischemic myocardial fibers lengthen along the same pressure-length curve; by contrast, there is a marked stiffening of the myocardium in the ischemic segment. (*Adapted from* Sasayama *et al.* [20].)

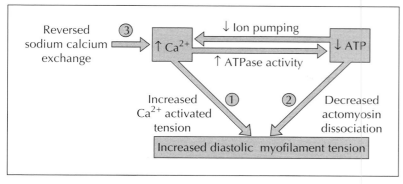

FIGURE 15-29. Increased calcium and decreased ATP as potential causes of acute ischemic diastolic dysfunction. There is a synergistic interaction between an increase in cytosolic calcium and a decrease in ATP availability to increase diastolic myofilament tension. This figure illustrates how an increased cytosolic calcium level or a decrease in ATP availability can

directly increase diastolic myofilament tension and cause or exacerbate ischemic diastolic dysfunction.

An increase in diastolic calcium can directly increase diastolic myofilament tension by binding to troponin C and/or can accelerate a decrease in ATP levels by activating a number of myocyte calcium ATPases. A decrease in ATP availability can directly increase diastolic tension by decreasing the rate or amount of actomyosin dissociation from the rigor complex state. A decrease in ATP availability can also impair the calcium removal from the cytosol by the sarcolemmal and sarcoplasmic reticular calcium ATPases. A decrease in ATP availability can also decrease the sarcolemmal sodium-potassium ATPase (sodium pump) activity, resulting in an increase in intracellular sodium, which increases intracellular calcium by means of sodium-calcium exchange. Thus either cytosolic calcium overload or a decrease in ATP availability can initiate a vicious cycle of calcium-ATP interactions that are synergistic in causing or exacerbating diastolic dysfunction. (*Adapted from* Apstein *et al.* [1].)

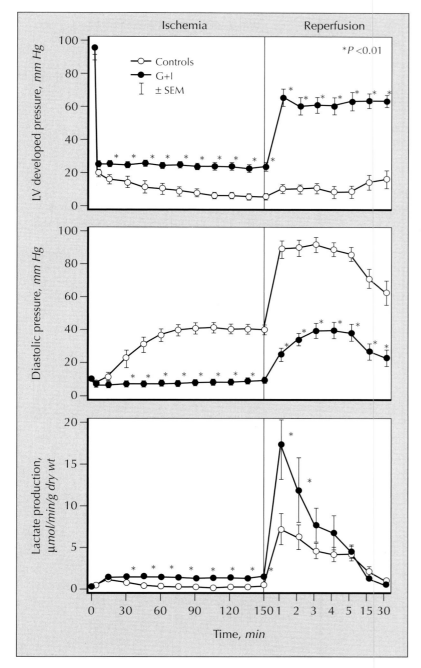

FIGURE 15-30. Prevention of ischemic diastolic dysfunction with increased glycolytic substrate. These graphs show left ventricular developed pressure, LV diastolic pressure, and lactate production of isolated isovolumic erythrocyte-perfused rabbit hearts exposed to 150 minutes of low-flow ischemia and 30 minutes of reperfusion, simulating an evolving myocardial infarction followed by reperfusion. After reduction of coronary perfusion pressure from 100 to 8 mm Hg coronary blood flow decreased to 11% to 13% of initial flow and a prompt decrease of developed pressure occurred. In the control group (controls: $n = 8$; *open circles*) glycolytic flux, as assessed by lactate production started to decrease after 30 minutes of low-flow ischemia concomitant with the decrease in developed pressure and the increase in diastolic pressure, which reflected an increase in diastolic chamber stiffness. In contrast, when glycolytic flux was enhanced by high glucose and insulin infusion (G + I; $n = 8$; *closed circles*) hearts maintained an increased lactate production throughout the ischemic period and showed a greater lactate washout during reperfusion. No increase in diastolic pressure occurred in G + I hearts during ischemia and hearts showed a better recovery of diastolic and systolic function during reperfusion. The G+I hearts had higher levels of ATP during ischemia, suggesting that a decrease in ATP is linked to the occurrence of acute ischemic diastolic dysfunction. (*Adapted from* Eberli *et al.* [21].)

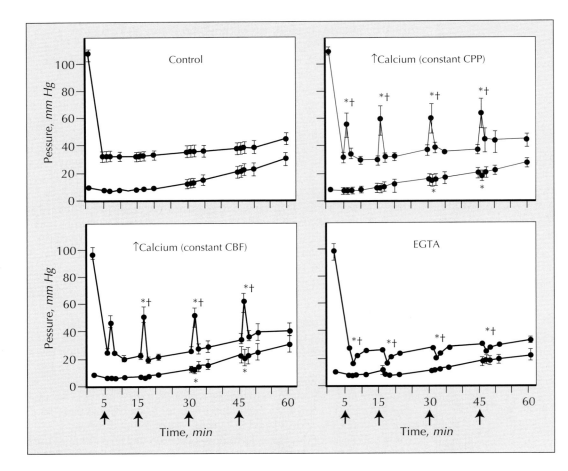

FIGURE 15-31. Lack of direct role for calcium in ischemic diastolic dysfunction. The effect of experimental calcium overload and of the calcium chelator, EGTA, on systolic pressure (*top line*) and diastolic pressure (*bottom line*) is shown during 60 minutes of low-flow ischemia in isovolumic rabbit hearts. The control group (*n* = 6) received 0.08 mL Na Cl 0.09% at 5, 15, 30, and 45 minutes (*arrows*), resulting in no change in hemodynamics. Experimental calcium overload (↑ Calcium) increased systolic pressure in the calcium group perfused at constant coronary perfusion pressure (CPP) (*n* = 6) and in the calcium group perfused at constant coronary blood flow (CBF) (*n* = 7) but did not increase diastolic pressure. EGTA bolus had a negative inotropic effect and no significant effect on isovolumic diastolic pressure (*n* = 6). Therefore, experimental calcium overload did not worsen and calcium removal did not attenuate the ischemic diastolic chamber stiffness increase. These results suggest that acute ischemic diastolic dysfunction is not directly mediated by a calcium activated tension. *Asterisk* indicates $P < 0.01$ vs preintervention. *Dagger* indicates $P < 0.01$ vs control. (*Adapted from* Eberli *et al.* [22].)

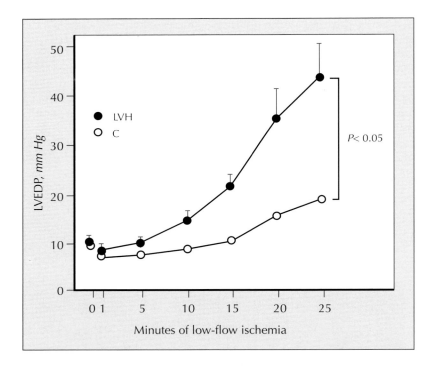

FIGURE 15-32. Exaggerated ischemic diastolic dysfunction with LV hypertrophy. Shown are the effects of low-flow global ischemia on LV end-diastolic pressure (LVEDP) in isolated isovolumic blood-perfused hearts from aortic-banded rats (LVH) and control (C) rats. The ischemic increase in isovolumic LVEDP was earlier and more severe in the hypertrophied hearts compared with controls despite similar levels of coronary flow per gram and myocardial ATP depletion. (*Adapted from* Lorell *et al.* [23].)

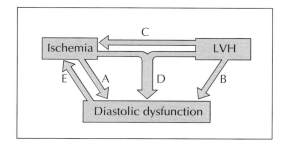

FIGURE 15-33. Interactions among LV hypertrophy (LVH), ischemia, and diastolic dysfunction. Ischemia and LVH can each cause diastolic dysfunction (*arrows A and B*). The presence of LVH predisposes to ischemia (*arrow C*). Hearts with LVH develop worse acute ischemic diastolic dysfunction than nonhypertrophied hearts, and the resultant exaggerated acute

ischemic diastolic dysfunction is superimposed on the stiff ventricle of LVH, resulting in a marked resistance to LV filling (*thick arrow D*). This exaggerated acute ischemic impairment of LV relaxation in the hypertrophied ventricle can markedly increase LV diastolic pressure, and exacerbate subendocardial ischemia by compression of the subendocardial vasculature (*arrow E*). Thus a vicious cycle is created in which LVH predisposes to ischemia, the ischemia causes an exaggerated impairment of relaxation in the heart with LVH, and this in turn worsens the severity of the subendocardial ischemia.

Why does LVH predispose to ischemia? Several mechanisms appear to be responsible. There is inadequate coronary growth relative to muscle mass and a resultant decreased capillary density. The increased wall thickness increases the epicardial-endocardial distance resulting in greater transmural dissipation of perfusion pressure and lower subendocardial perfusion pressure. Coronary vascular remodeling occurs with increased medial thickness and perivascular fibrosis. The increased LV mass and inadequate vascular growth results in altered coronary vascular resting tone (loss of coronary vasodilator reserve), so that there is a limited ability to increase myocardial perfusion in response to stress and an increase in oxygen demand; the vascular remodeling also contributes to the inability to increase coronary flow. Patients with chronic hypertension and hypertensive LVH have an increased incidence of coronary atherosclerosis. Last, an increased LV diastolic pressure exerts a compressive force against the subendocardium and restricts subendocardial perfusion.

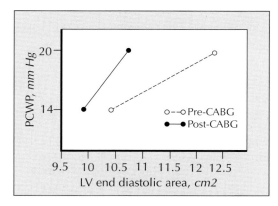

FIGURE 15-34. Acute increase in LV diastolic stiffness immediately after coronary artery bypass surgery. This figure shows the LV diastolic P-V relation of a representative patient before (pre) and immediately after (post) coronary artery bypass graft surgery (CABG). The pressure area relation is plotted. The pulmonary capillary wedge pressure is an index of LV end-diastolic pressure and the LV end-diastolic area determined by echocardiography is an index of LV diastolic volume. Thus, two points on the LV diastolic P-V curve are represented. Immediately after CABG, the LV end-diastolic area was smaller at each pressure level as reflected by a leftward shift of the pressure-area relation, indicating an increase in LV diastolic chamber stiffness. A similar leftward shift was observed in all 20 patients studied. (*Adapted from* McKenney *et al.* [24].)

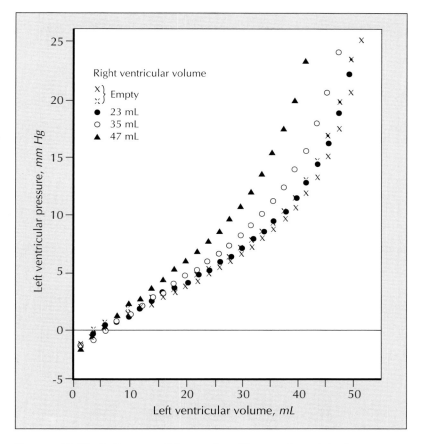

FIGURE 15-35. Influence of the pericardium and ventricular interaction on diastolic function. This figure shows LV diastolic pressure-volume (P-V) relation at varying levels of right ventricular filling in the dog. Note the upward shift at higher right ventricular volumes. (*Adapted from* Taylor *et al.* [25].)

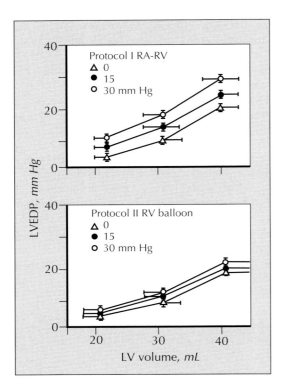

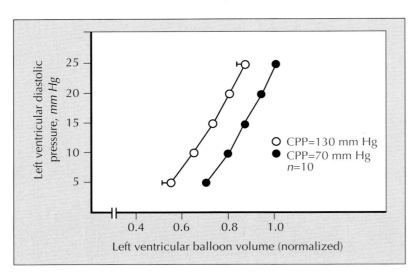

FIGURE 15-36. Effect of increased coronary venous turgor on LV diastolic stiffness. In these experiments, coronary venous pressure was increased by increasing the height of a blood reservoir connected to a cannula that opened in both the right atrium and right ventricle of a canine heart. The *top panel* shows that an increase in the RA-RV diastolic pressure over a range of 0 to 30 mm Hg was associated with a parallel upward shift of the LV diastolic pressure volume curve. An increase in RA and RV diastolic pressures increases intracavitary as well as coronary venous pressures. The *lower panel* reports experiments to assess the effect of an intracavitary increase in RV diastolic pressure. In the *lower panel*, an RV balloon was inflated over a pressure range of 0 to 30 mm Hg and the effect on the LV diastolic pressure-volume relation was measured. Distension of the RV balloon in the *lower panel* had much less of an effect than that which occurred when both the RV cavity and coronary venous pressures were increased, as shown in the *upper panel*. Thus, the difference between the *upper* and *lower panels* indicates the influence of an increase in coronary venous pressure on left ventricular diastolic distensibility.

These results demonstrate two mechanisms by which an increase in RV and RA pressure can increase LV diastolic chamber stiffness. An increase in RV volume to the limits of the pericardium can result in pericardial constraint of the LV as illustrated earlier. Additionally, because the coronary sinus empties into the RA, an increase in RA pressure will increase coronary venous turgor and LV stiffness. The clinical corollary of this phenomenon is that venodilators and diuretics that decrease RA and RV volume and pressure will improve LV diastolic distensibility and LV diastolic function. (*Adapted from* Watanabe *et al.* [26].)

FIGURE 15-37. Effect of increased coronary arterial turgor due to hypertension on LV diastolic stiffness. Isolated blood-perfused balloon-in-LV rabbit hearts were perfused at either a normal coronary perfusion pressure (CPP) of 70 mm Hg, or an elevated CPP of 130 mm Hg to simulate severe arterial hypertension. An LV diastolic P-V curve was measured by filling of the LV balloon at each CPP. LV balloon volumes were normalized to the largest volume obtained for each heart; that is, a value of 1.0 was assigned to balloon volume at an LV diastolic pressure of 25 mm Hg and a CPP of 70 mm Hg. During hypertensive coronary perfusion, the P-V curve was shifted significantly leftward, indicating an increase in LV diastolic chamber stiffness. At the higher CPP, LV wall thickness was also observed to increase by 20% above the value at the normal CPP. Thus, arterial hypertension has the effect of increasing LV wall turgidity and causing LV diastolic dysfunction. (*Adapted from* Wexler *et al.* [27].)

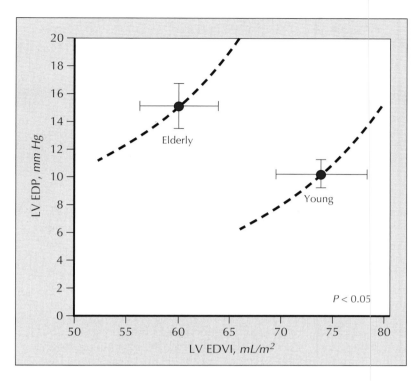

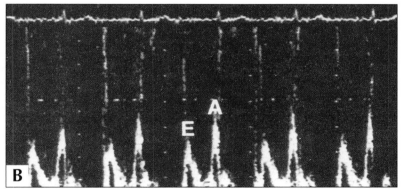

FIGURE 15-38. Diastolic dysfunction with normal aging. Left ventricular (LV) end-diastolic chamber stiffness is increased with normal aging. LV diastolic dysfunction increases with aging in both asymptomatic normal elderly people and as a cause of symptomatic congestive heart failure in the elderly. This figure reports the LV end-diastolic pressure-volume relation in 11 elderly normal (68 ± 5 years) and 15 young (31 ± 7 years) normal subjects who were screened by cardiac catheterization and were free of coronary artery disease, systemic hypertension, LV hypertrophy, or abnormality of LV systolic function and who did not have symptoms of congestive heart failure. As shown, the LV end-diastolic pressure volume (LV EDP) of the elderly subjects was significantly higher than that of the young ones, despite a smaller end-diastolic volume index (LV EDVI). The *dashed lines* indicate a shift of the pressure-volume relation upward to the left in the elderly subjects, indicating a reduction in passive LV diastolic compliance or increase in chamber stiffness. Such a shift indicates that an increase in pressure is required to distend and fill the LV during diastole, especially in late diastole.

Diastolic dysfunction is a major cause of CHF in the elderly. Delayed relaxation and increased LV stiffness both occur with normal aging. Hypertension, coronary disease, and diabetes frequently contribute to diastolic dysfunction in the elderly. (*Adapted from* Downes *et al.* [28].)

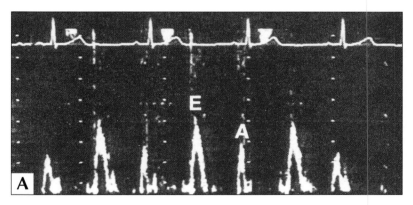

FIGURE 15-39. Delayed left ventricular (LV) relaxation with normal aging. Representative transmitral flow velocity patterns are shown. **A,** In the normal young subject, early filling (E wave) is more rapid than the late filling resulting from atrial contraction (A wave). **B,** Normal elderly subject. The reverse pattern is seen in a normal elderly subject in whom the peak E velocity was smaller than the peak A velocity.

This change in filling pattern implies an increased load on the left atrium. Left atrial contraction normally provides only a small contribution to total LV diastolic filling. However, when early diastolic filling is reduced, as occurs in the elderly, more of the burden of LV filling falls on the left atrium in late diastole. The left atrium can serve as a booster pump to maintain LV filling, and because LA pressure is only transiently increased during atrial contraction, mean LA and pulmonary venous pressures do not increase to cause pulmonary congestion. However, greater increases in LV stiffness, or chronic left atrial overload of long duration can lead to increased mean LA and pulmonary-capillary pressures and pulmonary congestion in the absence of LV systolic dysfunction; such a patient would present with the classic picture of congestive heart failure with normal systolic function, ie, primary diastolic dysfunction. (*From* Downes *et al.* [28]; with permission.)

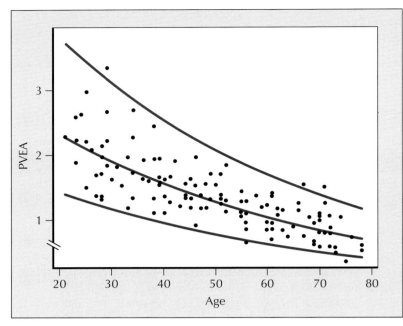

FIGURE 15-40. Effects of aging on transmitral flow velocity pattern. This figure reports the ratio of the peak velocity E/A (PVEA) of left ventricular (LV) filling as a function of age in a population of 127 randomly selected, rigorously defined, normal subjects from the Framingham heart study, evenly distributed by sex and age from the third to eighth decade. The *solid lines* indicate 95% confidence limits. With normal aging it is apparent that the pattern of diastolic filling shifts from rapid filling in early diastole in youth, to delayed filling in late diastole in the elderly. As noted previously, this change in filling pattern is associated with an increase in passive LV stiffness and probably represents a mild to moderate level of diastolic dysfunction in these elderly subjects despite a lack of symptoms. (*Adapted from* Benjamin *et al.* [29].)

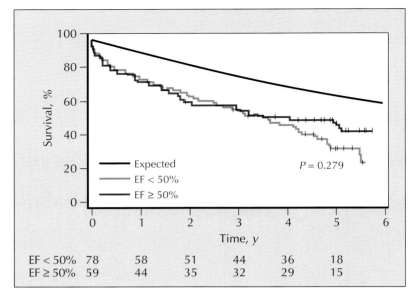

EF < 50%	78	58	51	44	36	18
EF ≥ 50%	59	44	35	32	29	15

FIGURE 15-41. Survival for CHF patients with systolic dysfunction (EF < 50%), diastolic dysfunction (EF > 50%), and an age- and sex-matched population without CHF. Either type of CHF had a significantly lower survival rate than the CHF-free population; there was no difference in survival between these diastolic and systolic dysfunction groups.

Two recent epidemiologic studies, the Rotterdam study and the Olmstead county study, have documented a high prevalence of CHF due to diastolic dysfunction among the elderly. All patients receiving a first diagnosis of CHF (*n* = 216) during 1991 in Olmstead county were included in this study. The new onset of CHF in the community setting largely occurred in the elderly, with a high prevalence of diastolic dysfunction. The Rotterdam study surveyed the health of all 5540 inhabitants of a Rotterdam suburb who were older than 55 years of age. Indices of diastolic dysfunction were not measured and the presence of diastolic dysfunction was inferred from the combination of symptomatic CHF with normal systolic function. This study documented a high prevalence of CHF due to diastolic dysfunction among the elderly. (*Adapted from* Senni et al. [30].)

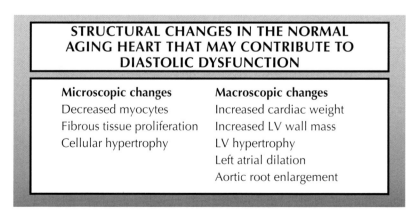

FIGURE 15-42. Structural changes in the normal aging heart that may contribute to diastolic dysfunction. (*Adapted from* Nixon and Burns [31].)

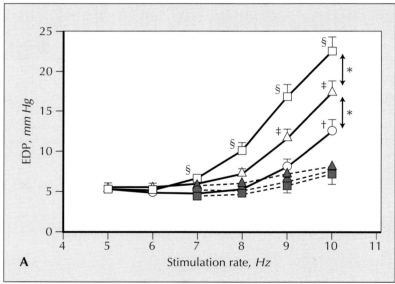

FIGURE 15-43. Basic mechanisms of impaired relaxation in the aging heart. The relationship between age-associated lusitropic (relaxation) impairment, heart rate, and β-adrenergic stimulation was assessed in adult (5 months), old (24 months), and senescent (34 months) isolated isovolumic (balloon-in left ventricle) blood-perfused mouse hearts. Hearts were paced from 5 to 10 Hz, returned to 7 Hz, exposed to isoproterenol, and paced again 7 to 10 Hz. **A**, The results for end-diastolic pressure (EDP). (*continued*)

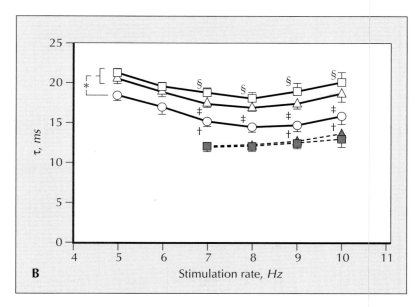

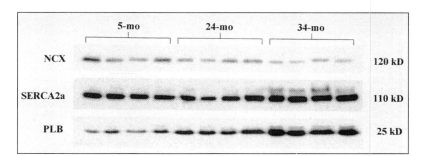

FIGURE 15-43. *(continued)* **B**, The time constant of LV relaxation, τ. before *(open symbols, solid lines)* and during *(closed symbols, dashed*

lines) isoproterenol administration at 5 months *(circles)*, 24 months *(triangles)*, and 34 months *(squares)* of age.

In this isovolumic model, shift in EDP reflects a change in position of the diastolic pressure-volume curve. With increasing heart rate, EDP was significantly increased in all three groups (**A**). In senescent hearts, the increased EDP was greater and occurred at lower heart rates than in old and adult hearts. Also the increased EDP in old hearts was greater than in adult hearts. The relationship between heart rate and τ is shown in **B**. τ was significantly prolonged in senescent and old hearts, compared with adult hearts, suggestive of a decreased LV relaxation rate with age.

Isoproterenol completely reversed the age-associated lusitropic impairments. These data suggest that impaired lusitropy in aging mouse hearts is related to a decreased rate of cytosolic calcium removal and that accelerating SR calcium reuptake via β-adrenergic stimulation can reverse this impairment. *Asterisk* indicates *P*<0.05 between groups indicated. *Dagger* indicates *P*<0.05, comparing before and during isoproterenol for 5-month-old hearts. *Double dagger* indicates *P*<0.05 for 24-month-old hearts. *Section symbol* indicates *P*<0.05 for 34-month-old hearts. *(Adapted from* Lim *et al.* [32].)

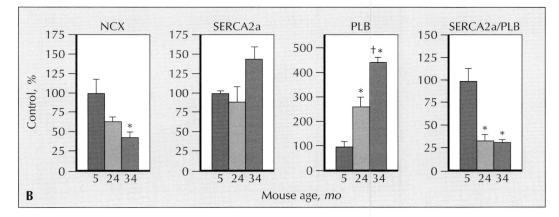

FIGURE 15-44. Calcium handling protein levels in old and senescent mouse hearts. The hearts described in Figure 15-43 were analyzed for their levels of the major calcium handling proteins, and the results are reported here. **A**, The original Western immunoblots against the Na-Ca^{2+} exchanger (NCX), sarcoplasmic reticulum Ca^{2+} ATPase (SERCA2a), and pentameric form of phospholamban (PLB) in 5-, 24-, and 34-month-old hearts. **B**, The Western immunoblots quantification results in 5-month-old, 24-month-old, and 34-month-old hearts. Because PLB inhibits SERCA2a, the ratio of the SERCA2a to PLB ratio (SERCA2a/PLB) was used as an index of SERCA2a activity. All data are expressed relative to the 5-month-old hearts.

Thus, aging was associated with a reduced protein level of Na^{+}-Ca^{2+} exchanger and increased phospholamban relative to SERCA2a, consistent with the slowed relaxation manifested by the old and senescent hearts. *Asterisk* indicates *P* < 0.05 relative to 5-month-old hearts. *Dagger* indicates *P* < 0.05 relative to 24-month-old hearts.) *(Adapted from* Lim *et al.* [32].)

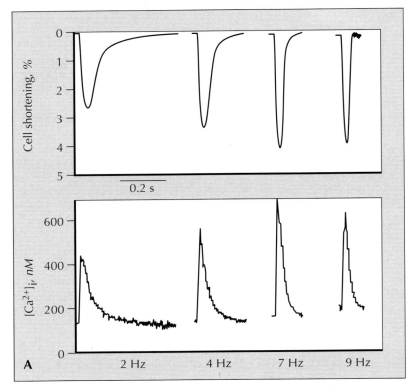

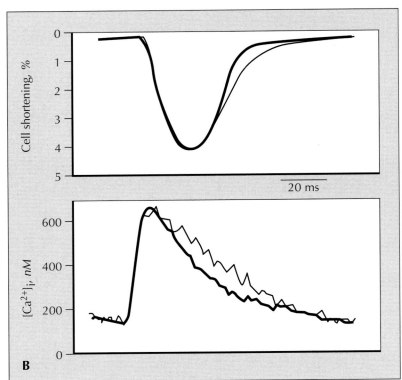

FIGURE 15-45. Effects of senescence on isolated heart cells. **A,**Averaged tracings of percentage cell shortening and $[Ca^{2+}]_i$, recorded at 37°C from a representative adult myocyte paced at 2, 4, 7, and 9 Hz. **B,** Normalized tracings of cell shortening (*top*) and $[Ca^{2+}]_i$ (*bottom*) from a representative adult (*thick line*) and senescent

(*thin line*) myocyte paced at 9 Hz. Tracings were normalized to peak value to show changes in time course. Cell shortening and $[Ca^{2+}]_i$ were acquired at 4.2 and 2 ms sampling rates, respectively. To reduce the signal-to-noise ratio, each tracing was depicted as an average of 10 original tracings. (*Adapted from* Lim *et al.* [33].)

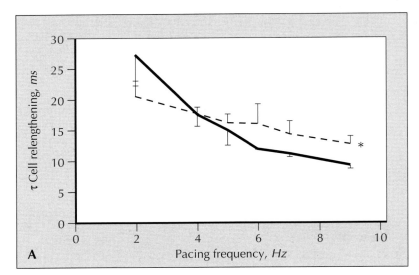

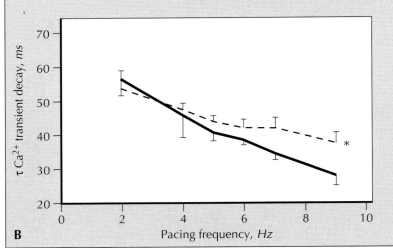

FIGURE 15-46. Slowed relaxation and calcium reuptake in senescent heart cells. **A,** Time constant (τ) of cell relengthening in adult (*solid line*; *n* = 4) and senescent (*dashed line*; *n* = 5) cardiomyocytes at increasing pacing rates. **B,** Time constant (τ) of the intracellular calcium transient decay in adult (*solid line*; *n* = 4) and senescent (*dashed line*; *n* = 5) at increasing pacing rates. Myocyte data from four adult and five senescent hearts were averaged and expressed as mean ± SEM. The *asterisk* indicates *P*< 0.05 between adult and senescent

curves Figures 15-45 and 15-46 illustrate direct cellular measurements of impaired calcium handling at higher heart rates that correlated with impaired cell relaxation. These results are consistent with the whole heart studies illustrated in Figure 15-43 and 15-44, and they define a basic mechanism that contributes to impaired relaxation and early diastolic LV filling with aging. (*Adapted from* Lim *et al.* [33].)

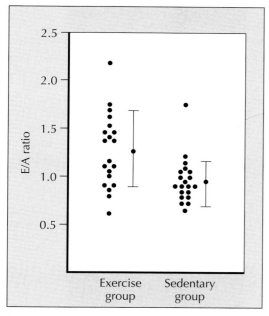

FIGURE 15-47. Improved left ventricular (LV) filling indices in older subjects with exercise training. This figure reports the peak early to late (E/A) velocity ratio for mitral valve inflow in two groups of older subjects (60± 6 years), a sedentary group, and an exercise group of long-distance runners who ran an average of 45 miles per week for an average of 15 years. The E/A ratio was significantly higher in the exercise group ($P = 0.001$). This result supports the idea that exercise training can blunt the progressive decrease in LV filling indices that occur with aging. (*Adapted from* Takemoto *et al.* [34].)

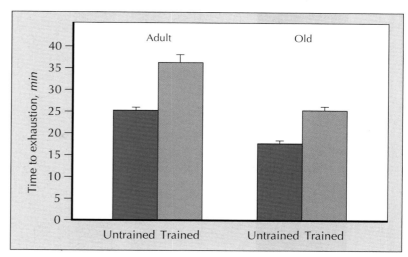

FIGURE 15-48. Exercise capacity in trained and untrained adult (6 months of age) and old (24 months of age) rats. Recent experimental studies have demonstrated that exercise training of old rats can improve their mitral inflow velocity profiles and exercise capacity. The training program consisted of 12 weeks of treadmill training (45 minutes per day, 5 days per week) compared with a sedentary cage life. In the absence of exercise training, the old rats had less exercise capacity than the adults. After exercise training, the old rats improved significantly and were comparable with the untrained adults, but the trained adults had the greatest exercise capacity. The 12 weeks of exercise training significantly increased maximal exercise capacity, defined as time to exhaustion on a standardized running protocol, in both age groups.

The exercise training produced a parallel response in left ventricular relaxation as assessed by mitral valve inflow velocities. With age, the early to late (E/A) wave ratio was decreased, but this index improved significantly, especially in the old rats. These results suggest that exercise training has the potential to improve diastolic function and exercise capacity in elderly individuals. $P< 0.01$ for effect of age; $P< 0.01$ for effect of training; $P<0.04$ for interaction. (*Adapted from* Brenner *et al.* [35].)

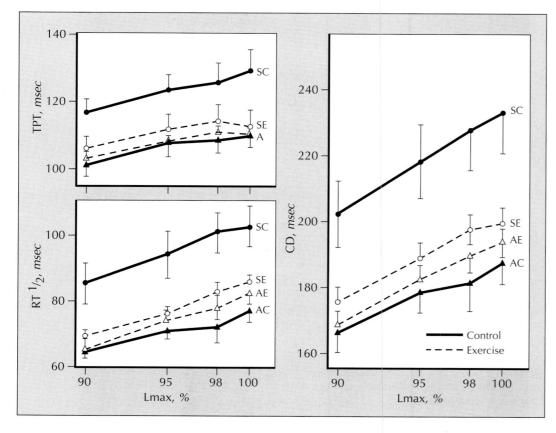

FIGURE 15-49. Chronic exercise improves relaxation in senescent rat hearts. Left ventricular (LV) trabeculae carnae muscle strips from adult (A) (3 to 4 month old) and senescent (S) (18 to 19 month old) rats, who underwent an 18- to 22-week exercise training program (E), or were sedentary controls (C). This figure reports results for the parameters of time to peak tension (TPT), time for 50% relaxation (RT1/2), and contraction duration (CD) over a range of muscle lengths.

Diastolic function is assessed by RT1/2. Note that the time for 50% relaxation (RT1/2) is prolonged for the senescent sedentary controls (SC). Chronic exercise training effectively reduced the slowed relaxation of the SC group and abolished the age difference among groups. This result shows that the effectiveness of exercise in modifying relaxation rate is highly dependent on the age of the animal, and that the slow relaxation that is characteristic of the senescent heart is not fixed, but can be modified by a mild chronic exercise protocol. (*Adapted from* Spurgeon *et al.* [36].)

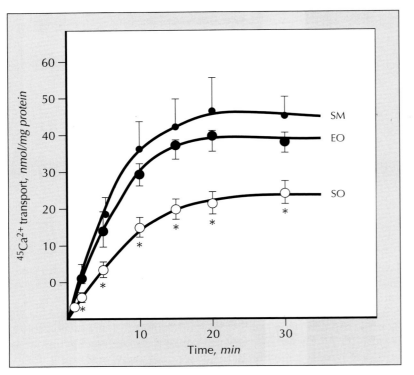

FIGURE 15-50. Enhanced calcium uptake of cardiac sarcoplasmic reticulum in exercise-trained old rats. This figure reports the rate of calcium transport by cardiac sarcoplasmic reticulum from sedentary mature (SM), sedentary old (SO), and chronically exercise old (EO) rat hearts. Chronic exercise improved calcium transport as indicated by the shift from SO to EO. There was a parallel improvement in muscle relaxation of isolated papillary muscle strips from these groups. Thus, an increased calcium transport by the cardiac sarcoplasmic reticulum may be one of the potential mechanisms underlying the improvement of myocardial relaxation with chronic exercise initiated during senescence. *Asterisk* indicates $P < 0.05$; SM or EO > SO. (*Adapted from* Tate *et al.* [37].)

CLINICAL FEATURES, PROGNOSIS, AND TREATMENT

COMMON CLINICAL FEATURES OF PURE DIASTOLIC DYSFUNCTION

Pulmonary congestion with a normal ejection fraction

Left ventricular hypertrophy

Myocyte hypertrophy and interstitial fibrosis

Exacerbation by ischemia

Hypertension (current or historical)

Responsible for 30% to 50% of CHF cases

Increased prevalence in the elderly

Common immediately after cardiac surgery

FIGURE 15-51. Common clinical features of pure (strain-independent) diastolic dysfunction.

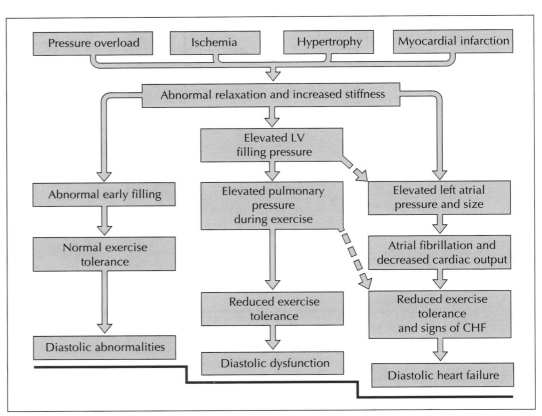

FIGURE 15-52. Natural history of diastolic heart failure. Abnormal relaxation and increased stiffness are associated with diastolic filling abnormalities and normal exercise tolerance in the early phase of diastolic dysfunction. When the disease progresses, pulmonary pressures increase abnormally during exercise with reduced exercise tolerance. When filling pressures increase further, left atrial pressure and size increase and exercise tolerance falls with clinical signs of congestive heart failure (CHF). (*Adapted from* Mandinov *et al.* [9].)

FEATURES OF LV SYSTOLIC AND DIASTOLIC DYSFUNCTION

	PURE SYSTOLIC DYSFUNCTION	PURE DIASTOLIC DYSFUNCTION	COMBINED DYSFUNCTION
Pulmonary congestion	No	Yes	Yes
Cardiac output	Low	Normal or increased	Normal or decreased
Ejection fraction	Depressed	Normal	Depressed
LV dilation	Yes	No*	Yes
Inotropic agents	Yes	No	Yes
Afterload reduction	Yes	No	Yes
Venodilators	No	Yes	Yes
Diuretics	No	Yes	Yes
Calcium antagonists	No	Yes	Questionable†

*In strain-dependent pure diastolic dysfunction, the LV size may be normal or slightly increased; by contrast, LV chamber dimensions are normal or small in the strain-independent forms of diastolic dysfunction.

†In combined systolic and diastolic dysfunction, the calcium channel blockers may be useful in the treatment of hypertension or angina.

FIGURE 15-53. Clinical features of systolic versus diastolic dysfunction. (*Adapted from* Levine and Gaasch [13].)

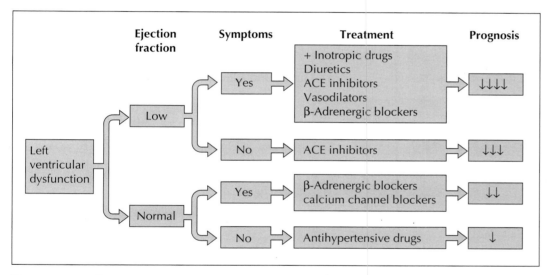

FIGURE 15-54. Diagnosis and treatment of congestive heart failure (CHF): systolic versus diastolic dysfunction. This scheme provides a separation of patients with systolic dysfunction (low ejection fraction) from those with diastolic dysfunction (normal ejection fraction). Within each category, treatment and prognosis are related to the presence or absence of symptoms. The *arrows* indicate relative prognosis (*eg*, four arrows indicate the worst prognosis). Thus, patients with LV systolic dysfunction and overt heart failure are treated with angiotensin-converting inhibitors and vasodilators in addition to the standard medical regimens using diuretics with digitalis. By contrast, symptomatic patients with a normal ejection fraction are best treated with calcium channel blocking agents and β-adrenergic receptor blocking agents. Asymptomatic patients in both categories also benefit from therapy. (*Adapted from* Gaasch [38].)

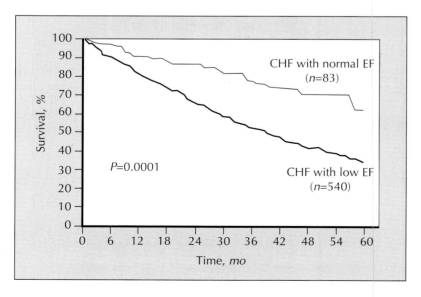

FIGURE 15-55. Survival curve of patients with congestive heart failure (CHF) with normal ejection fraction (EF) and presumed diastolic dysfunction or low EF (systolic dysfunction) from the VA Cooperative Study of heart failure (V-HeFT). In this study the normal EF was defined as 0.45 or greater. The average EF was 0.54 in the normal EF (diastolic dysfunction) group compared to 0.26 in the low EF (systolic dysfunction) group. The prognosis was significantly better in the diastolic dysfunction group, which had an annual mortality rate of 8% compared with 19% in the systolic dysfunction group. (*Adapted from* Cohn and Johnson [39].)

TREATMENT OF CONGESTIVE HEART FAILURE DUE TO DIASTOLIC DYSFUNCTION: ACUTE PULMONARY CONGESTION OR EDEMA

Reduce pulmonary capillary pressure
Avoid hypotension from excessive preload reduction in stiff LV
Correct any hypertension
Restore normal sinus rhythm and/or control rapid heart rate
Relieve ischemia

FIGURE 15-56. Treatment of acute pulmonary edema from diastolic dysfunction. Patients with diastolic dysfunction frequently have episodes of acute pulmonary edema, which may be life threatening. The treatment principles are outlined here. Pulmonary capillary pressure can be reduced by vasodilators such as intravenous nitroglycerin, which may also relieve any ischemia that contributes to LV stiffness. Rapidly acting diuretics, morphine, tourniquets and other standard care measures of treatment pulmonary edema (*eg*, oxygen) are also helpful. If atrial fibrillation is present, an attempt should be made to restore normal sinus rhythm to preserve the atrial contribution to ventricular filling.

Regardless of rhythm, any tachycardia should be controlled.

The stiff, noncompliant ventricle makes preload management difficult. A small increase in LV volume that would be tolerated without difficult in a normally compliant LV can result in a marked increase in pulmonary capillary pressure in a stiff LV and thereby precipitate pulmonary edema. Conversely, the stiff LV is abnormally sensitive to a lowering of filling pressure; due to its decreased distensibility and increased resistance to filling, the stiff LV requires a higher than normal filling pressure to maintain an adequate diastolic volume and stroke volume. If initial preload reduction results in hypotension, a normal blood pressure can usually be restored by discontinuing the vasodilators and increasing LV volume by leg raising or infusion of a small amount of saline.

GENERAL APPROACH TO THE TREATMENT OF DIASTOLIC DYSFUNCTION

GOAL OF TREATMENT	METHOD OF TREATMENT
1. Reduce venous pressure	Decreased central blood volume
	Diuretics
	Salt restriction
	Venodilation
	Nitrates
	ACE inhibitors
	Morphine
	Tourniquets
2. Maintain atrial contraction	Cardioversion of AF
	Sequential A-V pacing
3. Decrease heart rate	Digitalis in atrial fibrillation
	β-adrenergic blockers
	Verapamil, diltiazem
4. Prevent/treat ischemia	β-adrenergic blockers
	Calcium channel blockers
	Nitrates
	Coronary bypass or angioplasty
5. Improve ventricular relaxation	Systolic unloading
	Treat ischemia
	Calcium channel blockers (?)
6. Regression of hypertrophy	Antihypertensive therapy
	Surgery (AVR for aortic stenosis)

FIGURE 15-57. The goals and methods of long-term management. Chronic hypertension causes both myocyte hypertrophy and increased fibrosis. Experimental evidence suggests that antagonists of the renin-angiotensin-aldosterone pathway may decrease myocardial fibrosis, and such agents may be particularly useful in the long-term treatment of LV diastolic dysfunction for this reason, but clinical trials are lacking. Digitalis glycosides are not generally recommended for the treatment of CHF due to diastolic dysfunction in the absence of atrial fibrillation and LV systolic dysfunction. Maintenance of a relatively slow heart rate, and prevention of tachycardic episodes, is important in managing diastolic dysfunction. A slow heart rate reduces the risk of ischemia by decreasing myocardial oxygen demand and increasing the duration of diastole, which is the time in the cardiac cycle during which most coronary flow occurs. In cases in which LV relaxation is slow, a prolonged diastolic interval may permit more complete relaxation and improved LV filling at lower filling pressures. The patient's symptomatic response, especially with regard to relief of dyspneas with exertion, is a practical guide to optimizing drug therapy. (*Adapted from* Levine and Gaasch [13].)

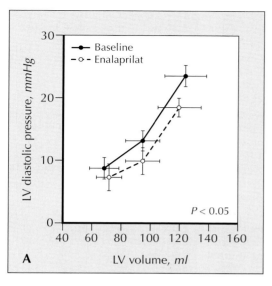

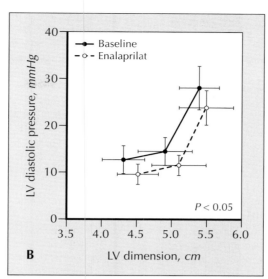

FIGURE 15-58. Effect of intracoronary enalaprilat on LV diastolic chamber stiffness in patients with LV hypertrophy from aortic stenosis. These graphs show the relations between LV diastolic pressure and LV volume and LV dimension in the aortic stenosis group, determined by ventriculography (n = 13) (*A*) and echocardiography (**B**), respectively. Measurements were performed simultaneously with LV micromanometer pressure measurements in all patients. Coordinates of pressure, volume, and dimension are averages at three diastolic points: early diastolic pressure nadir, mid-diastole, and end-diastole. In both groups there was a vertical downward shift with intracoronary enalaprilat indicating improved diastolic distensibility.

These observations support the hypothesis that the cardiac reninangiotensin system is activated in patients with concentric LVH and that this activation may contribute to diastolic dysfunction. *P* values indicate significance of the vertical downward shift for the relation (ANOVA for repeated measures). *Bars* indicate SEM. (*Adapted from* Friedrich *et al.* [40].)

ACKNOWLEDGMENT

The helpful advice of Drs. Herbert J. Levine and William H. Gaasch is gratefully acknowledged.

REFERENCES

1. Apstein C *et al.*: Exercise, diastolic function and dysfunction. In *Exercise and Heart Failure*. Edited by Balady GJ, Piña IL. Armonk, NY: Futura Publishing Company, Inc.; 1997:39–83.

2. Cheng CP, Igarashi Y, Little WC: Mechanisms of augmented rate of left ventricle filling during exercise. *Circ Res* 1993, 72:795–806.

3. Cheng CP, Noda T, Nozawa T, Little WC: Effect of heart failure on the mechanism of exercise induced augmentation of mitral valve flow. *Circ Res* 1993, 72:795–806.

4. Little WC, Cheng CP: Modulation of diastolic dysfunction in the intact heart. In *Diastolic Dysfunction of the Heart*, edn 2. Edited by Lorell BH, Grossman W. Boston: Kluwer Academic Publishers; 1994:167–176.

5. Labovitz AJ, Pearson AC: Evaluation of left ventricular diastolic function: clinical relevance and recent Doppler echocardiographic insights. *Am Heart J* 1987, 114:836–851.

6. Bonow RO: Radionuclide angiographic evaluation of left ventricular diastolic function. *Circulation* 1991, 84:1–208.

7. Cheng C-P, Igarashi Y, Little WC: Mechanism of augmented rate of left ventricular filling during exercise. *Circ Res* 1992, 70:9.

8. Udelson JE, Bacharach SL, Cannon RO III, Bonow RO: Minimum left ventricular pressure during beta-adrenergic stimulation in human subjects: evidence for elastic recoil and diastolic "suction" in the normal heart. *Circulation* 1990, 82:1174–1182.

9. Mandinov L, Eberli FR, Seiler C, Hess OM: Diastolic heart failure [review]. *Cardiovascular Research* 2000, 45:813–825.

10. Colucci WS, Braunwald E: Pathophysiology of heart failure. In Heart Disease, edn 6. Edited by Braunwald E, Zipes DP, Libby P. Philadelphia: WB Saunders; 2001:519.

11. Becker AE, Anderson RH: *Cardiac Pathology: An Integrated Text and Colour Atlas*. New York; Raven Press; 1983:1.7

12. Weber K, Brilla C: Pathological hypertrophy and cardiac interstitium: fibrosis and renin-angiotensin-aldosterone system. *Circulation* 1991, 83:1849–1865.

13. Levine HJ, Gaasch W: Clinical recognition and treatment of diastolic dysfunction and heart failure. In *Left Ventricular Diastolic Dysfunction and Heart Failure*. Edited by Gaasch WH, LeWinter M. Philadelphia: Lea & Febiger; 1994:439–454.

14. Zile MR: Diastolic dysfunction: detection, consequences, and treatment: II. Diagnosis and treatment of diastolic function. *Mod Concepts Cardiovasc Dis* 1990, 59:1.

15. Kitzman DW, Higginbotham MB, Cobb FR, *et al.*: Exercise intolerance in patients with heart failure and preserved left ventricular systolic function: failure of the Frank-Starling mechanism. *J Am Coll Cardiol* 1991, 17:1065–1072.

16. Carroll JD, Hess OM, Hirzel HO, Krayenbuehl HP: Dynamics of left ventricular filling at rest and during exercise. *Circulation* 1983, 68:59–67.

17. Carroll JD, Hess OM, Hirzel HO, Krayenbuehl HP: Exercise-induced ischemia: the influence of altered relaxation on early diastolic pressures. *Circulation* 1983, 67:521–528.

18. Pepine C, Wiener L: Relationship of anginal symptoms to lung mechanics during myocardial ischemia. *Circulation* 1972, 46:863–869.

19. Carroll JD, Carroll EP: Diastolic function in coronary artery disease. *Herz (Germany)* 1991, 16:1.

20. Sasayama *et al.*: Changes in diastolic properties of the regional myocardium during pacing-induced ischemia in human subjects. *J Am Coll Cardiol* 1985, 5: 599.

21. Eberli FR, Weinberg EO, Grice WN, et al.: Protective effect of increased glycolytic substrate against systolic and diastolic dysfunction and increased coronary resistance from prolonged global underperfusion and reperfusion in isolated rabbit hearts perfused with erythrocyte suspensions. *Circ Res* 1991, 68:466–481.

22. Eberli FR, Strömer H, Ferrell MA, *et al.*: Lack of direct role for calcium in ischemic diastolic dysfunction in isolated hearts. *Circulation* 2000, 102:2643–2649.

23. Lorell BH, Grice WN, Apstein CS: Impaired diastolic tolerance to low-flow ischemia in blood-perfused hypertrophied rat hearts. *Circulation* 1989, 80:II–97.

24. McKenney *et al.*: Diastolic function after bypass surgery. *JACC* 1994, 24:1189–1194.

25. Taylor RR, Covell JW, Sonnenblick EH, Ross J Jr.: Dependence of ventricular distensibility on filling of the opposite ventricle. *Am J Physiol* 1967, 213:711.

26. Watanabe J *et al.*: Effects of coronary venous pressure on left ventricular diastolic distensibility. *Circ Res* 1990, 67:923.

27. Wexler LF, Grice WN, Huntington M, *et al.*: Coronary hypertension and diastolic compliance in isolated rabbit hearts. *Hypertension* 1989, 13:598–606.

28. Downes TR, Nomeir A-M, Smith KM, *et al.*: Mechanism of altered pattern of left ventricular filling with aging in subjects without cardiac disease. *Am J Cardiol* 1989, 64:523–527.

29. Benjamin EJ, Levy D, Anderson KM, et al.: Determinants of Doppler indexes of left ventricular diastolic function in normal subjects (the Framingham Heart Study). Am J Cardiol 1992, 70:508–515.

30. Senni M, Tribouilloy CM, Rodeheffer RJ, et al.: Congestive heart failure in the community: a study of all incident cases in Olmsted County, Minnesota, in 1991. Circulation 1998, 98:2282–2289.

31. Nixon JV, Burns CA: Cardiac effects of aging and diastolic dysfunction in the elderly. In Left Ventricular Diastolic Dysfunction and Heart Failure. Edited by Gaasch WH, LeWinter M. Philadelphia: Lea & Febiger; 1994: 427–435.

32. Lim CC, Liao R, Varma N, Apstein CS: Impaired lusitropy-frequency in the aging mouse: role of Ca^{2+}-handling proteins and effects of isoproterenol. *Am J Physiol (Heart Circ Physiol)* 1999, 46:H2083–H2090.

33. Lim CC, Apstein CS, Colucci WS, Liao R: Impaired cell shortening and relengthening with increased pacing frequency intrinsic to the senescent mouse cardiomyocyte. *J Mol Cell Cardiol* 2000, 32:2075–2082.

34. Takemoto KA, Bernstein L, Lopez JF, *et al.*: Abnormalities of diastolic filling of the left ventricle associated with aging are less pronounced in exercise-trained individuals. *Am Heart J* 1992, 124:143–148.

35. Brenner DA, Apstein CS, Saupe KW: Exercise training attenuates age-associated diastolic dysfunction in rats. *Circulation* 2001, 104:221–226.

36. Spurgeon HA, Steinbach MF, Lakatta EG: Chronic exercise prevents characteristic age related changes in rat cardiac contraction. *Am J Physiol (Heart Circ Physiol)* 1983, 244:H513–H518.

37. Tate CA, Taffet GE, Hudson EK, *et al.*: Enhanced calcium uptake of cardiac sarcoplasmic reticulum in exercise-trained old rats. *Am J Physiol (Heart Circ Physiol)* 1990, 258:H431–H435.

38. Gaasch WH: Diagnosis and treatment of heart failure based on left ventricular systolic or diastolic dysfunction. *JAMA* 1994, 271:.

39. Cohn JN, Johnson G, and the Veterans Administration Cooperative Study Group: Heart failure with normal ejection fraction: the V-HeFT study. *Circulation* 1990, 81 (suppl III):III-48–III-53.

40. Friedrich SP, Lorell BH, Rousseau MF, *et al.*: Intracardiac angiotensin-converting enzyme inhibition improves diastolic function in patients with left ventricular hypertrophy due to aortic stenosis. *Circulation* 1994, 90:2761–2771.

INDEX

COLOR PLATES

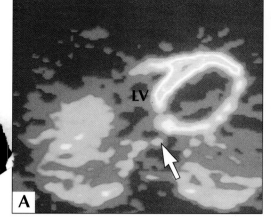

CHAPTER 3, Figure 3-7A, page 41

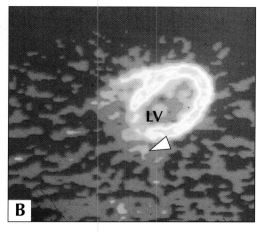

CHAPTER 3, Figure 3-7B, page 41

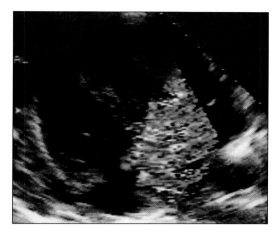

CHAPTER 3, Figure 3-9B, page 42

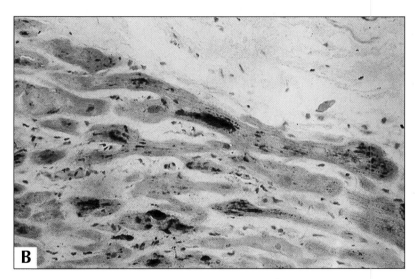

CHAPTER 3, Figure 3-39B, page 58

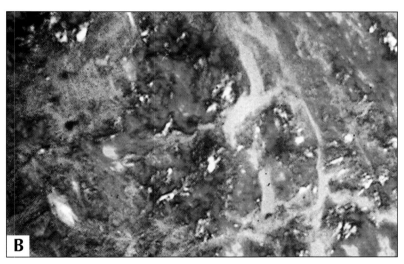

CHAPTER 3, Figure 3-41B, page 59

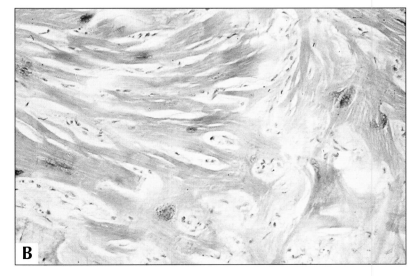

CHAPTER 3, Figure 3-43B, page 60

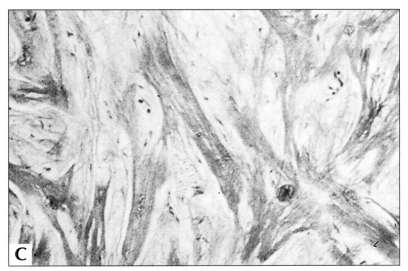

CHAPTER 3, Figure 3-43C, page 60

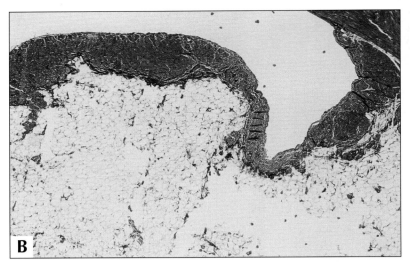

CHAPTER 3, Figure 3-45B, page 61

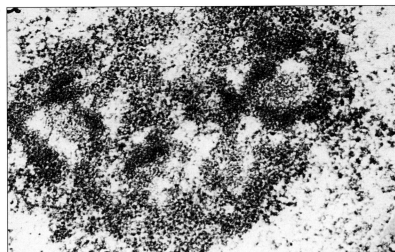

CHAPTER 4, Figure 4-22A, page 76

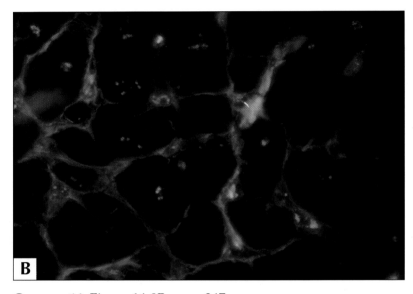

CHAPTER 14, Figure 14-9B, page 247

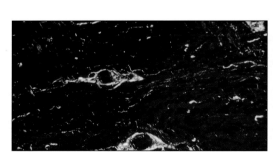

CHAPTER 15, Figure 15-16A, page 267

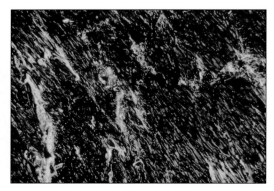

CHAPTER 15, Figure 15-16B, page 267